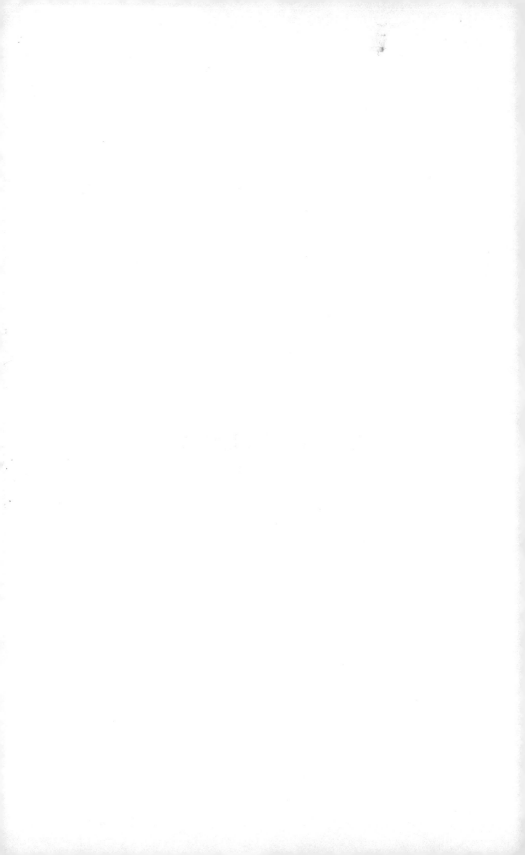

*N*The *ature* of Qualitative Evidence

To our colleagues,
In the spirit of a continuing dialogue

The Nature of Qualitative Evidence

edited by
Janice M. Morse
Janice M. Swanson
Anton J. Kuzel

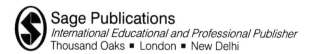
Sage Publications
International Educational and Professional Publisher
Thousand Oaks ▪ London ▪ New Delhi

BS

For information:

Sage Publications, Inc.
2455 Teller Road
Thousand Oaks, California 91320
E-mail: order@sagepub.com

Sage Publications Ltd.
6 Bonhill Street
London EC2A 4PU
United Kingdom

Sage Publications India Pvt. Ltd.
M-32 Market
Greater Kailash I
New Delhi 110 048 India

Printed in the United States of America

Library of Congress Cataloging-in-Publication Data

The nature of qualitative evidence / edited by Janice M. Morse,
   Janice M. Swanson, and Anton J. Kuzel.
      p.   cm.
   Includes index.
   ISBN 0-7619-2284-9 (cloth: alk. paper)
   ISBN 0-7619-2285-7 (pbk.: alk. paper)
      1. Qualitative research.   2. Medicine—Research—Methodology.
   I. Morse, Janice M.   II. Swanson, Janice M.   III. Kuzel, Anton J.
   R852 .N38 2000
   610'.72—dc21   00-011774

01   02   03   04   05   10   9   8   7   6   5   4   3   2   1

Acquiring Editor:	C. Deborah Laughton
Editorial Assistant:	Eileen Carr
Production Editor:	Denise Santoyo
Editorial Assistant:	Kathryn Journey
Typesetter/Designer:	Denyse Dunn/Marion Warren/Barbara Burkholder
Cover Designer:	Michelle Lee

5/18/05

Contents

Preface

In the past decade, two issues have led to increasing unease in qualitative inquiry. The first issue is the perceived weaknesses in qualitative methods and in the validity of understandings derived from their use. Put succinctly: How good is qualitative inquiry? The second issue, closely related to the first, is the concern about the practical application of such work, that is: What use is it? Or, more kindly, How can it be used?

Qualitative researchers made a concerted effort to respond to these implicit and direct challenges: A number of schemes emerged for the evaluation of the research per se and of the report, and these are discussed by Kuzel and Engel in Chapter 5. Various standards for the conduct of qualitative research have been developed, as were several journals dealing explicitly with qualitative inquiry. In response to the need for the advancement of qualitative methods, the International Institute for Qualitative Methodology (IIQM)(www.ualberta.ca/~iiqm) opened in 1998 and now sponsors annual multidisciplinary conferences. Graduate programs began acknowledging the role of qualitative inquiry, and, as a result, qualitative methods more often become a standard part of their programs. Granting agencies, responding to the new wave of qualitative methods, now place calls for proposals that include a component of qualitative methods. Given this astonishing progress in two decades, you may ask, "What is the problem here?"

Qualitative research still has a long way to go. Despite the advances in the explication of qualitative methods, the two basic questions remain in the minds of many. It is not difficult to find evidence for this assertion. "Pure" qualitative research remains difficult to get funded and, sometimes, to get published. Despite overwhelming demand by students, mentors remain in short supply. But most important, qualitative research is undervalued. Although we recognize that we cannot fully answer the "so what" question and make strong recommendations from our research, qualitative inquiry may inform and ultimately change clinical practice. However, qualitative researchers are still not comfortable with the emphasis on "directing" clinical practice. Thus, qualitative research has been accused of "going nowhere" (Hutchinson, 2001).

Compounding the problem of impotent inquiry was the rise of Evidence-Based Medicine in the form of the Cochrane Collaboration. This international movement reinforced the significance of clinical trials in medical research (and spilled over into other health sciences) to the extent that some medical funding agencies were using the *Cochrane Criteria* to evaluate proposals and allocate funding. The fact that the Cochrane Criteria were developed primarily as levels of evidence for determining the *efficacy of treatments* was missed by these committees: For them, real research was supposed to be large sample, randomized, experimental design. This has tended to delimit the definition of quality medical research to clinical trials, thereby making the *types of questions* qualitative research answers beyond the purview of health research and excluding it from funding. In fact, the Cochrane Criteria list four levels of evidence and place qualitative inquiry at the lowest level, in a category labeled "mere opinion."

What are these Cochrane Criteria? In 1972, Archie Cochrane published *Effectiveness and Efficiency,* in which standards for medical research were recommended. These are presented below, as summarized by Sackett (1993):

Level I. Randomized trials with low false positive (alpha) and/or low false negative (beta) errors. Low false positive studies demonstrate a statistically significant benefit from the treatment, while low false negative trials demonstrate either no effect from the treatment or no statistically significant difference between groups (usually multiple randomized controlled clinical trials conducted at a number of sites, with adequate controls). A *Grade A* recommendation for implementation would be supported by at least one (preferably more) Level I randomized trials.

Level II. Randomized trials with a high false positive (alpha) and/or high false negative (beta) errors. These are small randomized trials, with "uncertain results." These trials may have an interesting "positive trend" but not be statistically significant (alpha error), or conclude that the therapy was not efficacious (beta error). A *Grade B* recommendation will be supported by at least one Level II randomized trial. Although these results are not usually adequate for implementation, meta-analytic techniques may be used to analyze the results of two or more well-conducted studies but with small sample sizes to obtain statistically significant results and move these studies into a single Level I, Grade A, study.

Grade C consists of *Level III,* nonrandomized two-group concurrent cohort comparisons; *Level IV,* nonrandomized historical cohort comparisons, with the comparison group as a historical control, or those obtained from another institution; and *Level V,* where there are no controls, case study series and descriptive studies only. Level V recommendations also include those recommendations from expert committees. Grade C evidence is not recommended to inform practice (Sackett, 1993, pp. 487-488).

Cochrane did not intend these critieria to be used for *all* medical research. In fact, he presents the following example of a patient problem that was too complex for such methods of inquiry:

> The ward was full, so I put him in my room as he was moribund and screaming and I did not want to wake the ward. I examined him. He had obvious gross bilateral cavitation and severe pleural rub. I thought the latter was the cause of the pain and screaming. I had no morphia, just aspirin, which had no effect. I felt desperate. I knew very little Russian then and there was no one in the ward who did. I finally instinctively sat down on the bed and took him in my arms, and the screaming stopped almost at once. He died peacefully in my arms a few hours later. It was not the pleurisy that caused the screaming, but loneliness. It was a wonderful education about the care of the dying. I was ashamed of my misdiagnosis. [3887] (Sackett, 1996, Section I)

In the early 1970s, Cochrane did not know about research methods that could be used to investigate such problems, for qualitative methods were not commonly used in medicine at that time. Clearly, experimental design was unsuitable when not enough was known about the problem itself, not enough was known in order to develop or test an intervention, the problem was too complex, or too many variables were present to use single interventions. Therefore, the Cochrane Criteria should be used to address problems in medicine that focus only on the efficacy of treatments.

Yet, the parameters of Evidence-Based Medicine have been less clearly established. Sackett writes as recently as 1995 that "ultimately randomized trial of different strategies for interacting with patients" may be appropriate. He uses the term "care" loosely, writing: "Evidence based medicine is the conscious, explicit, and judicious use of current best evidence in making decisions about the *care* of individual patients" (Sackett & Rosenberg, 1996, p. 71, italics added). Although the use of "care" in the above sentence does not restrict care to "treatment," Sackett and Rosenberg note that Evidence-Based Medicine is the integration of "individual clinical expertise [proficiency and judgment] with the best available external evidence from systematic research" (p. 71). They continue: "Increased expertise is reflected . . . especially in more effective and efficient diagnosis and *in the more thoughtful identification and compassionate use of individual patients' predicaments, rights, and preferences in making clinical decisions about their care*" (p. 71, italics added). Thus, while we are not questioning the pertinence of the use of Cochrane's Criteria for the determination of the former, that is, more effective and efficient diagnosis—and we would add therapy—the latter, "the identification and compassionate use of patients' predicaments, rights, and preferences," are not the purview of experimental trials. They are the appropriate domain of social science research methods, best addressed by qualitative methods and, to a lesser extent, by quantitative methods, or by the triangulation of qualitative and quantitative methods.

What should qualitative researchers do? Two recourses were apparently left to qualitative researchers: We could ignore the Cochrane movement, determining that it was not pertinent to qualitative research, and continue to feel slighted and misunderstood at grant-funding time, clutching our rejection slips, and discounting these actions as the result of ignorance or hegemony. Or we could attempt to move the discipline forward by responding to the doubts about qualitative methods, critically examining qualitative inquiry from the perspective of evidence, and helping to find practical ways for clinicians to use qualitative inquiry.

We chose the second route. This book is the result of two think tanks addressing these issues and culminating in this volume. We do not have all the answers, as the edict wryly notes, but at least we are clearer about the questions, and in the spirit of this series, we have scattered our discussions throughout the text.

The book is organized in five sections. In the first section, The Nature of Evidence, Ross Upshur explores the nature and characteristics of evidence and describes the status of qualitative research as evidence. A model of evidence integrating both meaning and measurement is proposed. He then links the qualities of evidence with processes of inference and then with the "best explanation." Irena Madjar and JoAnn Walton, in Chapter 2, "What Is Problematic About Evidence?" discuss evidence, first by describing the Cochrane Collaboration movement and the levels of evidence used in Evidence-Based Medicine. Then they introduce other sources of evidence, focusing on examples using qualitative research.

The second section addresses The Nature of the Question. The issue of "Who Decides What Counts as Evidence?" is further explored by Lynne Ray and Maria Mayan. They consider various audiences (health care organizations, insurers, the health professions, regulators, the medical industry, the legal system, and consumers), each with their own agenda. Ray and Mayan then link externally constructed research priorities, research design, and the use of research evidence with the consequences for the public. In Chapter 4, Janice Swanson explores the role of questions and questioning when conducting a qualitative study. She examines the linkage between the type of question and the subsequent research design and method. Finally, she explores in depth getting from experience to theory-generating research, including the differences between the nature of the clinician's, the participant's, and the decision maker's questions.

Standards have always been a foremost concern in qualitative inquiry and have been an issue in qualitative research for more than two decades. The third section addresses The Nature of Standards. Anton Kuzel and John Engel thoughtfully explore published criteria and standards and present astute and sensitizing questions for the review of qualitative inquiry. Next, in Chapter 6, Sally Thorne reveals the implicit assumptions underlying disciplinary agendas for qualitative inquiry. The differing perspectives create tensions within the hospital and the research arena and, unfortunately, result in discrediting parallel professions. The section closes with Chapter 7 on participatory action research by Nancy Gibson, Ginger Gibson, and Ann Macaulay. These authors propose ethical and practical standards for evaluating evidence that is co-created with a community.

Extending standards of inquiry to the nature of analysis and interpretation, Chapters 8 and 9 explore how evidence is constructed within a qualitative project and how findings continue to be verified beyond the initial study. Lynn Meadows and Janice Morse, in Chapter 8, examine strategies developed to ensure verification of the project, reviewing such techniques as bracketing, sampling, and saturation. Next, they evaluate the validity of a qualitative project, using such strategies as inter-rater reliability (when is it appropriate?), and finally, they demonstrate techniques to promote reliability.

In Chapter 9, Morse explores techniques that continue to verify the validity of a study once the project is completed. This includes such techniques as conducting complementary projects, or triangulating projects, implementing the findings, and evaluating the results.

The final section, The Nature of Utilization, consists of three chapters: Janice Swanson addresses "The Nature of Outcomes," Kärin Olson writes about "Using Qualitative Research in Clinical Practice," and Carole Estabrooks discusses the barriers and facilitators to utilization in "Research Utilization and Qualitative Research." These three perspectives complement each other to illustrate the complexity of producing a study that is not only methodologically sound and verifiable, but useful as well.

As with the previous books in these series, we used some of the audiotaped conversations at the think tanks as Dialogues between chapters. Readers in the past have told us that they like these insights—they can see our disagreements and even our mistaken ways of thinking. We hope that the Dialogues will once again create a greater sense of participation and intimacy for the reader. This book completed a long and arduous task. It began 4½ years ago, when we very wrongly thought we could tackle the problem of qualitative evidence using an e-mail discussion group. Now, nearing completion of the project, the editors feel obligated to many people. First and foremost, we thank our colleagues, our authors, who good-naturedly tackled the monstrous problem. Perhaps we made progress—we will let you, our readers, decide. We thank our graduate students, who listened to our prattle without smirking and gently guided our thinking with astute and

well-timed comments. We thank Don Wells and Irene Sywenky, our technical editors, who patiently nudged the last words out of us and pulled it together in a respectable form. Finally, we are indebted to the Alberta Heritage Foundation for Medical Research, which sponsored our think tanks. This book was completed under the auspices of the International Institute for Qualitative Methodology at the University of Alberta.

Janice M. Morse
Janice M. Swanson
Anton J. Kuzel

References

Cochrane, A. L. (1972). *Effectiveness and efficiency.* London: Abingdon, Berks, Burgess.

Hutchinson, S. A. (2001). The development of qualitative health research: Taking stock. Keynote presentation at QHR 2000, the Sixth Annual International Qualitative Health Research Conference, Banff, Alberta, Canada. *Qualitative Health Research 11*(4).

Sackett, D. L. (1993). Rules of evidence and clinical recommendations. *Canadian Journal of Cardiology, 9*(6), 487-489.

Sackett, D. L. (Ed.). (1996). *Cochrane Collaboration. Cochrane Collaboration Handbook.* Retrieved from the World Wide Web: http://hiruet.mcmaster.ca/cochrane/handbook/cchb_00_.htm, Section I.

Sackett, D. L., & Rosenberg, W. M. C. (1996). Evidence based medicine: What it is and what it isn't. *British Medical Journal, 312,* 71-72.

I

The Nature of Evidence

Dialogue:

Introducing Evidence

KUZEL: The original purpose of this book was to give the reader a sense of qualitative inquiry in the everyday arena of health care. When people ask me about the place of qualitative research in everyday practice, I can spiel off things, but I never feel very coherent about it. So I am looking forward to getting help from all of you in framing and articulating a more coherent response!

ESTABROOKS: But there is a problem with evidence. We no longer talk about straightforward "research-based practice," but about "evidenced-based practice." Now in the beginning, the Cochrane Collaboration equated evidence with the fairly restricted notion of research. But if we really want to address "evidence," it is a much broader concept than we could tackle in this book, because it's an enormous area—much greater than the Evidence-Based Practice movement. I would like to see it clarified: In this book we are talking about qualitative research findings. Evidence is a very broad concept under which research is a slice.

Now, are we undertaking *all* of evidence, or are we undertaking the evaluation and dissemination of research?

MADJAR: Again, this has to do with our audience. Are we talking to *clinicians,* or are we talking to *researchers?* Because if we are only talking to other researchers, people will be largely looking for *research evidence* in order to develop policy and so on.

ESTABROOKS: But to talk about "evidence" is a far bigger project than this book can manage, in my mind. For evidence is many things besides research. And I wouldn't classify evidence as quantitative or qualitative. I don't think it even works. But in terms of research, we have qualitatively derived research findings and quantitatively derived research findings.

What is the "evidence" we are taking about? We have to make explicit a broader notion of evidence. Evidence, as you know, is art, it's experience, it's intuition, it's history, it's literature, it's many, many, many, many things. To make that explicit when we say what this book is about may be a very useful thing.

OLSON: And it would put clinicians at ease, too. It would be a relief to them to know they could use something other than *p* values.

SWANSON: I think maybe using Jan's [Morse] model from the last meeting, where she had that pie, and other forms of evidence are three quarters of the pie. And then there was research evidence, and a slither of that was qualitative. In terms of clinicians and policy makers—they don't use research a whole lot. A window of opportunity comes along and bingo, snap! They are not going to use meta-analysis and meta-synthesis to get into that window of opportunity. Come on—that's been written about.

MEADOWS: It seems to me that we are doing research, and we need to demonstrate that rigor. At the same time, we are trying to talk clearly and provide information to those who may not understand the method but do research that is of use for clinicians.

MADJAR: But this is a political statement. If it wasn't for Cochrane, we would not be writing this book—it would not be quite the same kind of issue. Now we can be defensive about that, or we can be actually quite aggressive about that. Or we can try and be balanced and provide a well-thought-out statement that says: The current debate about evidence has a tendency to be very much into experimental design, and that has tremendous implications for how the health services will develop in the future, what the policy makers are going to do, what the legislators are going to do, what the research allocations are going to be. It has the potential to influence where the priorities are going to be placed, where the research funds will go, and so on. And for all sorts of reasons, it is important that the debate about the role of qualitative inquiry be opened up.

So we must start this book by saying that. Then this book must set out to make, in a very positive way, a case for qualitative research: that it is *research*, that it is *systematic*, that it does produce evidence, and that such evidence needs to be taken seriously, because it is relevant to clinical practice.

KUZEL: But this book is not a rejoinder to Cochrane, but rather a putting of Cochrane in context, and playing out the rest of the story.

1

The Status of Qualitative Research as Evidence

ROSS E. G. UPSHUR

> But facts do not make history; facts do not even make events. Without meaning attached, and without understanding of causes and connections, a fact is an isolate particle of experience, is reflected light without a source, planet with no sun, star without constellation, constellation beyond galaxy, galaxy outside the universe—fact is nothing.
>
> Russell Banks (1997, p. 339)

For all the attention devoted to the varied manifestations of evidence-based health care, there is a dearth of reflection on the nature of evidence itself. Perhaps this is because the concept has been so successfully appropriated and uprooted from its original meaning and fastened tightly to the enterprise of research. The purpose of this chapter is to open up for consideration the nature and structure of evidence. I will commence with a discussion of the problems of defining and characterizing evidence. Following this, I will describe a model of evidence. A discussion concerning the nature of reasoning in practice and linking the model to practice will follow. This will be illustrated with examples drawn from qualitative research in primary care. Finally, I will offer some thoughts on the challenges posed by the Cochrane Collaboration.

Do We Need a Definition of Evidence?

Current approaches in philosophical analysis eschew the attempt to provide essential definitions of terms but rather, in the wake of Wittgenstein, attempt to illuminate how the meaning of a term relates to the context of its use. However, a standard gambit in scientific discourse is to taxonomize the object of discussion so that its ontological status is unquestioned. In what ensues I will try to balance both perspectives. I will commence with a brief discussion of etymology and some definitions of evidence.

The etymology of the word *evidence* is rooted in the concept of experience, relating to what is manifest and obvious, apparent to sight. The origins of the word, then, are deeply connected to sense experience. The *Oxford English Dictionary* (1971) indicates several senses relevant to our considerations:

1. The quality or condition of being evident
2. Manifestation
3. That which makes evident, mark, trace
4. Ground for belief; that which tends to prove or disprove any conclusion. (p. 909)

Evidence has central standing as a key concept in jurisprudence and law. Legal definitions of evidence stress its probative function: Evidence consists of the varied sources of information such as witnesses, documents, concrete objects which are submitted to a court "for the purpose of inducing beliefs in the minds of the court or the jury." A quotation from a legal dictionary—Oran's *Dictionary of the Law* (2000, online)— makes this point clear:

1. Any species of proof or probative matter, legally presented at the trial of an issue, by the act of the parties and through the medium of witnesses, records, documents, exhibits, concrete objects, for the purpose of inducing beliefs in the minds of the court or the jury as to their contention.
2. All the means by which any alleged matter of fact, the truth of which is submitted to investigation, is established or disproved.

An important point that emerges from legal concepts of evidence is that the same evidence can be interpreted in different ways as either corroborating or refuting the matter at hand. It is inherent in legal concepts of evidence that a univocal understanding of evidence is infrequent. Hence, there is the need for adjudication and argument. Indeed, the weighing of evidence is contingent on context. Depending on the seriousness of the matter at hand, the weight of evidence varies. Thus, in matters of criminal law, such as murder, evidence should lead to proof beyond a reasonable doubt, whereas in torts, the evidence is adjudicated according to the balance of probability.

In health care and medicine, evidence is conceived in a scientific context. Goodman and Royall (1988) have defined scientific evidence as follows: "Evidence is a property of data that makes us alter our beliefs about how the world around us is working. Another way to say this is that evidence is the basis upon which we derive inferences" (p. 1568). A recent editorial in *The Canadian Medical Association Journal* explicitly seeks to define scientific evidence: "In its simplest form, the available scientific evidence consists of the published report of a single piece of original research" (Miettinen, 1998, p. 215).

Evidence-Based Medicine advocates do not define evidence per se, but rather characterize the process of evidence-based care as "the conscientious, explicit and judicious use of best evidence in making health care decisions" (Sackett, Rosenberg, Gray, Haynes, & Richardson, 1996, p. 71). Evidence in this sense is that which is produced by a scientific study. The approach advocated by Evidence-Based Medicine creates a hierarchy of evidence on the basis of the rigor of study design.

From the definitions cited, it is clear that evidence, in some way, is conceptually linked to notions such as proof, belief, and rationality. The definitions advanced by Goodman and Royall (1988) and Miettinen (1998) contribute the concepts of research, probability, and inference. The definition advanced by Sackett et al. (1996) uses language with moral overtones (conscientious, judicious) and logical connotations (explicit).

In the constructions of Miettinen (1998) and Goodman and Royall (1988), evidence assumes the form of a probability statement. When evidence is constrained to being a probability, it can be managed by the probability calculus and, therefore, is inherently quantitative. As Miller and Safer (1993) have argued, this effectively rules out qualitative sources as being capable of standing as evidence. Nonquantitative dimensions of both research and practice are of immense importance in health care. Therefore, there is a need to conceptualize evidence in a manner that admits qualitative considerations as evidence.

To summarize, evidence is an observation, fact, or organized body of information offered to support or justify inferences or beliefs in the demonstration of some proposition or matter at issue. The determinants of belief in health care may arise from either quantitative or qualitative grounds. There is no a priori reason to exclude qualitative research from assuming the status of evidence so far as qualitative research can change or modify beliefs.

The central questions in terms of the status of qualitative research as evidence (and here I will restrict myself to the context of clinical practice and not the theory of knowledge) focus on when, in what contexts, and for what purposes can one regard qualitative studies as "best evidence." The goal of Evidence-Based Practice is to integrate research with practice. Hence, my task in the remainder of this chapter is not to enter the debates about qualitative versus quantitative research, about which methods to employ, or any of the many important theoretical discussions. Rather, my goal, more limited, humble, and likely yet incomplete, is to sketch out a justification for the manner in which qualitative research can inform practice that goes beyond simple dichotomies such as fact/value, subjective/objective, and hypothesis generating/hypothesis testing. The first task is to reconstruct a model of evidence that integrates qualitative research.

A Synthetic Model of Evidence

Qualitative research, including narrative approaches to medicine, has recently received increased attention in the mainstream medical journals. The *British Medical Journal* ran a series of articles outlining the fundamental tenets of qualitative research and recently included a series called "Narrative-Based Medicine" (Greenhalgh & Hurwitz, 1999). Qualitative approaches have informed nursing research for the better part of the past twenty years and have been a major component of research in primary care. However, the first proponents of Evidence-Based Medicine were, for the most part, specialists in internal medicine with a particular interest in clinical epidemiology. Hence, the impetus for Evidence-Based Medicine derived from a tradition wedded to quantitative approaches committed to more or less reductionist, positivist, and physicalist worldviews. Although there is some suggestion of a recognition of the importance of qualitative research by Evidence-Based Medicine proponents (see, for example, the editorial by Sackett & Wennberg, 1997), the status of qualitative research in the hierarchy of evidence articulated by Evidence-Based Medicine is not acknowledged[1] or is relegated to a less reliable form of research (Gray, 1997).

This indicates that qualitative research is still problematic for certain traditions.

The task then becomes to build a model of evidence that is inclusive enough to accommodate qualitative and quantitative research modalities. This model should place each on common ground and equal footing. Also, given that the concept of evidence can only be restricted to research findings by stipulative definition, the model of evidence must be able to incorporate evidence derived from experience.

Such a model was created under the auspices of HEALNet, which is a Canadian network of researchers in the health, social, and applied sciences. It is a member of the Canadian Networks of Centres of Excellence program that is a partnership between Canadian universities, Industry Canada, and the Canadian research granting councils. HEALNet's research mission is to optimize the use of the best evidence in decisions made about workplace health and at all levels within the health care system. As part of its mandate, HEALNet commissioned a project to investigate the nature and structure of evidence.

Setting the Coordinates

A model of evidence can be created within boundaries set in logic, statistics, epidemiology, epistemology, and interpretive social sciences. A description follows of the elements of a framework within which we can locate different conceptions of scientific evidence and map their interrelationships.

Toulmin (1976) identifies a set of contrasting distinctions within which to situate medical knowledge. The distinctions are also applicable to evidence as related to the broader field of health care. I have added four additional distinctions. The distinctions developed in the next section will set the limits of the possible interpretations or characterizations of evidence. It will therefore allow for the identification of areas of agreement and disagreement. Rather than viewed as dichotomies (either/or), these distinctions should be seen as poles of contrast, recognizing that there is a dynamic tension between the two poles of the distinctions and interaction between them. The explicit importance of these distinctions will emerge when the concepts of inference are taken up in greater detail.

11 Distinctions

1. Abstract and concrete
2. Mathematical and historical
3. Theoretical and practical
4. Pure and applied
5. General and particular
6. Collective and personal
7. Descriptive and prescriptive
8. Predictive and interpretive
9. Algorithm and judgment
10. Inference and decision
11. Disinterested and interested.

The adjectives on the left side characterize one conception of scientific evidence and its desired characteristics. It stems from the explanatory or Galilean conception of science (Vineis, 1997). For many disciplines, scientific evidence is characterized by its abstract nature. This is most readily understood by reflecting on mathematical or statistical models. Newtonian mechanics is a perfect example of this kind of scientific model. It is abstract, it employs mathematical language (therefore transcending the particularities of specific natural languages); it is general in its application (it applies to all physical objects of a certain size range), universal in scope (that is, one can make the calculations from another planet or galaxy), and compels assent from those who understand its logic. Abstraction requires the elimination of particular detail but therefore allows more general or universal application. The results of the mathematical predictions are thought to hold true regardless of whether the individual making the predictions is alive or present to witness the event. Predictive capacity and explanatory power are the hallmarks of this vision of science. Quantitative measurement is the usual expression of meaning. Precision and accuracy are virtues. This model of scientific reasoning exerts tremendous influence and is the model of science to which emerging sciences aspire. This conception of science animates pure sciences such as physics and chemistry. In health care, general laws like inheritance and chemical and thermodynamic properties of energy metabolism are illustrative examples.

Most abstract and general evidence comes from fundamental laboratory research.

The contrasts on the right side illustrate the contextual or hermeneutic dimensions of evidence. Clinical encounters are concrete, dealing with this individual at this particular time, in a specific embodiment of language and culture, and within a historical horizon of knowledge. The salient features of this form of evidence are its narrative structure and contextuality. The concern is with the understanding of meaning rather than quantities or properties of objects. Epistemologically, it is also rooted in empiricism, but is not necessarily quantified reasoning. It is empirical because it relates to the evidence of the senses of the perceiver (in this case, the clinician).

The salient issue with regard to these preconditions is their very conditionality. The aim of explanatory science in health care is to discern causal structure in order to predict accurately what will occur subsequent to the occurrence of a set of initial conditions. In this sense, the general concepts of cause and effect, and the evidence that such relationships are known, are conditional. Many of the means by which evidence is presented in the literature are attempts to characterize the extent to which the cause and effect relationship is understood. Numbers needed to treat, confidence intervals, and p values are various ways in which we can express our confidence in predicting outcomes under certain conditions. As the methods used are probabilistic, they fall short of the certitude and generality as promised by the Galilean conception of science.[2]

The important point to establish in this analysis is that evidence in health care is neither exclusively abstract, mathematical, and general nor narrative and particular, but is a mediation and interaction of both types of knowledge.[3] The issues become problematic only when one wishes a monolithic conception of evidence, that is, a single criterion to reliably distinguish truth from falsehood.[4] Clearly, in the complex world of medical care, it is unlikely that one criterion or form of reasoning will be effective in all instances. The universalizing tendency of early conceptions of EBM needs to be tempered with the idiosyncrasies that are embedded in human life, and especially in the client/health care system interaction. It is necessary, however, to give an account that clarifies how the differing roles of evidence can be weighted in different contexts and at different levels of health care.

Linking the Distinctions: A Simplified Model of Evidence

How do the two different definitions of evidence relate to each other? The set of contrasts drawn here and their interrelation can be conceptualized and described in a model, such as a schematic representation that depicts the poles of evidence (see Figure 1.1). The anchors of the axes demarcate the poles of evidence. The vertical axis depicts the range of methodologies used in health care research. It shows that methodology is central to how observations are collected, aggregated, analyzed, and interpreted.

The horizontal axis sets out the domain or context of evidence. It demonstrates that evidence has personal connotations related to the capacity to change, alter, or support beliefs. The personal dimensions of evidence are most clearly manifest in the clinical realm and at the microallocation level, where health care worker/patient interactions are focused on the distinct and unique aspects of an individual and his or her care.[5] The horizontal axis represents the level of aggregation to which the evidence may be applied. It represents the continuum from the individual to population.

The figure, then, creates four quadrants in the evidence universe: qualitative/personal; qualitative/general; quantitative/general; quantitative/personal. In the initial taxonomic structure, the quadrants will be characterized in isolation as distinct entities. It is in the subset relationship where the similarities and differences, conflicts and concordances, between different concepts of evidence become apparent.

What the model intends to communicate is that there are competing views about evidence; some are contrary to others, but there is also considerable overlap. In logical terms, there is a fuzzy set relationship at the interstices. The borders blur in certain areas.

The model is a very abstract representation of evidence scaled down to its elements. Table 1.1 sets out the model in more detail. It provides illustrative examples of the types of evidence that predominate in each quadrant, the reasoning style, and disciplinary manifestations, and gives examples from the literature. Thus, the table links the abstract descriptive model to the concrete manifestations and uses of evidence.

Quadrant 1: Qualitative/Personal

The first quadrant in the ideal model depicts evidence as primarily personal and qualitative. Evidence emerges from the particular and

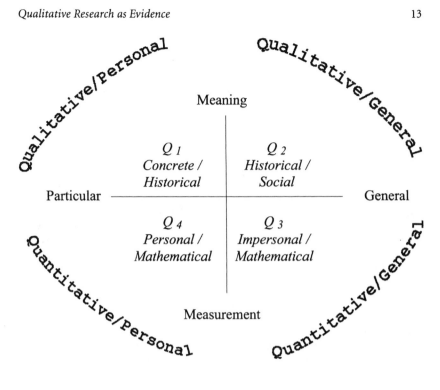

Figure 1.1 Conceptual Basis of the Taxonomy of Evidence

historical nature of the perceptions, beliefs, and attitudes of persons. This evidence is expressed through narratives. The form of reasoning that predominates is practical and goal oriented.

This form of evidence is very closely analogous to legal concepts of evidence in that it is very case and individual focused. The clinical encounter is an exemplification of this form of evidence, and the case report is its research manifestation. The patient history and physical examination, the laboratory and other diagnostic tests, the treatment plan and follow-up, are all part of this quadrant, as are the varying beliefs, attitudes, preferences, predispositions, perceptions, and "epistemological frames" brought forth by both health care provider and patient. This form of evidence predominates at the "micro" level. In terms of research typology, the array of techniques associated with qualitative research belong here: in-depth interviews, focus groups, and textual analysis.

TABLE 1.1 Relationship of Evidence Quadrants and Evidential Features

	Illustrations	Evidence Type	Reasoning Style	Disciplinary Manifestation
Q₁ Qualitative/ Personal	Attitudes Perceptions Signs and Symptoms	Concrete Particular Historical	Narrative	Nursing Clinical Medicine Ethnography Humanities
Q₂ Qualitative/ General	Policies Consensus Statements Community and Social Goals	Historical Social	Narrative	Administration Social Sciences Epidemiology
Q₃ Quantitative/ General	Traditional Evidence Hierarchy	General Mathematical	Quantitative	Clinical Epidemiology Bench Sciences Statistics
Q₄ Quantitative/ Personal	Bayesian Decision Theory Quality of Life	Particular Mathematical	Quantitative	Economics Political Science Statistics

In positivistic conceptions of evidence, this quadrant would be largely abjured and denigrated. Indeed, some theorists of Evidence-Based Medicine are explicit in stating that the kind of reasoning found in Quadrant 1 is an obstacle to evidence-based decision making (Gray, 1997). However, insofar as the social sciences have a bearing on health care and stand as scientific disciplines in their own right, the approaches used and the data derived from such studies have scientific status, and therefore the results must be considered as evidence.

The theoretical frameworks associated with this quadrant come from the humanities and social sciences. Hermeneutics, semiology, social constructivism, critical theory, ethology, ethnomethodology, and postmodernism are all represented here.

Quadrant 2: Qualitative/General

As one moves along the horizontal axis, the context of evidence shifts from a purely personal to more aggregate levels. In the ideal model, the most "impersonal" domain would be the population level, where the interests of any particular individual and his or her health concerns are subsumed by population considerations. Hence, the vertical axis represents the transition from the micro through the meso to the macro levels of organization and delivery of health care. In Quadrant 2, the managerial perspective emerges, as does the set of sciences devoted to the study of health care in its organizational manifestations (Lomas, 1991; Lomas, Sisk, & Stocking, 1993; Naylor, 1995). The cultural, social, and gender dimensions of evidence emerge more prominently in this quadrant. It is important to recognize that competing views of evidence and preferred action emerge here. Hence, the concept of consensus and the application of "political" rationality (negotiated agreement upon ends, goals, and goods) are manifest in this quadrant.

Historical and social forms of evidence are employed in this domain. It is qualitative in the sense that in this domain, the voices of multiple stakeholders, all armed with evidence and its preferred interpretation, come into interaction. Policy analysis, organizational decision making, planning, and implementation are the practical applications.

Quadrant 3: Quantitative/General

In this domain, traditional concepts of scientific evidence emerge. Quantitative data derived through the application of recognized study designs (in the case of evidence-based decision making, the emphasis is on epidemiological study design) constitute the basis of evidence. It is impersonal in the sense that the evidence is intended to be general in application and not subject to bias or group or self-interest. It is expressed quantitatively and usually, though not invariably, employs statistical measures as the means of representing outcomes of interest. Most of the evidence hierarchy as articulated by Sackett, Richardson, Rosenberg, and Haynes (1997) and Haynes, Sackett, Gray, Cook, and Guyatt (1996, 1997) fits in this quadrant. In this model, the strength of evidence is linked to the methodological quality of the study design, with preference given to designs with the most rigor relative to the research question at hand. On the basis of methodological considerations, the evidence is then graded hierarchically. This approach applies to average populations and patients and favors data over theoretical considerations.

The standard of rationality and proof in this quadrant tends to be more closely aligned with mathematical standards in the emphasis on rules and algorithms. Contextual modification is not explicitly emphasized, as it represents a potential form of bias.

Quadrant 4: Quantitative/Personal

The fourth quadrant of the ideal model seeks to capture the quantification of personal beliefs and attributes. The most clearly elaborated manifestation of this feature is found in the development of Bayesian methods of reasoning. The important point here is to acknowledge the growing importance of this approach and to highlight its distinctness from other approaches.

The approach to evidence in this quadrant is mathematical, and the standard of rationality calculative. Decision theory, econometric approaches, and quality of life scales that embody time trade-offs or standard gambles are all manifestations of this approach. The disciplines of statistics, economics, political science, and quality of life research are the most significant disciplinary manifestations.

Applying the Model:
Identifying Arguments and Contexts

Evidence functions within the set of reasons asserted to support belief in a specific proposition. These propositions can be as varied as the world itself. Indeed, a proposition is merely a statement about beliefs concerning the truth, falsity, or probability of states of affairs in the external world. The set of propositions that relate to evidence and health care is large but not infinite. The important point to recognize is that any information, quantitative or qualitative, does not have meaning unless placed in propositional form related to some context of application. For it to be expressed, it must be formulated as a statement. Odds ratios, p values, and confidence intervals alone have no meaning. Evidence has meaning only insofar as it is used in some context with regard to some claim. Hence, evidence can be regarded as playing a role in the context of an argument (Dickinson, 1998; Horton, 1998).

An argument, in the sense intended here, is an attempt to use a sequenced set of reasons to bring about agreement concerning the truth or falsity of states of affairs in the world. Arguments usually consist of a sequence of statements (propositions) leading to a conclusion (as to what is to be accepted as true, or what is to be done). The premises are intended to justify or lead to the conclusion, and the conclusion should follow from the premises or be entailed by them.

Consequently, an argument is a form of persuasive rational discourse used to resolve "uncertainty, instability, or conflict" (Walton, 1998). Evidence is proffered in arguments as probative, that is, having the status of truth, or compelling assent, or belief in the state of affairs described. For example, if the results of a randomized controlled trial comparing an antibiotic to a placebo in the treatment of otitis media in children are statistically significant (at a conventional level of significance) and clinically relevant (by whatever predetermined set of clinically relevant standards), and the study passes scrutiny by critical appraisal standards, then, at some level, one should be persuaded of its effectiveness. Whether this demonstration serves to be conclusive enough to change practice, though, is another matter entirely. Studies, then, are rhetorical devices intended to persuade readers of the probity of the data.[6]

Arguments and Inference

Arguments are assessed on the basis of the validity of inference and truth (or probability) of the explicitly asserted premises. Inferences are constitutive of the intellectual practice of reasoning. Reasoning consists of the evaluation of the logical relations that exist between propositions about states of affairs in the world. There are three types of inference:

1. *Deductive* Deductive inferences are logical demonstrations of the relationship between premises and conclusions. The conclusion is said to follow from or be entailed by the premises with certainty, that is, the conclusion is a logical consequence of the premises. Deductive inferences can be certain or apodictic (admit no exception). An example of a deductive inference is Pythagoras's theorem. In general, deduction

moves from rule and case to result. The two sets of inferences below illustrate deductive reasoning.

All beans in this bag are white.
These beans are from this bag.
Therefore these beans are white.

All children with fevers have viral infections.
This child has a fever.
Therefore this child has a viral infection.

2. *Inductive* Inductive inferences build from particular instances to general lawlike descriptions. Conclusions from inductive premises, while not logically necessary, are to follow with either high probability or high plausibility. Induction moves from case and result to rule. Inductive inference is typically described as the goal of empirical science.

These beans are from this bag.
These beans are white.
Therefore all the beans from this bag are white.

These children have fevers.
These children have viral infections.
Therefore all children with fevers have viral infections.

3. *Abductive* Abductive reasoning accepts conclusions not on the basis of its lawlike character or on the basis of entailment but on the grounds that it provides an adequate or best explanation of the available evidence. Abductive reasoning is used extensively in health care. Abduction moves from rule and result to case, that is, one moves from the facts to the possible explanation of the facts.

Most of the beans in this bag are white.
This handful of beans is from this bag.
Probably most of this handful of beans are white.

This child has a fever.
Most children with fevers have viral infections.
Probably this child has a viral infection.

Nondeductive inferences, such as inductive or abductive inferences, are rarely simply true or false; rather, they admit to degrees of probability. Consequently, they are defeasible, that is, capable of being overturned by either evidence from subsequent studies or further consideration. Not surprisingly, abductive inference is also termed as inference to the best explanation (Upshur, 1997).

> Inference to the best explanation takes the following logical form:
> D is a collection of data (facts, observations, data etc);
> H explains D (that is, if true, H would explain D);
> There are no other hypotheses that can explain D as well as H does,
> Therefore H is probably true. (Walton, 1996, p. 259)

Linking Evidence and Inference: Some Characteristics of Evidence

Evidence provided by empirical studies, either qualitative or quantitative, has important essential features that require explication. To conflate the concept of evidence with the concept of truth will lead to serious misunderstanding. As Oreskes, Shrader-Frechette, and Belitz (1994) have argued persuasively, the concept of truth is illusive in open systems.

Evidence in health care has the following four qualities:

1. Provisional
2. Defeasible
3. Emergent
4. Incomplete

Evidence from health care research, particularly clinical and epidemiological studies, is provisional and defeasible. This means that it never attains absolute certainty and can be revised in light of new evidence. Consequently, the occurrence of definitive studies is comparatively rare. This is a common feature encountered in the interpretation of health information.

Similarly, qualitative studies are provisional and defeasible. It is a rare study that provides unequivocal interpretations. However, due to the concern with meaning, the qualitative tradition may be more ac-customed to the lack of finality of interpretations.

An excellent example of the provisional nature of medical evidence is peptic ulcer disease. In thirty years, the etiology and management of this disease have undergone dramatic and profound changes. In the 1970s, textbooks proclaimed the need for white diets and postulated stress as an important element of causation. In the 1980s, with the introduction of cimetidine, hypersecretion and the use of H_2 blockers were, respectively, the cause and treatment. In the late 1990s, Helicobacter pylori was the favored etiologic agent, and eradication with triple therapy the preferred treatment.

This is but one example of the way that new research findings have dramatically altered the manner in which a disease entity is understood, with major consequences for diagnosis, treatment, and patient educa-tion. This is not to argue for the existence of paradigm shifts, but rather to assert that there is something inherently protean about scientific research. If evidence were not defeasible, that is, revisable in the light of new information, new findings could not be accommodated in the context of prior beliefs. Hence, one salient feature of medical evidence is its inherent provisional nature. Research evidence is rarely an eternal truth or a constant (outside of certain basic biologic laws). This is a major barrier to both the public and professional dissemination of research evidence, as there seems to be a dissonance between the actual evolution of scientific knowledge and the public's preconceptions about what science is. Rather than being a producer of fixed truths, scientific research is dynamic. The dynamism and changeability of medical science in particular is a barrier to the straightforward dissem-ination of research evidence into practice. Indeed, clinicians' conserva-tism and reluctance to change practice, so much bemoaned by the ad-vocates of EBM, may be understandable, given the contrariness that seems apparent in much research evidence.

This contrariness occurs because evidence is emergent and therefore is expected to change with time. There is always the possibility that even the best evidence can be overturned in the course of time. Ex-cellent evidence-based therapies can be superseded by newer ones, but more important, some evidence-based therapies should be re-placed. For example, isoniazid (INH) is used for the prophylaxis of tuberculosis (TB) infection. Several excellent randomized trials unequiv-ocally establish its effectiveness in the prevention of TB. It is granted a

Grade A recommendation in *The Canadian Guide to Clinical Preventive Health Care* (Canadian Task Force, 1994), indicating the highest form of endorsement. However, compliance with this medication is poor, largely for two reasons. The duration of therapy is long (6 to 12 months), and there are potential side effects. Clinically ill people are poorly compliant, so it is no surprise that clinically well people are similarly noncompliant. Consequently, despite the impeccable status of INH as an evidence-based intervention, INH prophylaxis stands in need of improvement. Excellent evidence does not necessarily translate into excellent or successful therapy. Diagnostic and screening tests likewise can be superseded. For this reason, despite the existence of good evidence, research will continue, and standards of best evidence will change with time.

How does this relate to the concept of inference that has been outlined? Quite simply, it illustrates that any use of research evidence entails the use of abductive forms of inference. If the issue of empirical research is not eternal truths, then the practical reasoning that follows from it is neither deductive nor inductive. What this establishes is that the use of evidence in practice is not premised on its being derived from quantitative or qualitative methodology but rather on how reasonable it is to apply the results in a particular context.

Qualitative Research and Inference to the Best Explanation

I teach EBM to medical students and first- and second-year residents in family medicine. I routinely employ qualitative studies as part of our efforts. My favorite session uses two papers: a qualitative study that compares the perceptions of physicians who prescribe antibiotics for sore throats (Butler, Rollnick, Pill, Maggs-Rapport, & Stott, 1998) and a systematic review and meta-analysis that shows the lack of effectiveness of antibiotics in acute upper respiratory illness (Fahey, Stocks, & Thomas, 1998). Antibiotic resistance has become a major public health concern, and physician overuse of antibiotics has been implicated in the rapid increase of drug resistance. Evidence also indicates that physicians prescribe antibiotics with full knowledge of their lack of effectiveness. What can explain this?

The session incorporates the two methodological poles of evidence. The meta-analysis has two wonderfully persuasive peto-grams: one shows the lack of benefit of antibiotics in acute respiratory disease in comparison to placebo, and the other demonstrates that antibiotics cause significantly higher rates of adverse effects as compared to placebo.

The qualitative study seeks to explore the issue further. The findings are quite illuminating:

- Physicians state that they know antibiotics are useless, express dismay at themselves for "not following the evidence," and fail to elicit the chief reason for the patient's consultations. They express a fear that doctor-patient relationships will be jeopardized if antibiotics are not prescribed.
- Patients rarely make their expectations explicit in regard to antibiotics, and the desire for antibiotics is not the primary reason for seeking medical attention: reassurance and information may be more important.

The two papers create a compelling portrait. The meta-analysis clearly shows a lack of benefit associated with antibiotic use and an increase of harm. A simple interpretation of the study would be that practitioners ought not to prescribe them. The qualitative study indicates that in full knowledge of this, clinicians regularly prescribe antibiotics. What the qualitative study highlights is the mismatch of expectations between physician and patient. This finding is immediately applicable to practice. I ask my residents whether they explicitly seek information concerning patient expectations in their consultations. Invariably the answer is no. I further ask if, on the basis of this study, they believe it is reasonable or justified to do so. They invariably answer yes. To the important question of whether they would do so in practice, they usually answer they would. Whether they do or not is another matter.

This example illustrates how qualitative research can be immediately transferred into practice. The results of the study give sufficient grounds for changing a belief that is reasonable and justifiable by any standard of adjudication. What makes this study so compelling is the way in which it illuminates experiences that are common for all primary care physicians. The results are reconcilable with their clinical experience.

The question of the applicability of the results of any research study relates only partially to the methodology of the study itself, but more profoundly to whether or not it is reasonable in the intended context. Evidence is only part of what makes a course of action reasonable. Hence, the best explanation to which evidence can be used varies according to context. Once this is clear, and once misconceptions about evidence and the nature of clinical reasoning are removed, qualitative research results are unproblematically granted the status of evidence.

The Cochrane Collaboration

The mission of the Cochrane Collaboration is to be an organization that aims to help people make well-informed decisions about health care by preparing, maintaining, and promoting the accessibility of systematic reviews of the effects of health care interventions.

The Collaboration is built on nine principles:

1. collaboration
2. building on the enthusiasm of individuals
3. avoiding duplication
4. minimizing bias
5. keeping up-to-date
6. ensuring relevance
7. ensuring access
8. continually improving the quality of its work
9. continuity

That the central focus of the Cochrane Collaboration has been restricted to systematic reviews is both a benefit and a burden. The way the current versions of the evidence hierarchy are structured, pride of place is given to randomized control trials and systematic reviews. The process of integrating and summarizing results from sources such as observational studies is technically demanding and, in the eyes of some commentators, futile. It may be that an attempt to systematically analyze and commensurate qualitative studies is a form of conceptual confusion. Qualitative studies are not designed, as are trials, to isolate an effect from a discrete intervention. In essence, a Cochrane-like Collaboration for qualitative research intends toward the opposite pole, a map of the range of possible meanings and perceptions. Such an endeavor could encompass what is most admirable about the Cochrane Collaboration, which is the enthusiasm and dedication of the work groups to produce an evidence synthesis. Such an international collaboration is possible for qualitative researchers, but the results would be very different from the traditional Cochrane group.

Conclusions

In this chapter, I have argued that there is a need to understand the concept of evidence more broadly and that the means by which evidence is introduced into practice also needs to be reconstituted. A model of evidence that integrates issues of meaning and measurement and the context of application was advanced and described. The concept of inference was revisited, and I argued that if one views the use of evidence as an expression of abductive reasoning, then there is no tension between qualitative and quantitative modes of research when applied in practice. An example from clinical practice was used to illustrate the points. Finally, some thoughts on the role of the Cochrane Collaboration were advanced.

Notes

1. See, for example, the Levels of Evidence at http://cebm.jr2.ox.ac.uk/docs/levels.html as of June 6, 2000 (Centre for Evidence-Based Medicine, 1999).

2. Indeed, very little in biological science will come close to the Newtonian model. It is important to note that the Newtonian model is also constrained by the larger theoretical structure of quantum theory. For a deeper discussion of these issues, please see John Barrow (1998).

3. Aristotle, the Greek philosopher, characterized the interaction of the universal and particular types of knowledge as the exercise of practical reasoning. The exercise of sound practical intelligence that is able to fuse the universal and particular in practical reasoning is called phronesis. Indeed, the definition of EBM that invokes virtues of conscientiousness and judiciousness are very close to Aristotle's concept of phronesis.

4. This is the philosopher's quest, best epitomized by Leibniz's conception of a universal language or *mathesis universalis,* which was a language capable of deciding all disputes. Calculus was to provide this service of being the impartial, objective adjudicator of knowledge claims. Leibniz envisioned a time when all disputes could be resolved through calculation.

5. This leads to an apparent paradox in that personal attributes, such as beliefs and values, may in fact be more stable than scientific evidence. As shall be demonstrated, scientific evidence has a protean and dynamic nature that may be at variance with the need for stable belief about efficacy. This apparent paradox was first thoroughly explored by C. S. Peirce.

6. It is well recognized that published studies present the best side of data: the statistical model of the best "fit," figures formatted for maximal visual effect. The space limitations imposed by journals illustrate the "edited" and "molded" nature of published evidence, which is winnowed considerably before presentation. For an account of visual biases, see Tufte (1983, 1997).

References

Banks, R. (1997). *Affliction*. Toronto: McLelland and Stewart.

Barrow, J. D. (1998). *Impossibility: The limits of science and the science of limits*. New York: Oxford University Press.

Butler, C. C., Rollnick, S., Pill, R., Maggs-Rapport, F., & Stott, N. (1998). Understanding the culture of prescribing: Qualitative study of general practitioners' and patients' perceptions of antibiotics for sore throats. *British Medical Journal, 317*(7159), 637-642.

Canadian Task Force on the Periodic Health Examination. (1994). *The Canadian Guide to Clinical Preventive Health Care*. Ottawa: Minister of Supply and Service Canada.

Centre for Evidence-Based Medicine, Levels of Evidence and Grades of Recommendations. (November 19, 1999). Retrieved June 6, 2000, from the World Wide Web: http://cebm.jr2.ox.ac.uk/docs/levels.html

Dickinson, H. D. (1998). Evidence-based decision-making: An argumentative approach. *International Journal of Medical Informatics, 51*(2-3), 71-81.

Fahey, T., Stocks, N., & Thomas, T. (1998). Quantitative systematic review of randomised controlled trials comparing antibiotic with placebo for acute cough in adults. *British Medical Journal, 316*(7135), 906-910.

Goodman, S. N., & Royall, R. (1998). Evidence and scientific research. *American Journal of Public Health, 78*(12), 1568-1574.

Gray, J. A. M. (1997). *Evidence-based healthcare*. New York: Churchill Livingstone.

Greenhalgh, T., & Hurwitz, B. (1999). Narrative based medicine: Why study narrative? *British Medical Journal, 318*(7175), 48-50.

Haynes, R. B., Sackett, D. L., Gray, J. M., Cook, D. J., & Guyatt, G. H. (1996). Transferring evidence from research into practice: 1. The role of clinical care research evidence in clinical decisions. *ACP Journal Club, 125*(3), A14-A16.

Haynes, R. B., Sackett, D. L., Gray, J. M., Cook, D. J., & Guyatt, G. H. (1997). Transferring evidence from research into practice: 2. Getting the evidence straight. *ACP Journal Club, 126*(1), A14-A16.

Horton, R. (1998). The grammar of interpretive medicine. *Canadian Medical Association Journal, 159*(3), 245-249.

Lomas, J. (1991). Words without action? The production, dissemination, and impact of consensus recommendations. *Annual Review of Public Health, 12,* 41-65.

Lomas, J., Sisk, J. E., & Stocking, B. (1993). From evidence to practice in the United States, the United Kingdom, and Canada. *Milbank Quarterly, 71*(3), 405-410.

Miettinen, O. S. (1998). Evidence in medicine: Invited commentary. *Canadian Medical Association Journal, 158*(2), 215-221.

Miller, S. I., & Safer, L. A. (1993). Evidence, ethics and social policy dilemmas. *Education Policy Analysis Archives, 1,* 1-13.

Naylor, C. D. (1995). Grey zones of clinical practice: Some limits to evidence-based medicine. *Lancet, 345*(8953), 840-842.

Oran's *Dictionary of the Law*. (2000). Retrieved March 4, 2000, from the World Wide Web: www.rfpwire.com/pathfind/orans/.orans.asp.

Oreskes, N., Shrader-Frechette, K., & Belitz, K. (1994). Verification, validation, and confirmation of numerical models in the earth sciences. *Science, 263,* 641-646.

Oxford English Dictionary (Compact Edition). (1971). New York: Oxford University Press.

Sackett, D. L., Richardson, W. S., Rosenberg, W., & Haynes, R. B. (1997). *Evidence-based medicine.* New York: Churchill Livingstone.

Sackett, D. L., Rosenberg, W. M., Gray, J. A., Haynes, R. B., & Richardson, W. S. (1996). Evidence-based medicine: What it is and what it isn't. *British Medical Journal, 312*(7023), 71-72.

Sackett, D. L., & Wennberg, J. E. (1997). Choosing the best research design for each question. *British Medical Journal, 315*(7123), 1636.

Toulmin, S. (1976). On the nature of the physician's understanding. *Journal of Medicine and Philosophy, 1,* 32-50.

Tufte, E. R. (1983). *The visual display of quantitative information.* Cheshire, CT: Graphics Press.

Tufte, E. R. (1997). *Visual explanations: Images and quantities, evidence and narrative.* Cheshire, CT: Graphics Press.

Upshur, R. (1997). Certainty, probability and abduction: Why we should look to C. S. Peirce rather than Godel for a theory of clinical reasoning. *Journal of Evaluation in Clinical Practice, 3*(3), 201-206.

Vineis, P. (1997). Proof in observational medicine. *Journal of Epidemiology and Community Health, 51*(1), 9-13.

Walton, D. (1996). *Argument structure: A pragmatic theory.* Toronto: University of Toronto Press.

Walton, D. (1998). *The new dialectic: Conversational contexts of argument.* Toronto: University of Toronto Press.

Dialogue:

The Form of Evidence

UPSHUR: This is an effort to investigate what evidence is and how it could be understood. It is my perception from teaching undergraduate medical students, from rounds, and from teaching courses at the university that historically, there is nowhere in the curriculum where they get any exposure to qualitative research and qualitative findings. When the residents come to me [for instructions], I encourage them to broaden what they admit as evidence into their thinking, I encourage them to bring qualitative papers to the table, because they don't really know how to deal with it. They need some reassurance that they can take this form of research and use it. And that is what I find problematic.

It comes to residents as something foreign, as most of them have years of biomedical training. Interestingly enough, things are changing now. We are incorporating qualitative research into an Evidence-Based Medicine component of a course, and we are also putting qualitative methods into a second-year research course, so it is getting into the curriculum. You can make an argument that qualitative research is in some sense more useful than a meta-analysis in certain situations, so I have to get them from shying away from using it.

2

What Is Problematic About Evidence?

IRENA MADJAR
JO ANN WALTON

> The social structure of scholarly work and its rhetorical practices have
> given rise to the belief, even among the most sophisticated, that there is a
> fundamental difference between the concept and role of "facts" in science
> and in history. It is by no means clear that such a fundamental difference
> exists, and there are serious questions about the evidence on which that
> belief is based.
>
> R. C. Lewontin (1994, p. 478)

Sooner or later, most of us will consult a physician or spend time in a
clinic or hospital where we will come in contact with a range of health
professionals. When we depend on them for diagnosis, care, and intervention, we would like to think that the knowledge these health workers have is up-to-date, reliable, and based on solid evidence. However
skeptical we may be about the "sales pitch" related to other services and
products we buy—from soft drinks to cars—as patients we need to
believe that medically prescribed treatments are based on scientifically
tested evidence. We certainly do not want care based on personal whims,
outdated ideas, or the latest marketing push by a pharmaceutical
company. In other words, when our health or that of people close to us
is at stake, we look for help that is both scientifically sound and provided in an atmosphere of trust.

But what constitutes evidence in this context, and how may focusing
on different sources and forms of evidence influence people's experience of illness and treatment? What is the evidence that does and ought
to underpin professional health practice, and what are the standards by
which we may weigh different forms of evidence?

In this chapter, we take the stance that "facts" alone do not constitute evidence. Rather, along with authors such as Chandler, Davidson, and Harootunian (1994), we accept that (a) evidence does not exist in a vacuum but is contextual, in the sense that "facts can only become evidence in response to some particular question" (Chandler et al., 1994, p. 1), and (b) the rules and standards by which facts are given the status of evidence are themselves products of historical and social processes, including conventions and ideologies. As such, they are subject to change and redefinition.

Furthermore, we contend that the complexities of human experience and of clinical practice call for consideration of a range of issues and, thus, a range of evidence. It includes evidence derived from personal experience, cultural understandings, and psychosocial and moral concerns that are an integral part of the illness experience and of therapeutic encounters between patients and health workers. Finally, we wish to propose that just as evidence does not arise in a vacuum, neither can it be used in isolation from other contextual considerations.

However valuable the evidence on the efficacy of an intervention, the decision to prescribe it to a particular person cannot be divorced from a host of other considerations. As Carr (1996) argues in relation to the care of people with schizophrenia, application of evidence is a matter of balancing, often with extraordinary difficulty, and a matter of consideration of

> all the relevant neurobiological, medical, pharmacological, neuropsychological, cognitive, intrapsychic, behavioral, interpersonal, familial, and sociocultural phenomena, the myriad factors involved in the human experience of schizophrenia; assignment of appropriate *weighting* to each of these (not all factors are equally salient in all cases); and then *integrating* them in a clinical formulation for the purposes of planning and conducting treatment. (p. 54)

There is no intervention that can "cure" schizophrenia or ensure that future psychotic episodes are prevented. So, apart from the question of what constitutes adequate evidence upon which to base treatment-related decisions, this situation highlights another relevant issue: What outcome indicators should be used to measure the effectiveness of pharmacological and other types of interventions in this context?

Chronic mental illnesses and pain (especially persistent chronic pain) present particularly pertinent examples of the complexity of human experience and of what may therefore be regarded as adequate evidence for sound clinical practice. These conditions arise from complex and often poorly understood etiologies and may be treated through a variety of interventions. At the same time, the effects and measurable outcomes of the conditions themselves, and the prescribed interventions, are poorly developed. Just as important, both pain and chronic mental illness affect people at different life stages and under very different circumstances, with varying impact on the patients and those around them and with a range of illness and coping trajectories arising from the complex interplay of all the variables.

Given this complexity, a clinician wishing to apply the results of a well-designed clinical trial, or even a meta-analysis of a series of such trials, cannot be sure how the individual patient will respond to the recommended treatment. Application of research-derived evidence is not simply a matter of being informed of the latest research findings and following "the rules." It requires a great deal more. It involves knowledge of the individual patient and his or her lifestyle, needs, wishes and preferences, comorbid problems and current therapies, past history, and responses to previously prescribed therapies. In this context, one must ask what is the best evidence that ought to guide clinical practice. Should some types of evidence be privileged over other sources of necessary and useful knowledge?

The Rise of the Evidence-Based Medicine Movement

Modern medicine, along with related disciplines such as nursing, physical therapy, and dietetics, has increasingly come to claim the status of science. As basic and applied research has proliferated, and new knowledge of genetics, molecular biology, biochemistry, pathophysiology, pharmacology, and other therapeutics developed, the view of medicine as science has spread into the community. Results of medical research are often reported as scientific "breakthroughs," and media reports of "miracle cures" are common. This has led to what Moynihan (1998) has called "one of the most widespread misunderstandings in the community" (p. 5): the perception that all medicine is scientific and that treatments and interventions provided by today's physicians and surgeons are proven through scientific research.

One of the effects of this misunderstanding has been the ever rising expectations by the community, at least in the relatively affluent Western societies, of what modern medicine can deliver. Such expectations have been tempered somewhat by anecdotal reports of failed therapies and the challenges of living either with chronic and degenerative conditions for which there are no "miracle cures" or with troublesome and unpleasant symptoms for which there are no effective and reliable interventions. Some suggest that such concerns, along with resistance to increasingly brief and impersonal doctor-patient consultations, have led to the growing popularity of complementary and alternative health practitioners offering more "natural" and "holistic" approaches to treatment of many common ailments (Blair, 1997; Moynihan, 1998).

A further issue that needs to be recognized is that of health economics, with its questions about the costs of health care and the distribution of scarce health service resources. As the dean of the Faculty of Medicine at the University of Sydney, Professor Stephen Leeder (1998, in the Foreword to Ray Moynihan's *Too Much Medicine?*), put it, "Health is so precious. Medicine is so expensive" (p. v). Calls for cost containment in health service delivery are widespread and raise legitimate questions about funding of unnecessary and ineffective treatments along with the broader issues of allocation of scarce resources.

The relatively recent rise of the evidence-based movement in medicine and health care[1] is a response to many of these issues. While the emphasis on scientific and evidence-based clinical practice goes back much further, the movement and its support structure of international Cochrane Collaboration centers and groups is a phenomenon of the 1990s. Although the general population remains largely unaware of the developments in this field, the Evidence-Based Medicine movement has become international, and the debate arising within and between various health professional groups is lively and in danger of becoming polarized (Blair, 1997; Closs & Cheater, 1999; DiCenso, Cullum, & Ciliska, 1998; Kerridge, Lowe, & Henry, 1998; Mitchell, 1997, 1999; Moynihan, 1998; Mulhall, 1998).

Its proponents argue that Evidence-Based Medicine, defined as "the conscientious, explicit, and judicious use of current best evidence in making decisions about the care of individual patients" (Sackett, Rosenberg,

Gray, Haynes, & Richardson, 1996, p. 71), has the capacity to improve the quality of decision making in clinical practice, the effectiveness of treatments, and the outcomes of care. In addition, Evidence-Based Medicine should lead to the elimination of inappropriate and ineffective interventions and to the more effective use of resources (Sackett & Rosenberg, 1995; Sackett et al., 1996).

Evidence-Based Medicine is also advocated as a way of overcoming the difficulties busy clinicians have in accessing relevant evidence and assessing the relative merits of research results that are reported in increasing numbers of papers published in an ever growing number of professional journals.

While scientific evidence may be lacking in some areas, in other areas the problem is one of dissemination of research evidence and its adoption in clinical practice. In the area of pain management, for example, a great deal of research evidence is available—over 16,000 randomized clinical trials (RCTs) alone, reported in over 900 journals (Jadad, 1999). But the volume of literature notwithstanding, studies assessing pain management continue to report inadequate or inappropriate interventions, and patients continue to experience inadequately relieved pain (Carr & Goudas, 1999; Fox, Raina, & Jadad, 1999; Hall-Lord, Steen, & Larsson, 1999; Warfield & Kahn, 1995; Wolf, 1999).

Thus, meta-analyses of reports of clinical trials are seen as a reliable way of summarizing findings from a series of studies and making the evidence and recommendations for clinical practice more readily accessible by busy clinicians (Sackett, 1995). A further benefit of systematic reviews and meta-analyses is the use of such evidence by patients when making decisions about the choice of intervention; for example, the use of epidural or parenteral analgesia in labor and delivery (Jadad, 1999).

The Nature of Evidence

Few would argue that until the rise of the Evidence-Based Medicine movement, the practice of medicine and the other health professions was completely unscientific. Rather, what is now being called into question is the definition of scientific evidence itself, and with it the hitherto accepted standards of what ought to count as fact or evidence for sound clinical practice. The standards are being redefined, as they have been at various other times in history (Chandler et al., 1994), and the status of some types of knowledge is being elevated to that of evidence, fact, or proof providing a more confident basis for clinical decisions and actions.

Proponents of Evidence-Based Medicine and health care acknowledge that evidence from experimental research cannot be applied directly to individual clinical situations. Nevertheless, they call for abandonment of the traditional approach to clinical practice with its apparent reliance on reflection and intuition developed through clinical experience, on understanding of underlying pathophysiology, and on consultation with local or international experts (Sackett, 1995). The findings of single research studies, even well-designed RCTs, have also come to be regarded as inadequate. Even though all these sources of knowledge are seen as important, they are regarded as providing an insufficient basis for clinical practice.

The authority of individual clinical expertise is recognized as important in the diagnostic process (history taking, physical examination, and ability to make a diagnosis), in applying the results of research to individual patients, in understanding patients' emotional needs, and in demonstrating caring and compassion but not in determining the choice of therapy (Sackett, 1995, pp. 62-63). For this, the "best available external clinical evidence" is needed; it consists of "clinically relevant research . . . into the accuracy and precision of diagnostic tests . . . , the power of prognostic markers, and the efficacy and safety of therapeutic, rehabilitative, and preventive regimens" (Sackett et al., 1996, p. 72).

Thus, while the importance of other forms of knowledge and evidence is acknowledged, the emphasis is predominantly on research evidence derived from RCTs and on systematic reviews and meta-analyses of the findings of experimental research. The standards for evaluation of evidence adopted by the Cochrane Collaboration, the United States Preventive Services Task Force, and the Australian National Health and Medical Research Council clearly privilege some forms of evidence over others.

Although the specific wording may differ, most tables of "strengths" or "levels" of evidence use the following classification:

Level/Type I: evidence obtained from systematic review(s) of relevant (and multiple) randomized controlled trials (with meta-analysis where possible)

Level/Type II: evidence obtained from one or more well-designed randomized controlled trials

Level/Type III: evidence obtained from well-designed nonrandomized controlled trials; or from well-designed cohort or case-control analytical studies, preferably multicenter or conducted at different times

Level/Type IV: evidence obtained from well-designed nonexperimental research (preferably from different centers)

Level/Type V: represents the opinions of respected authorities based on clinical experience, descriptive studies, or reports of expert committees

Some sources use only four levels, combining either Levels III and IV or Levels IV and V (see, for example, Gray, 1997; National Health and Medical Research Council, 1999).

It may be argued that Level I evidence and the RCTs from which it is derived provide "the best available external clinical evidence" (Sackett et al., 1996, p. 72) for the effectiveness of specific therapeutic interventions such as drugs or surgical procedures. Few patients would want to begin a course of medication without being able to assume that the drug had been tested and found to be effective. Few clinicians would want to prescribe or administer a course of therapy whose effectiveness was unknown and whose side effects and risks were undocumented. Given the time lag between the production of research evidence and its incorporation into textbooks and adoption in practice, the call for more appropriate ways of providing evidence for clinical decision making is timely and very much needed. The call for similar standards of evidence to be applied to investigative and diagnostic tests and procedures is also well founded. Many tests and procedures are time consuming, invasive, uncomfortable, or even painful for the patient. Many are also costly. Knowing how accurately they assist in the diagnostic process should lead to a more judicious use of such procedures.

But perhaps we need to return to the beginning. What is the question that we are trying to answer? If the question is "What is the effectiveness of Drug X for the treatment of Condition Y?" then experimental evidence from well-designed randomized trials will provide the answer. This holds true even though currently available evidence from past trials may have its flaws and limitations. Even the strongest proponents of Evidence-Based Medicine recognize that RCTs have their shortcomings (imprecise results due to small sample sizes, biased results due to tendency to exaggerate benefits of treatment, and publication bias [Jadad, 1999]). In principle, however, RCTs and subsequent procedures of systematic review and meta-analysis provide the highest level of evidence for the overall effectiveness of specific individual clinical interventions.

The situation becomes much more ambiguous when a single name is given to a complex overall approach (a good example is case management in the mental health field). Using the accepted practices of randomized controlled clinical trial (or meta-analysis of a series of studies) to evaluate an overall approach leaves open a whole series of questions about how much confidence can be placed in whether the outcomes can be attributed to the intervention (Repper & Brooker, 1998). This is because such conventional techniques for testing outcomes do not explore exactly what the intervention itself consists of. As Pincus, Zarin, and West (1996) point out, evaluating complex health care services requires our "peering into a black box." Yet, neither the randomized controlled trial nor meta-analyses of such studies encourage us to examine the complex processes involved in health service delivery modes.

An example is the recent Cochrane review of case management for people with severe mental disorders (Marshall, Gray, Lockwood, & Green, 1998). The authors identify a series of different models of case management that are then analyzed together, the conclusion being that "case management is an intervention of questionable value, to the extent that it is doubtful whether it should be used by community psychiatric services" (p. 2). In a further review, a distinction is made between case management and assertive community treatment. The latter is judged to be "a clinically effective approach to managing the care of severely mentally ill people in the community" and one that, if well targeted, can "substantially reduce the costs of hospital care whilst improving outcome and patient satisfaction" (Marshall & Lockwood, 1999, p. 2). Given the striking differences between the two reviews, it seems that there is much more that could and should be uncovered about what goes on in individual cases, and what *exactly* it is that is effective in the assertive community treatment model.

If, rather than asking "What is the effectiveness of Drug X for the treatment of condition Y?" our question relates to a particular patient, then it can no longer be limited to the issue of average effectiveness. A clinician may need to ask a series of questions: "What are all the factors underlying this patient's condition? How does the presence of Condition Y relate to other health problems this patient is experiencing? If Drug X has been tested on middle-aged adults with Condition Y in its more advanced stages, what effects will it have on this elderly patient whose condition is still mild but who is also being treated for two other chronic conditions? How willing is this patient to accept the side effects (and risks, if any) of Drug X? What does Condition Y and its alleviation mean to this person, and how does it fit in with this person's life goals and priorities? Given all these factors, is any therapy necessary or advisable for this person at this time?" The two sets of questions illustrate the crucial difference between the considerations pertinent to the researcher and those that are critical to the clinician.

RCTs are conducted with clearly delineated and delimited patient groups. Older adults, those who are too ill or unable to communicate in the language of the researchers, people with cognitive or communication impairments, and many others are frequently excluded from RCTs. Issues of generalizability have to be balanced against the need for internal validity. Individual differences are discounted or controlled through randomization and large sample sizes. Extreme scores may be disregarded or excluded from calculations, with aggregate data relating to the average patient—a statistical construction bearing limited resemblance to the actual persons encountered in clinical practice. RCTs focused on therapeutic effectiveness seldom include questions about participants' experience of the prescribed therapy, their preferences, or levels of satisfaction. In the end, even the narrowly defined questions of effectiveness of specific treatments produce answers that are difficult to apply in clinical practice (Blair, 1997; Hellman & Hellman, 1991; Repper & Brooker, 1998).

Clinical practice is different. It involves individual people: complex; idiosyncratic; living with a host of other concerns; enmeshed in habits and relationships that in one way or another affect their illness and its therapy; and bringing with them personal, family, and cultural values, preferences, motivations, needs, abilities, and expectations. Dealing with individual patients requires scientific evidence and a great deal more.

Recognition of the problems arising from narrowly designed clinical trials has led some medical researchers to recommend broadening the range of people traditionally recruited into clinical trials. Some suggest presenting findings for specific categories of participants according to characteristics such as age, sex, and the presence of other conditions or use of therapies (Glasziou, Henry, O'Connell, and others, reported by Moynihan, 1998, p. 232). Others advocate greater emphasis on the evaluation of outcomes of routine care patients receive in a range of clinical settings (Harvey, reported by Moynihan, 1998, p. 233), thus bringing the research evidence closer to the context in which it will be applied. Descriptive and correlational surveys and longitudinal studies are also relevant, providing important contextual information about the prevalence and trends in morbidity among different groups of population, consumer perceptions of their health care needs, and factors that impact on their health and well-being (Brown, Dobson, & Mishra, 1998; Byles, Feldman, & Mishra, 1999; Harris, Byles, Mishra, & Brown, 1999). But is this enough?

The simple answer to this question has to be "no." Although the evidence from RCTs is clearly important, both those who advocate the new evidence-based approach (DiCenso et al., 1998; Sackett, 1995; Sackett et al., 1996) and those who express the need for caution (Kerridge et al., 1998; Mitchell, 1997, inter alia) agree that application of any evidence requires clinical experience, wisdom, care, understanding, and compassion. Where is the knowledge to underpin "the conscientious, explicit, and judicious use of current best evidence" (Sackett et al., 1996, p. 71) to come from?

Other Sources of Evidence

Health economists may be surprised "by the degree to which medicine is still an art," "the importance of communication and coordination among the different providers of care and the families involved," or the relevance of "the nonclinical aspects of the patient's situation" in deciding on an approach to treatment (Walter, Hurley, Labelle, &

Sackett, 1990, pp. 616-617). For clinicians, however, dealing with such issues is a matter of everyday practice.

Selecting the most effective intervention is only a part of it. Understanding the patient and the situation calls for different kinds of knowledge and the preparedness to use more than one model of decision making (Stein, 1991). Such knowledge is not derived from probabilistic thinking. It is accessible through systematic inquiry, subject to reasoned appraisal, and forms an essential component of clinical practice. What is problematic in the current push for Evidence-Based Practice is that, although acknowledged as valuable, such knowledge is taken for granted and seldom discussed in any detail or recognized as a source of important (if different) evidence (Gray, 1997; Sackett et al., 1996).

It is as though education in randomized trial design and conduct of systematic reviews and meta-analyses are all that is needed. The mostly unspoken assumption is that the rest—personal and cultural understanding, ethical reasoning, clinical wisdom—is unproblematic. Yet, as Malterud (1995) points out, "Clinical interaction requires the understanding of particulars to be integrated with the understanding of universals" (p. 187). The explicit scientific evidence has to be integrated with the personal biography of the patient, and interventions have to be negotiated in a way that makes them meaningful and acceptable to him or her.

Qualitative research has the capacity to inform clinical practice by deepening our understanding of human experience and of phenomena that exemplify that experience. It does this by creating awareness of idiosyncrasies and patterns in human behavior and by providing descriptions and theories of the processes involved in becoming ill, recovering, healing, and learning to cope with chronic illness, disability, or frailty, and with the beginning and the end of life. It also provides a means by which we can explore the components that make up complex interventions (and few health interventions are as simple as the administration of Drug X for Condition Y), thus helping us to better understand what elements might be contributing to particular desired outcomes or detracting from them.

Qualitative research may provide important evidence of the cultural similarities and differences that make some therapeutic interventions more or less appropriate for particular patients. Stein (1991), for example, illustrates the need for specific cultural understanding in order to see the inappropriateness of prescribing group rehabilitation therapy (an integral part of the "North American biomedical rehabilitation culture," p. 15) for Slavic American women after a stroke. The ethnographic approach he employs allows Stein to balance the biomedical evidence against cultural and situational factors—evidence of a different kind but of equal importance. To prescribe therapy that the patient finds meaningless or demeaning is to not only fail to help the patient but to also add to the burden of that person's illness and disability.

The aim of the researcher designing RCTs is to remove individual and contextual differences in order to provide answers to carefully formulated research questions and produce generalizable findings. The clinician must recontextualize such findings and reassess their relevance in a particular situation. The aim of the clinician is to understand the concerns of a particular patient and his or her family and to respond to those concerns in a way that is not only scientifically appropriate but is also appropriate to the needs and wishes of the patient.

Clinical practice involves the application of scientific evidence in the choice of appropriate treatment, but it is also concerned with life stories of individual patients and the narratives they tell as they describe, interpret, and try to find meaning in their situation. Clinicians need to listen to the stories their patients present, since, as Greenhalgh and Hurwitz (1999) suggest, "Understanding the narrative context of illness provides a framework for approaching a patient's problems holistically, as well as revealing diagnostic and therapeutic options" (p. 48). To borrow from an anthropological classic, the clinicians "work by the light of local knowledge" (Geertz, 1983, p. 167).

Individual narratives, biographical and autobiographical accounts of illness experiences, can also act as important contextualizing evidence— as sensitizing reminders of the dangers of generalizing and failing to understand the real need of the patient. Such sensitivity cannot be learned from decontextualized data. It is learned from clinical experience, from examples presented by other clinicians, from patients, and from qualitative research and other written accounts of observed experiences. The following example from Arthur Frank's reflections on his and others' experiences of illness (Frank, 1991), quoted at length here, shows what can happen when biomedical evidence of the effectiveness of a "typical" intervention is not balanced with contextual evidence.

> Too few people, whether medical staff, family or friends, seem willing to accept the possibility that depression may be the ill person's most appropriate

response to the situation. I am not recommending depression, but I do want
to suggest that at some moments even fairly deep depression must be accepted as part of the experience of illness.

A couple of days before my mother-in-law died, she shared a room with a
woman who was also being treated for cancer. My mother-in-law was this
woman's second dying roommate, and the woman was seriously ill herself. I
have no doubt that her diagnosis of clinical depression was accurate. The
issue is how the medical staff responded to her depression. Instead of trying
to understand it as a reasonable response to her situation, her doctors
treated her with antidepressant drugs. When a hospital psychologist came
to visit her, his questions were designed only to evaluate her "mental status."
"What day is it? Where are you and what floor are you on? Who is Prime
Minister?" And so forth. His sole interest was whether the dosage of antidepressant drug was too high, upsetting her "cognitive orientation." The hospital needed her to be mentally competent so she would remain a "good
patient" requiring little extra care; it did not need her emotions. No one attempted to explore her fears with her. No one asked what it was like to have
two roommates die within a couple of days of each other and how this affected her own fear of death. No one was willing to witness her experience.
(pp. 65-66)

However effective an intervention is, it may not be the best therapeutic strategy in a specific situation, and it seldom is the only one. For
health professionals open to learning, Frank's description tugs at their
conscience and draws forth remembrances of similar "misreadings" of
a person or a situation. It would be wrong to assume, however, that
individual illness narratives are the only type of qualitative evidence
health professionals need and can draw on to guide their practice.

Qualitative research, such as ethnography, grounded theory, or
phenomenology, involves extended periods of time in observation and
dialogue with study participants and can provide explanations of
complex individual and collective dynamics of human motivation and
action. It can also move beyond individuals and family groups to examine how economic and social conditions influence the space that
illness and disability occupy in people's lives and the choices people
make that contribute to illness and to the seeking or not seeking of
professional help. Such research provides evidence that often challenges
the taken-for-granted understanding that nurses, physicians, and other
health workers have of human behavior and human aspirations.

Tourigny (1998) provides a vivid example of such research; the findings are surprising and shocking even to her as an ethnographer who has spent months in the field working closely with her study participants. Her findings relate to a small number of African American young people living in inner-city Detroit. Although aware of the risks of HIV/AIDS and witnessing the devastation of the disease through care of a family member affected by it, they nevertheless made a deliberate choice to "acquire" HIV. Tourigny's explanation of the intentional nature of the young people's behavior derives from her knowledge of the poverty and despair of inner-city life and challenges our inclination to interpret these actions as some kind of "momentary aberration." According to Tourigny, for them, "AIDS seems to offer one way of accessing some semblance of care. It also provides the attraction of self-erasure without imposing the immediacy of death" (p. 164). What should be the therapeutic aims when these clients seek professional help? And how should the effectiveness of clinical interventions be measured in this situation?

Tourigny's research highlights two important issues in the consideration of evidence for clinical practice. One is the need for openness to questions that existing knowledge and theories may constrain us from asking. The young people in Tourigny's study were auxiliary participants, invited into the study because they were the family caregivers of AIDS patients involved as primary respondents. It was only through prolonged contact, the open nature of research dialogues, and the trust that had developed between the respondents and the researcher that they volunteered the information about the true nature of their own situation. One strength of qualitative research is that it can produce new and unexpected data, evidence we did not know was there.

The second issue highlighted by Tourigny's study is the moral dimension in human inquiry and in clinical practice. The way research and clinical questions are constructed often privileges the voices of those who ask them. Unless opportunities are also offered for other questions to be asked and for other voices to be heard (especially those of service users), the "evidence" produced is predetermined, and other, potentially critical discourses are silenced. Qualitative research, with its focus on the processes and the context of human experience, provides a means by which that experience can be explored and understood in ways that allow research participants to provide their own meanings and explanations and to challenge the outsiders' views or theories.

As Green and Britten (1998), for example, point out, it is through qualitative research that we have gained an understanding of the balancing that people with asthma undertake in relation to taking prescribed medication and managing their lives. Rather than being seen as a question of mere compliance with medical directives, the taking of medication is more accurately seen as a balancing of multiple factors, including one's personal identity as a "healthy" person, subjective interpretations of symptoms and physiological indicators such as peak flow measures, need for personal control, and development of explanatory frameworks that reflect one's own lived reality. Effectiveness of medication is neither the most important nor the only consideration.

All definitions of what ought to count as evidence are at least in part ideologically driven. As Lewontin (1994) suggests, "Facts make a theory, but it takes a theory to make facts, and occasionally, but only occasionally, this dialectic becomes disturbingly clear to the practitioners of science" (p. 485). What is clear about the current debate on evidence in the health sciences is that the positions adopted by various writers have as much to do with ideological orientations as any "facts" of their respective sciences. It may be appropriate, therefore, to reiterate the truism that clinical practice depends on a broad spectrum of knowledge, and one can seldom engage in it without some kind of moral commitment. Thus, the range of evidence needed for responsible clinical practice must be broader than that generated through experimental research and presented in summarized guidelines.

What the current debate on evidence for clinical practice needs is a more open dialogue between people who are concerned with clinical research, practice, and the goal of better patient care, but who nevertheless approach the question of relevant knowledge from different philosophical and epistemological perspectives. One measuring stick cannot do justice to all evidence. The complexity of human experience and of clinical practice should act as a strong counterweight to the temptations of reductionism. We should resist suggestions that human suffering and compassionate care should be subjected to the same experimental manipulations as new drugs and judged primarily by their outcomes (as implied by Sackett, 1995).

Our argument in this chapter is not that evidence-based health care is in itself problematic. Far from it. Rather, we suggest that the potential exists for a wider range of evidence to be recognized as relevant and helpful. Qualitative research methods, which at present are not well accepted in the move toward evidence-based health care, have the potential to provide useful, research-based information of real relevance to clinical problems. In health services, qualitative research methods "focus . . . on the appropriateness of care and aid understanding of the basis of lay and clinical behavior" (Popay, Rogers, & Williams, 1998, p. 349). This kind of understanding, provided by systematic qualitative inquiry, is of a higher order than the anecdotal evidence often employed in clinical practice (Green & Britten, 1998). As such, it offers answers to the kinds of questions that the gold standard evidence of randomized controlled trials simply does not address.

In the Preface to his book *The Enigma of Health* (1996), philosopher Hans-Georg Gadamer states, "The physics of our century has taught us that there are limits to what we can measure" (p. vii). There is a need to clarify the basis upon which researchers, clinicians, and policy makers decide what ought to be measured. There is also much in the human experience of health and illness that cannot and, just as important, should not be measured. Rather, we should use all means, including those of qualitative inquiry, to develop well-grounded understandings and theories that can nurture more informed and more sensitive clinicians and lead to effective and appropriate health care.

Note

1. Sackett (1995) distinguishes these terms (problematically, for nurses and other health clinicians) by defining "the new approach [as] 'evidence-based medicine' when applied by individual clinicians to individual patients, and [as] 'evidence-based health care' when applied by public health professionals, administrators, and policy-makers to groups of patients and populations" (p. 61).

References

Blair, L. (1997). Short on evidence: Evidence-based medicine in the witness box. *Canadian Family Physician, 43,* 427-429.
Brown, W., Dobson, A., & Mishra, G. (1998). What is a healthy weight range for middle aged women? *International Journal of Obesity, 22,* 520-528.

Byles, J., Feldman, S., & Mishra, G. (1999). For richer, for poorer, in sickness and in health: Older widowed women's health, relationships and financial security. *Women & Health, 29*(1), 15-30.

Carr, D. B., & Goudas, L. C. (1999). Acute pain. *The Lancet, 353,* 2051-2058.

Carr, V. (June 20-22, 1996). Getting the balance right in a more restrictive environment. *Proceedings of the Symposium on Schizophrenia* (pp. 53-58). University of Newcastle, NSW, Australia.

Chandler, J., Davidson, A. I., & Harootunian, H. (Eds.). (1994). Editors' introduction. In *Questions of evidence: Proof, practice, and persuasion across the disciplines* (pp. 1-8). Chicago: University of Chicago Press.

Closs, S. J., & Cheater, F. M. (1999). Evidence for nursing practice: A clarification of the issues. *Journal of Advanced Nursing, 30*(1), 10-17.

DiCenso, A., Cullum, N., & Ciliska, D. (1998). Implementing evidence-based nursing: Some misconceptions. *Evidence Based Nursing, 1*(2), 38-40.

Fox, P. L., Raina, P., & Jadad, A. R. (1999). Prevalence and treatment of pain in older adults in nursing homes and other long-term care institutions: A systematic review. *Canadian Medical Association Journal, 160,* 329-333.

Frank, A. W. (1991). *At the will of the body: Reflections on illness.* Boston: Houghton Mifflin.

Gadamer, H.-G. (1996). *The enigma of health* (J. Gaiger & N. Walker, Trans.). Stanford, CA: Stanford University Press.

Geertz, C. (1983). *Local knowledge: Further essays in interpretive anthropology.* New York: Basic Books.

Gray, J. A. M. (1997). *Evidence-based health care: How to make health policy and management decisions.* London: Churchill Livingstone.

Green, J., & Britten, N. (1998). Qualitative research and evidence based medicine. *British Medical Journal, 316,* 1230-1232.

Greenhalgh, T., & Hurwitz, B. (1999). Why study narrative? *British Medical Journal, 318,* 48-50.

Hall-Lord, M. L., Steen, B., & Larsson, G. (1999). Postoperative experiences of pain and distress in elderly patients. *Aging, 11*(2), 73-82.

Harris, M. A., Byles, J., Mishra, G., & Brown, W. J. (1999). Screening for cervical cancer: Health care, isolation and social support. *Health Promotion Journal of Australia, 8*(3), 167-172.

Hellman, S., & Hellman, D. S. (1991). Of mice but not men: Problems of the randomized clinical trial. *New England Journal of Medicine, 324,* 1585-1589.

Jadad, A. (April 17, 1999). *Evidence-based practice and pain management.* Paper presented at the 20th Annual Scientific Meeting of the Australian Pain Society, Perth, WA. (Cassette Recording. Perth: Quickopy Audio Recording Services).

Kerridge, I., Lowe, M., & Henry, D. (1998). Ethics and evidence based medicine. *British Medical Journal, 316,* 1151-1153.

Lewontin, R. C. (1994). Facts and the factitious in natural sciences. In J. Chandler, A. I. Davidson, & H. Harootunian (Eds.), *Questions of evidence: Proof, practice, and persuasion across the disciplines* (pp. 478-491). Chicago: University of Chicago Press.

Malterud, K. (1995). The legitimacy of clinical knowledge: Toward a medical epistemology embracing the art of medicine. *Theoretical Medicine, 16,* 183-198.

Marshall, M., Gray, A., Lockwood, A., & Green, R. (1998). Case management for people with severe mental disorders (Cochrane Review). In *The Cochrane Library, Issue 4,* 1998. Oxford: Update Software.

Marshall, M., & Lockwood, A. (1999). Assertive community treatment for people with severe mental disorders (Cochrane Review). In *The Cochrane Library, Issue 1,* 1999. Oxford: Update Software.

Mitchell, G. J. (1997). Questioning evidence-based practice for nursing. *Nursing Science Quarterly, 10*(4), 154-155.

Mitchell, G. J. (1999). Evidence-based practice: Critique and alternative view. *Nursing Science Quarterly, 12*(1), 30-35.

Moynihan, R. (1998). *Too much medicine?* Sydney: Australian Broadcasting Corporation Books.

Mulhall, A. (1998). Nursing, research, and the evidence. *Evidence Based Nursing, 1*(1), 4-6.

National Health and Medical Research Council. (1999). *Acute pain management: Scientific evidence.* Canberra: Commonwealth of Australia.

Pincus, H. A., Zarin, D. A., & West, J. C. (1996). Peering into the "black box": Measuring outcomes of managed care. *Archives of General Psychiatry, 53*(10), 870-877.

Popay, J., Rogers, A., & Williams, G. (1998). Rationale and standards for the systematic review of qualitative literature in health services research. *Qualitative Health Research, 8*(3), 341-351.

Repper, J., & Brooker, C. (1998). Difficulties in the measurement of outcome in people who have serious mental health problems. *Journal of Advanced Nursing, 27*(1), 75-82.

Sackett, D. L. (1995). Applying overviews and meta-analyses at the bedside. *Journal of Clinical Epidemiology, 48*(1), 61-66.

Sackett, D. L., & Rosenberg, W. M. C. (1995). On the need for evidence-based medicine. *Journal of Public Health Medicine, 17*(3), 330-334.

Sackett, D. L., Rosenberg, W. M. C., Gray, J. A. M., Haynes, R. B., & Richardson, W. S. (1996). Evidence based medicine: What it is and what it isn't. *British Medical Journal, 312,* 71-72.

Stein, H. F. (1991). The role of some nonbiomedical parameters in clinical decision making: An ethnographic approach. *Qualitative Health Research, 1*(1), 6-26.

Tourigny, S. C. (1998). Some new dying trick: African American youths "choosing" HIV/AIDS. *Qualitative Health Research, 8*(2), 149-167.

Walter, S. D., Hurley, J. E., Labelle, R. J., & Sackett, D. L. (1990). Clinical rounds for non-clinicians: Some impressions. *Journal of Clinical Epidemiology, 43*(6), 613-618.

Warfield, C. A., & Kahn, C. H. (1995). Acute pain management: Programs in U.S. hospitals and experiences and attitudes among U.S. adults. *Anaesthesiology, 83,* 1090-1094.

Wolf, A. R. (1999). Tears at bedtime: A pitfall of extending paediatric day-case surgery without extending analgesia (Editorial). *British Journal of Anaesthesia, 82*(3), 319-320.

II

The Nature of the Question

Dialogue:

Articulating a Theoretical Framework

THORNE: The way I understand theory in the social sciences, it really is intended to do something much larger than simply describe a phenomenon. For health science researchers, an interpretive description can often constitute a sufficient theory that will meet the criterion of credibility. I'm not wanting to advocate that health science researchers pay more serious attention to their theoretical linkages, because I actually do think that it might constrain them. When they do it—for example, when health professionals have had advanced degrees in the social sciences and they've had a lot of pressure in that direction—you can sometimes see the tension coming through in both the way they structure their findings and analyze them. Their focus can shift as if the real point of their science was to make a contribution to the theory.

KUZEL: I understand what you are saying, but I'd want to come back to recognizing that the questions people have are inherently linked to values and to theories of some sort. So making those explicit at some point in the research process is a generally good principle.

THORNE: Although I generally agree with you, people have assumed that the requirement for articulating a theoretical framework for the purposes of research means essentially naming a particular theory. Simply saying that the general wisdom in clinical medicine is that "these kinds of patients have these kinds of fears and anxieties so I am going to study them" isn't quite considered as strong. And from my point of view, that would be as legitimate a form of inquiry, probably even more so in certain circumstances. I think the specific relationship of a social science project to the social science is quite different from the relationship of a health science project to the work of theory development. It may simply be inquiry and knowledge. I really do think that in the applied spheres, finding out that there appears to be a common pattern is often a sufficient answer to a question. My reading is that people prematurely take their small study and say this proves the usefulness of the theoretical structure they used, which is not a useful way to think about this kind of inquiry.

MADJAR: To me there is a world of difference between somebody who deliberately decides to stay away from existing theory and to explore something in a more open way because they are aware of the limitations of theory or the constraining nature of theory, and somebody who actually doesn't do their theoretical work out of sheer intellectual laziness.

THORNE: I absolutely agree with you, and I think Jan Morse's chapter also comments on this problem very nicely.

3

Who Decides What Counts as Evidence?

LYNNE D. RAY
MARIA MAYAN

Context and Intent of the Discussion

Health care professionals and agencies are expected to demonstrate that the care they provide does make a difference for the population receiving care. In the early 1990s, health professionals observed an increasing interest in outcomes research (National Center for Nursing Research, 1991). Now, evidence-based health care is gaining prominence. Nursing has witnessed the development of institutes such as the Centre for Evidence-Based Nursing in the United Kingdom, McMaster's Nursing Effectiveness, Utilization and Outcomes Research Unit in Canada, and the Joanna Briggs Institute for Evidence-Based Nursing and Midwifery in Australia. A new journal, *Evidence-Based Nursing,* parallels similar journals for medicine, mental health, health management, and policy. As Hayward and colleagues noted (1996), evidence of positive outcomes has become the currency of health care exchange, and calls for evidence inform all levels of decision making.

From an Evidence-Based Practice perspective, professionals and organizations are asked, "What evidence do you have that the care you provide improves, maintains, or promotes the health of your target population?" Or "What evidence are you using to decide what is the most appropriate care for an individual or population?" (Butcher, 1998; Gilbert & Logan, 1996; Gray, 1997). Evidence-Based Practice is about research utilization and decisions regarding future care. Whether health professionals are generating or using evidence, there are critical presuppositions that often remain unchallenged.

Author's Note: Adapted from Ray, L. D. (1999). "Evidence and Outcomes: Agendas, Presuppositions, and Power." *Journal of Advanced Nursing, 30*(5), 1017-1026. Used with permission of Blackwell Science Ltd.

One of the major challenges in generating and using evidence is to negotiate among the multiple notions of what constitutes a meaningful difference in health status. This chapter analyzes and critiques the presuppositions and power relations that shape how criteria for effectiveness are derived and subsequently maintained. Raising such a question is a reflection of the current historical, political, and economic contexts. As well, current philosophic and methodologic debates have led to what has been called a crisis of legitimation and representation (Lather, 1993; Seidman, 1994). Critical and reflexive debates are challenging the presuppositions and power relations that have informed prior research and praxis (Lather, 1991; Longino, 1990; Smith, 1990).

Specifically, this chapter begins by examining how clinical researchers must negotiate the agendas of diverse audiences while maintaining a program of research that is true to the needs of the population they work with. It will then describe the presuppositions and power relations that shape the generation and utilization of evidence in health care. It concludes with a discussion of the consequences for researchers and the public.

Audiences and Agendas

Current efforts to generate and use health-related evidence are a product of the intersecting and often competing agendas held by different audiences. Audiences can be grouped into eight major categories: health care organizations (public and for profit), insurers (tax-based and for profit), the health professions, the research community (funding agencies and researchers), regulators, the "medical-industrial complex" (Navarro, 1984), the legal system, and consumers (health plan purchasers and the public). Figure 3.1 represents these audiences. In this illustration, the relative power, voice, or influence held by each of these audiences is represented by the width of each pie slice. The power that each audience has will vary according to the structures and mechanisms of their nation's health care system and the nation's socially determined priorities. Figure 3.1 represents the relative power that different audiences have in Canada's health care system.

The public's power is significantly smaller than the power of other audiences. Our argument is that the public audience is purposefully excluded and discredited in the creation and utilization of evidence in health care. The values underlying prevailing presuppositions and

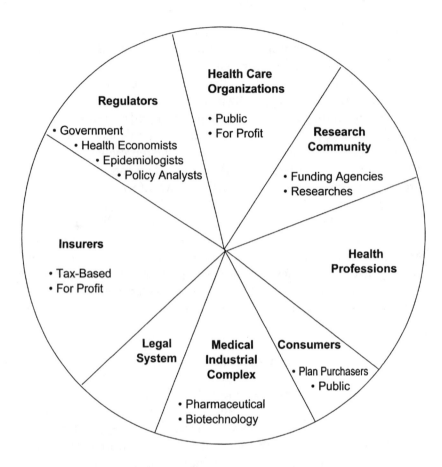

Figure 3.1 Categories of Audiences

power relations exclude the public from all stages of the research process. As well, compared to other audiences, the public is motivated by different agendas. Specifically, the public is motivated by a unique agenda of personal need for health services. Other audiences are motivated according to the following five agendas: fiscal accountability, risk and liability, quality care, social and moral responsibility, and professional effectiveness. These agendas are represented in Figure 3.2 and are outlined next.

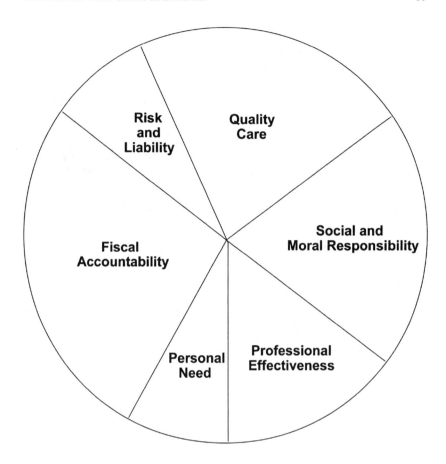

Figure 3.2 Types of Agendas

Fiscal Accountability Whether a health system is publicly funded and managed within a limited budget, or is for profit and managed with the goal of maximized profit, evidence of positive outcomes play a role in fiscal accountability. In a for-profit system, evidence of positive outcomes is used as a competitive tool when marketing to insurers, health plan purchasers, and the public (Jones, 1997). Tanenbaum (1996) claimed that private health organizations use effectiveness research to make marketing appear more legitimate.

For insurers and health care organizations in a tax-based system, evidence of positive health outcomes provides a means of arbitrating among competing demands for health services (Butcher, 1998). In the first half of the 1990s, the outcomes movement was promoted as a means of determining which services were ineffective or too costly and which were cost effective (Crane, 1991). Program funding that was once dependent on the preferences of politicians and bureaucrats and on allocation patterns of the previous year increasingly required evidence of positive outcomes for continued funding (Fulton, 1993; Moritz, 1995).

Risk and Liability Because of the fiscal restraint and health care restructuring of the 1990s, the principal use of evidence was limited to proving that cost containment was successful without affecting the quality of health care (Ware, 1995). The original intent of risk management was preventative, but when applied in a context of fiscal restructuring, the risk and liability agenda shifted to a narrow application of economic theory (Davis & Howden-Chapman, 1996) and a harm reduction orientation to health research. Under strong political and financial pressures, the paramount agenda is defending cost control over any other kind of health objective (Gray, 1998).

Quality Care The claim that evidence of positive outcomes is required to ensure quality health care is ubiquitous. In the late 1980s, health accreditation organizations started shifting from an emphasis on structure and process to a greater emphasis on outcomes. Now, quality care is framed as evidence-based care, and the questions about quality are left open to a broad range of interpretations. Who decides what constitutes quality? Who arbitrates among competing claims of quality care? What forms of evidence are legitimate? How should research evidence, clinical expertise, resources, and patients' preferences be weighted when making decisions about optimal quality care (DiCenso & Cullum, 1998)? Presupposed answers to these questions vary markedly among audiences.

Social and Moral Responsibility Audiences who have a social and moral responsibility agenda tend to be more closely aligned with the perspectives of the public or consumers. Researchers, as an audience that uses critical or interpretive methods and becomes intimately aware of patients' and families' stories, often take this position (e.g., Anderson, 1996; McKeever, 1996; Wuest, 1997). A growing number of organizations and lobby efforts stem from an alliance between clients and professionals. Such efforts are usually framed under the rubric of advocacy and are held up as models of excellent professional practice (Benner, DeCoste, & Clark, 1990; Gadow & Schroeder, 1996). Critics of client-professional alliances argue that professionals and patient advocates use the social and moral responsibility agenda to protect and advance their personal and economic interests (Estroff, 1993). They argue, for example, that the quest for an increase in services is not for the well-being of patients, but to create jobs and ensure job security. Critics such as health care insurers and regulators often highlight the advancement of personal and economic interests to criticize and discredit public lobby efforts.

Professional Effectiveness The future of professions rests on their ability to demonstrate the effectiveness of their practice. Research evidence can be used to demonstrate the value, cost effectiveness, and unique contribution of specific professional groups (Griffiths, 1995; Kitson, 1997). In nursing, this includes skill mix research—the association between different levels of nurse education and patient outcomes (Mitchell, Ferketich, Jennings, & American Academy of Nursing Expert Panel on Quality Health Care, 1998). Other initiatives in the United States have involved classifying nursing outcomes in a format that fits with current classification systems for nursing diagnoses and interventions (Bowles & Naylor, 1996; Johnson & Maas, 1997; Maas, Johnson, & Moorhead, 1996; Martin & Scheet, 1995; Micek et al., 1996). In the context of health care restructuring and/or in a managed care system, nursing has been compromised because there are few data on the types of services that nurses provide or the contributions they make to patient outcomes (Jones, 1997). Cost-effective contributions have become the currency by which professional groups maintain their positions in health care agencies, and consequently, more research on effectiveness of particular professions is needed to influence health care policy and provide a rationale for funding choices (Scott & Moneyham, 1995).

Multiple Agendas: Reconcilable or Incommensurable? This overview of competing agendas raises questions of just how many audiences can be satisfied through a single program of research. Is there a degree of incommensurability that makes it impossible to relate the multiple perspectives through a common logical framework that would permit differences among them to be unambiguously settled (Guba, 1992)? Or are there questions that are equally meaningful among various audiences? Are there common criteria by which the evidence can be judged? Answers to these questions lie not in face-value agendas but in the hidden presuppositions and the power imbalances between audiences.

Presuppositions and Power Relations

In considering what presuppositions are operating in health care research, it is useful to consider the hermeneutic claim that there are no presuppositionless interpretations. Even scientific interpretations and approaches are governed by the concrete situation of the researcher (Bernstein, 1991). Each discipline has its linguistic, conceptual, and methodological traditions that serve to locate researchers as they frame their questions and interpretations.

In addition to the taken-for-granted preunderstandings that researchers work from, critical theorists draw attention to the relations of power that constitute the available options in any situation. Power has been framed in many ways: as the ability to define and direct, as the freedom to choose, as the ability to withhold, and as a repressive agent. Foucault (1980) offered this view: "Power . . . only functions in the form of a chain. It is never localized here or there, never in anybody's hands, never appropriated as a commodity or piece of wealth. Power is employed and exercised through a net-like organization" (p. 98). This interconnected view of power complements the notion of multiple audiences and accountabilities that delineate the options available to researchers. The presuppositions and power relations that shape the way criteria for effectiveness are derived and subsequently maintained include disciplinary socialization and language of researchers, externally constructed research priorities, methodological superiority of the randominized clinical trial (RCT), and definitional authority for problems.

Disciplinary Socialization and Language of Researchers

As researchers act from within their different professional locations, they use the language and presuppositions of their scholarly community to determine where the "problem" lies and to structure their arguments and explanations (Sullivan, 1993). Each discipline has its research topics and conventions that are self-perpetuating (Good & Good, 1993) and become part of the taken-for-granted life-world of the researcher (Bernstein, 1991). For example, researchers concerned with the struggles of families with chronically ill members will frame their questions from the perspective of stress and coping if influenced by psychology (primarily following Lazarus & Folkman, 1984). From a sociological perspective, similar concerns are commonly framed as managing (Anderson & Elfert, 1989; Corbin & Strauss, 1988; Knafl, Breitmayer, Gallo, & Zoeler, 1996; Robinson, 1993). Authors in other scholarly communities use the term *suffering* (Frankenberg, 1993; Kleinman, 1992; Morse & Carter, 1996). These variables are not inherent essential qualities of the caregiving experience (Conkey, 1991). Rather, they are culturally constructed, with scholarly communities acting as bearers of the codifying discourse (Foucault, 1980).

The argument that supports framing questions with consistent concepts is one of consistency and comparability within and between studies and databases. Enthusiasm for concept analysis (Rodgers, 1989; Walker & Avant, 1988), meta-analysis (Lynn, 1989; Reynolds, Timmerman, & Stevenson, 1992), and minimal data sets (Hogston, 1997; Johnson & Maas, 1997; Martin & Scheet, 1995; Ryan & Delaney, 1995) serve to further structure and institutionalize the way researchers view their study population and frame their questions. These strategies do achieve focus, consistency, and the statistical power of large databases. However, conceptual and methodological conformity also reproduces the status quo and dictates the boundaries of inquiry (Smith, 1990; Wuest, 1994). Innovative or divergent conceptualizations are marginalized or excluded when conformity is the priority.

Language plays a critical role in professional socialization due to its power to carry and create epistemological codes and traditions (Gadamer, 1975; Lather, 1991). Although some view this as helpful in establishing the professional identity (Toulmin, 1972), others fear the dangers of conceptual overdeterminism in prefiguring knowledge (Lather, 1991; Richardson, 1991). The organizing capacity of language is becoming more apparent in an era of computerized databases. Not only do such databases structure the way we present knowledge (so that it is retrievable), but they also determine who has access to certain scholarly discourses. For example, when research-funding bodies index their scientific reviewers according to MEDLINE's MESH headings, reviewers who do not practice within the traditional medical model are left without a language to classify their areas of expertise.

In addition to the traditional medical model, the economic model of health care has insurmountable linguistic power. In this model, health care is viewed as a commodity and is described through language such as objectivity, supply and demand, efficiency, value-free, cost effectiveness, and risk minimization for third-party payers (Melhado, 1998). In contrast, a social conflict or collective welfare model focuses on social solidarity and distributive justice (Melhado, 1998) and has a completely different language set. Although both models are attempting to explain and describe the best operations of a health care system, the dominance of the economic model and its language determines what is valued and legitimized. Policy makers rely on the economic model, to the exclusion of other models, as it most closely matches their values (Melhado, 1998) or disciplinary socialization.

Other examples of linguistic power are the national databases on health services and expenditures. Jones (1997) argued that American nurses should adopt a standardized nursing language and develop a nationwide infrastructure that will demonstrate nursing's contribution in a managed care environment. In Canada, Hayward et al. (1996) advised that health professionals must speak the language of evidence to be heard. In New Zealand, Davis and Howden-Chapman (1996) noted that for research to be translated into policy, it must be couched in the language of institutional analysis. These examples illustrate the power of audiences' linguistic conventions in shaping the generation and utilization of evidence in health care.

Externally Constructed Research Priorities

Not only does the scientific community construct its terms, but it also formalizes the boundaries of acceptable (fundable and publishable) inquiry and sets priorities within those boundaries. Conkey (1991) used the notion of a "research cone" as a heuristic that locates both implicitly and explicitly acceptable research foci. She claimed that those who control the point of the cone "control that which comes after; they control knowledge, and anyone writing about subsequents must pass through—or at least reference—this point" (p. 112). One needs only to do a MEDLINE search using the term *outcome* to see the vast diversity of articles that have referenced the term. The use of the words *outcome* or *evidence-based* conveys a timeliness and acceptability of one's research.

The most formalized means by which prioritization occurs is through consensus surveys and conferences such as the American congressionally mandated conference to develop a research agenda for outcomes research for the Agency for Healthcare Research and Quality and the American Academy of Nursing invitational conference on outcome measures and care delivery systems (Mitchell, Heinrich, Moritz, & Hinshaw, 1997). Although such consensus panels reduce fragmentation and clarify focus, it may also be argued that they serve as a "mode of discourse that gives expression to rank, order, definition, and distinction" (Greiner, 1993, p. 6). The questions become "Whose account is being privileged?" and "What knowledge remains unprivileged, unworthy of being characterized as a relevant outcome?" (Richardson, 1991). It is encouraging to see that some direction-setting panels include public audiences among researchers, clinicians, program planners, and policy makers (Bastian, 1994; Patterson & Blum, 1993).

The constructed research priorities best known to researchers are the specific calls for proposals that designate circumscribed topics for investigation. Erben, Franzkowiak, and Wenzel (1992) asked whether researchers control what they want to control, or whether the scientific control mechanisms control intentions. In the case of funding, the latter seems the case; the power of funding bodies to structure inquiry cannot be underestimated. Another consideration is the needs of decision makers. The topics they need to have researched may not coincide with the topics of interest to researchers or funders (Frenk, 1992).

Methodological Superiority of the RCT

The orthodox consensus within the medical research community holds that the RCT is unquestionably the strongest research tool in terms of its warrant for causal inference. The preference for the RCT is predicated on the desire to maximize internal validity. Promulgation of RCTs is institutionalized in the funding priorities of research institutes (see, for example, Cazares & Beatty, 1994) and in the levels of evidence defined by the Cochrane Collaboration (Gray, 1997). This definition of what counts as evidence is narrow in the extreme. It does support clinical decision making, as it represents only a portion of the clinical situations and questions that health care practitioners face.

What counts as evidence in a clinical trial is different from what counts as evidence in other situations (Butcher, 1998). One problem is that the more tightly controlled a study is, the less likely will it constitute a representative sample of any natural population. Highly controlled trials tell us little about the use and acceptance of treatments or services in ordinary circumstances (Moritz, 1995; Tanenbaum, 1994). Another problem is that the presuppositions informing practice in different clinical areas differ. Hayward et al. (1996) give the example of public health. In many public health situations, social diffusion of information may be the desired intervention; in an RCT, this is considered contamination. To answer the questions that are relevant to all audiences requires a full range of research methods and units of analysis (Batterham, Dunt, & Disler, 1996).

The RCT debate reflects an essential tension between those who privilege the universal versus the particular, the generic versus the contextualized, and efficacy versus effectiveness. This tension may be a function of audiences and their location. Patients, families, and, to some extent, clinicians experience illness from a highly contextualized contingent world. Their narrative model of illness is individual, episodic, and emplotted (Frankenberg, 1993). In contrast, the work of policy makers and epidemiologic researchers preclude attention to the localized experience. By first privileging a particular method or unit of analysis, the options of what may count as evidence will be delimited. Proceeding without questioning the permissible methods will only reproduce the status quo.

Definitional Authority for Problems

Much of what is defined as problematic in the health evidence literature relates to specific methods issues. Rarely do authors discuss health research from a philosophical or even theoretical perspective. Ware (1995) observed that health care organizations may enthusiastically embrace data collection related to health outcomes without a clear understanding of how they will use the data. Similarly, decisions of what to treat as an outcome are often determined by availability of instruments, databases, or the statistical requirements for meta-analysis. Investigators making design decisions in this manner may have no knowledge of the conceptual presuppositions that have informed earlier work.

One presupposition that pervades much research is the notion that the professional perspective and method is always the accurate one. For example, Newacheck, Stoddard, and McManus (1993) warned that data obtained from household interviews must be considered in light of reporting error, ascertainment error, underreporting, and over-reporting. The methodological problem is assumed to lie with the families rather than the researcher's construction of what is problematic. As a public representative on research review panels, Bastian (1994) noted that many researchers' claims of objectivity in their analyses suggested that they were unaware of the value-laden elements of what they did at each step in the research process. Consumers and professionals may well see "threats to validity" in completely different places.

Another example of a professionally defined problem is that of compliance or adherence. From a professional perspective, the problem is "Why aren't patients or families following my prescribed treatment regimen?" From the family perspective, the problem is often "Why are these professionals expecting us to do something that ignores our priorities and life circumstances?" (Buchmann, 1997; Hess, 1996; Playle & Keeley, 1998). As Genovich-Richards (1997) argued, noncompliance may be a sad commentary on the lack of creativity and the inflexibility of health professionals to fully engage the public and understand their health preferences. Some research has even shown that patients and professionals disagree on the severity of symptoms experienced by patients and use different criteria to determine effectiveness of treatments (Feine, Awad, & Lund, 1998). "Evaluating health care from the standpoint of the patient is not yet a universally accepted idea" (Ware, 1995, JS29). Consequently, the designation of what is problematic depends on who is defining the problem, on the implicit assumptions about who has definitional authority, and on the network of power from which the respective individuals are operating.

Consequences for the Researcher

Each researcher, by virtue of being embedded in his or her disciplinary, historical, political, and economic contexts, starts from a preset range of research options. Among these preset options is the tendency for method and instruments to direct decisions in various aspects of a study.

Research Designs Directed by Method and Instruments

Outcome selection reflects fundamental decisions about what counts as health (Hayward et al., 1996). Unfortunately, clinicians and researchers with the task of documenting health outcomes frequently start with the question "What instruments can I use?" or "What databases already exist that I can use?" To start with, these questions not only put the methodological cart before the horse, but they also represent an atheoretical position. Concepts and variables are selected according to available instruments rather than sound theoretical or clinical rationale. The statistical requirements for different modeling and analytic techniques can strongly affect decisions about what is or is not researched (McAllister, 1994). Until outcomes research is conducted with prior attention to theoretical organization and integration of findings, clinical utilization of these findings will be jeopardized.

There are several reasons why health care research may start at the question of instrumentation. Timelines may be very short and prohibit either the development of new measures or the time-consuming analysis of interpretive data. Health care demonstration projects often have very short time frames in which to produce and adequately capture any positive outcomes. Because research teams could include clinicians, administrators, insurers, pharmaceutical or biotechnology firms, and researchers, each with markedly different agendas and methodological expertise, the quickest and easiest option is to start by finding an instrument. Conceptual congruence and validity become secondary. Even the population being studied may be defined so that it matches the population for which normed instruments are available (Perrin et al., 1993).

When analysis and obtaining statistical significance are the primary concerns, they too may define and direct a study. Inclusion criteria may have as much to do with reducing within-subject variability and subsequently decreasing p values as with the clinical or theoretical definitions of the population. The same holds for sample size: given a sufficiently large sample, a null hypothesis of no treatment effect can always be rejected (Slakter, Wu, & Suzuki-Slakter, 1991). Therefore, those with access to large populations and sufficient funding to support lengthy data collection are in a better position to demonstrate statistically significant outcomes. Whether statistical significance actually represents clinical significance has been a long-standing topic for debate (Cohen, 1990; French, 1997; LeFort, 1993; Rosnow & Rosenthal, 1989; Slakter et al., 1991; Smith, 1983). Batterham et al. (1996) argued that variables can be selected because they change readily, not because they represent an improvement in the underlying issue. Regardless, statistical significance, available instruments, and abbreviated timelines continue to structure much of what is done in health care research.

Responsibility for Ensuring Informed Use of Research Evidence

In an era of health care restructuring, investigators are acutely aware of the potential for their findings to be used in justifying programming decisions. Greene (1992) argued that the clinical researcher is responsible for how his or her findings are read, understood, and acted upon or not, and for who benefits and who does not as a result of the inquiry. "Responsible inquiry must attend to its consequences as part of its intent" (p. 42). This challenge to investigators is particularly difficult, since both the science of studying health outcomes and the use of these outcomes for Evidence-Based Practice and policy decisions are new.

The potential for misunderstanding of statistical conclusions, naive utilization of outcomes, and selective use of findings are all increased in a methodologically immature field. For example, questions of how to capture meaningful improvements in people's lives have yet to be answered. Even though failure to demonstrate positive outcomes in any given study may be a function of evolving methodological sophistication, rather than an ineffective service, such findings may still be used to justify program cuts.

Regulators and insurers may place little credence in claims of methodological inadequacy:

> Intervention studies originate from a bias: the conceptually, empirically, or otherwise justified intellectual desire to document the presumed efficacy of some nursing interventions over other ones. Statistically significant results on more or all patient outcomes are believed to advance knowledge, thus equating new knowledge with statistically significant knowledge. In contrast, nonsignificant results tend to be "explained away" as being due to methodological or conceptual flaws. (Abraham, Chalifoux, & Evers, 1991, p. 78)

Such critiques illustrate that not only may the survival of a service or program be at stake but also the researchers' ability to publish results that are not positive or at least encouraging (Abraham et al., 1991) and their ability to receive subsequent funding.

Stetler (1994) describes how research utilization may be symbolic or political by using research to legitimate a current program. This may be done by choosing methodologically weak studies or presenting only the research that supports the preferred decision. The inability to distinguish between design inadequacy and an ineffective program remains a major problem for health care researchers, and safeguards to ensure informed use of research evidence need to be both epistemological and political (Batterham et al., 1996).

Consequences for the Public

Suppressed Agency

The public, as health care consumers and as participants in health research, is the audience with the least access to the social processes through which claims to legitimacy are made (Davis & Howden-Chapman, 1996; Kushner & Rachlis, 1997). At one time, it was the patient or family that determined what counted both as professional competence and as therapeutic success (Sullivan, 1993). This sense of agency has been eroded over the years to such an extent that some professionals are outraged at the notion of patients or families having a voice in setting health policy. Resistance to patient or family involvement persists: "There is an anti-medical doctor movement which seeks to take away the control of health from medical doctors and give it not only to doctors of osteopath, chiropractors, nurses, and public health scientists but also to an empowered American population" (Greenberg, 1992, p. 535).

In principle, Evidence-Based Practice requires that the impact of care on people's lives become the center of health care (Bastian, 1994). The new journal *Evidence-Based Health Policy and Management* includes a section on evidence-based patient choice. This is a good start, but to fully support patient or family decision making, the shift in orientation will need to occur at the beginning of the research process, not at the utilization stage.

Mechanisms of Exclusion

There are two mechanisms by which the public can be excluded from the research process. First, from the standpoint of *who* is being studied, and second, from the standpoint of *what* is being studied. In the first instance, one way the public is denied access to direction setting in research is through the definition of categories for inclusion and exclusion in research. For example, with populations that are difficult to define, like children with chronic health conditions, the researcher makes a decision about whether to define the research sample by medical diagnosis, age, technology dependence, or cognitive capacity. Gender has often been a source of exclusion. For example, women were often excluded from studies of cardiovascular disease. These decisions have far-reaching implications, as they will determine who has evidence to support decision making at a funding and policy level. Those who are studied are given a voice by virtue of being studied.

Second, the research question chosen dictates *what* will be studied. For example, it is common for studies with the chronically ill to address questions regarding functional status or days hospitalized. However, studies have shown that patients understand their health in a holistic manner and that they consider their symptoms, disease, and treatment problems in the context of all dimensions of their life when rating their overall health. To understand the public's perspective, we need a much broader understanding of outcomes (Ware, 1995). The methodologic priorities of the research community can create distance from public audiences and vest researchers with priorities that may or may not be consistent with public interests (Bastian, 1994).

Discredited Knowledge

When the public assumes responsibility for the care of family members, they become quasiprofessionals. Their responsibilities often exceed those of more qualified paid professionals (Pierce & Frank, 1992), and their specific knowledge of their family member's condition exceeds that of most professionals. As unpaid labor, these families, primarily women, represent an essential and unacknowledged component of health care delivery (Bridges & Lynam, 1993; Keating, Fast, Fredrick, Cranswick, & Perrier, 1999; McKeever, 1996; Wuest, 1993).

Rather than highlighting family caregivers' expertise, much of the research can be framed under the rubric of asking family caregivers to rationalize their actions. The onus of accountability is unidirectional and follows a gradient of relative power. The most striking examples are found in the compliance literature (e.g., Chigier, 1992; Koocher, McGrath, & Gudas, 1990; VanSciver, D'Angelo, Rappaport, & Woolf, 1995). Rather than acknowledging caregiving families' purposeful, constructive, and self-sustaining actions to modify care regimens so that they work within the family context (Buchmann, 1997; Playle & Keeley, 1998; Thorne, 1990; Wuest, 1993), families are portrayed as willfully disobedient, incapable, or both. Their situated and practical knowledge has been disqualified as inadequate or naive, "located low down on the hierarchy, beneath the required level of cognition or scientificity" (Foucault, 1980, p. 82).

As various audiences embark on the task of capturing evidence to guide health care, families are likely to be left out of the evidence discourse, just as they were not included in planning care regimens. Even though the latter has produced the "problem" of noncompliance, lack of family participation in the outcomes discourse is likely to result in nonsignificance. "It is a rare study that asks . . . what the clients think. . . . If the clinician deprives the clients of control over what is clinically significant, then clinical significance is called that only because it denotes significance for the clinician" (Baer, 1988, p. 222). Just as families should have a voice in determining salient outcomes, so should they receive credit for their role in achieving positive outcomes.

Methodological Approaches
to Support Public Inclusion

Multiple audiences and agendas shape health care research and evidence-based decision making. New definitions of scholarship emphasize accountability to the public who will be most affected by research findings (Sandelowski, 1996). Achieving this accountability means rebalancing the agendas and relative power of the various audience groups. It requires that investigators reflect on the presuppositions that inform their questions and consider what decisions the public needs to make in managing their own health, and what evidence the public needs for informed decisions.

It is vital that researchers examine the methodological choices they are making, either actively or passively, and carefully consider the consequences of those choices. One of the methods researchers may choose to ensure that they are true to the needs of the people they work with is participatory action research. This method involves a group of people coming together (i.e., health care professionals, patients, family members) as participants, and not "objects," in the research process. The group's task is to reflect on the needs, resources, and constraints within the present setting, to examine ways of improving the present setting, and then to put in place mechanisms of improvement. At the heart of this method is the production of knowledge and solutions to improve a situation by working with those who experience the problem (i.e., health care professionals, patients, family members). This group has ownership of the process—what questions are asked and how they are pursued. No one person or subgroup enters the research with the questions predetermined (Smith, 1997; Chapter 7, this volume).

Participatory action research ultimately moves all of those involved in the research from "what is" to "what could be" or, in this case, hearing and acting on the voices of patients and their family members. Thus, participatory action research is a way to ensure patient or family agency and ensure that their voices count in what is considered professional competence, therapeutic success, and necessary policy changes. The methods of exclusion (who and what are studied) are also addressed by participatory action research. The people involved in the process and experiencing the problem will themselves define categories of inclusion and exclusion. Moreover, because they are part of developing the research questions, participants are part of determining what will be studied. Finally, because people's experiences and knowledge are not considered supplemental or inadequate, but essential to the research process, their knowledge is not discredited—it is fundamental to every step taken during the research and to the resulting outcomes.

Employing a participatory method and making those who are receiving care an inherent part of the research process is one of the best ways to make the public agenda more central. It is also one of the best ways health care professionals and agencies can demonstrate that the care they provide does make a difference for those receiving care. Health care research and Evidence-Based Practice will not be relevant to the public unless their agendas become more central than they are now.

References

Abraham, I. L., Chalifoux, Z. L., & Evers, G. C. M. (1991, September). *Conditions, interventions, and outcomes: A quantitative analysis of nursing research (1981-1990)*. Paper presented at the Patient Outcomes Research: Examining the Effectiveness of Nursing Practice, Rockville, MD.

Anderson, J. M. (1996). Empowering patients: Issues and strategies. *Social Science and Medicine, 43*(5), 697-705.

Anderson, J. M., & Elfert, H. (1989). Managing chronic illness in the family: Women as caretakers. *Journal of Advanced Nursing, 14*, 735-743.

Baer, D. M. (1988). If you know why you're changing a behavior, you'll know when you've changed it enough. *Behavioral Assessment, 10*, 219-223.

Bastian, H. (1994). *The power of sharing knowledge: Consumer participation in the Cochrane Collaboration*. Retrieved June 26, 1998, from the World Wide Web: www.updatesoftware.com/ccweb/cochrane/powershr.htm.

Batterham, R. W., Dunt, D. R., & Disler, P. B. (1996). Can we achieve accountability for long-term outcomes? *Archives of Physical Medicine and Rehabilitation, 77*, 1219-1225.

Benner, P., DeCoste, B., & Clark, L. (1990). Dialogues with excellence: The many faces of advocacy. *American Journal of Nursing, 90*, 80-82.

Bernstein, R. J. (1991). *Beyond objectivism and relativism: Science, hermeneutics, and praxis*. Philadelphia: University of Pennsylvania Press.

Bowles, K. H., & Naylor, M. D. (1996). Nursing intervention classification systems. *IMAGE: Journal of Nursing Scholarship, 28*(4), 303-308.

Bridges, J. M., & Lynam, M. J. (1993). Informal carers: A Marxist analysis of social, political, and economic forces underpinning the role. *Advances in Nursing Science, 15*(3), 33-48.

Buchmann, W. F. (1997). Adherence: A matter of self-efficacy and power. *Journal of Advanced Nursing, 26*, 132-137.

Butcher, R. B. (1998). Foundations for evidence-based decision making. In National Forum on Health (Ed.), *Canada health action: Building on the legacy: Vol. 5, Making decisions: Evidence and information* (pp. 259-294). Ottawa: Éditions Multimondes.

Cazares, A., & Beatty, L. A. (Eds.). (1994). Scientific methods for prevention intervention research. National Institute on Drug Abuse. *NIDA Research Monograph 139*. Rockville, MD: U.S. Department of Health and Human Services.

Chigier, E. (1992). Compliance in adolescents with epilepsy or diabetes. *Journal of Adolescent Health, 13*, 375-379.

Cohen, J. (1990). Things I have learned (so far). *American Psychologist, 45*(12), 1204-1312.

Conkey, M. W. (1991). The political economy of gender in archaeology. In M. diLeonardo (Ed.), *Gender at the crossroads of knowledge: Feminist anthropology in the postmodern era* (pp. 102-139). Berkeley: University of California Press.

Corbin, J. M., & Strauss, A. (1988). *Unending work and care: Managing chronic illness at home*. San Francisco: Jossey-Bass.

Crane, S. C. (1991, September). *A research agenda for outcomes research.* Paper presented at the Patient Outcomes Research: Examining the Effectiveness of Nursing Practice, Rockville, MD.

Davis, P., & Howden-Chapman, P. (1996). Translating research into health policy. *Social Science and Medicine, 43*(5), 865-872.

DiCenso, A., & Cullum, N. (1998). Implementing evidence-based nursing: Some misconceptions. *Evidence-Based Nursing, 1*(2), 38-40.

Erben, R., Franzkowiak, P., & Wenzel, E. (1992). Assessment of the outcomes of health interventions. *Social Science and Medicine, 35*(4), 359-365.

Estroff, S. E. (1993). Identity, disability and schizophrenia. In S. Lindenbaum & M. Lock (Eds.), *Knowledge, power and practice: The anthropology of medicine and everyday life* (pp. 247-286). Berkeley: University of California Press.

Feine, J. S., Awad, M. A., & Lund, J. P. (1998). The impact of patient preference on the design and interpretation of clinical trials. *Community Dentistry and Oral Epidemiology, 26,* 70-74.

Foucault, M. (1980). *Power/knowledge: Selected interviews and other writings 1972-1977.* New York: Pantheon Books.

Frankenberg, R. (1993). Anthropological and epidemiological narratives of prevention. In S. Lindenbaum & M. Lock (Eds.), *Knowledge, power and practice: The anthropology of medicine and everyday life* (pp. 219-242). Berkeley: University of California Press.

French, B. (1997). British studies which measure patient outcome, 1990-1994. *Journal of Advanced Nursing, 26,* 320-328.

Frenk, J. (1992). Balancing relevance and excellence: Organizational responses to link research with decision making. *Social Science Medicine, 35*(11), 1397-1404.

Fulton, J. (1993). *Canada's health system: Bordering on the possible.* (Vol. 1 International Health Policy Series). Washington, DC: Falkner & Gray.

Gadamer, H.-G. (1975). *Truth and method.* New York: Seabury Press.

Gadow, S., & Schroeder, C. (1996). Ethics and community health: An advocacy approach. In E. Anderson & J. McFarlane (Eds.), *Community as partner: Theory and practice in nursing* (2nd ed., pp. 123-137). Philadelphia: J. B. Lippincott.

Genovich-Richards, J. (1997). The customer: Perspectives and expectations of quality. In C. G. Meinsenheimer (Ed.), *Improving quality: A guide to effective programs* (2nd ed., pp. 133-146). Gaithersburg, MD: Aspen.

Gilbert, R., & Logan, S. (1996). Future prospects for evidence-based child health. *Archives of Disease in Childhood, 75,* 465-473.

Good, B. J., & Good, M.-J. D. (1993). "Learning medicine": The construction of medical knowledge at Harvard Medical School. In S. Lindenbaum & M. Lock (Eds.), *Knowledge, power and practice: The anthropology of medicine and everyday life* (pp. 81-107). Berkeley: University of California Press.

Gray, G. (1998). Access to medical care under strain: New pressures in Canada and Australia. *Journal of Health Politics, Policy and Law, 23*(6), 906-947.

Gray, J. A. M. (1997). *Evidence-based health care: How to make health policy and management decisions.* London: Churchill Livingston.

Greenberg, M. (1992). Impediments to basing government health policies on science in the United States. *Social Science and Medicine, 35*(4), 531-540.

Greene, J. C. (1992). The practitioner's perspective. *Curriculum Inquiry, 22*(1), 39-45.

Greiner, D. S. (1993, March). *Justifying truth claims.* Paper presented at the Fourth Annual Critical and Feminist Perspectives in Nursing Conference, School of Nursing, Atlanta, GA.

Griffiths, P. (1995). Progress in measuring nursing outcomes. *Journal of Advanced Nursing, 21,* 1092-1110.

Guba, E. G. (1992). Relativism. *Curriculum Inquiry, 22*(1), 17-23.

Hayward, S., Ciliska, D., DiCenso, A., Thomas, H., Underwood, E. J., & Rafael, A. (1996). Evaluation research in public health: Barriers to the production and dissemination of outcomes data. *Canadian Journal of Public Health/Revue Canadienne de Santé Publique, 87*(6), 413-417.

Hess, J. D. (1996). The ethics of compliance: A dialectic. *Advances in Nursing Science, 19*(1), 18-27.

Hogston, R. (1997). Nursing diagnosis and classification systems: A position paper. *Journal of Advanced Nursing, 26,* 496-500.

Johnson, M., & Maas, M. (1997). *Nursing outcomes classification (NOC).* St. Louis, MO: Mosby.

Jones, L. D. (1997). Building the information infrastructure required for managed care. *IMAGE: Journal of Nursing Scholarship, 29*(4), 377-382.

Keating, N., Fast, J., Fredrick, M., Cranswick, K., & Perrier, C. (1999). *Eldercare in Canada: Context, content, and consequences.* Ottawa: Statistics Canada.

Kitson, A. (1997). Using evidence to demonstrate the value of nursing. *Nursing Standards, 11*(28), 34-39.

Kleinman, A. (1992). Local worlds of suffering: An interpersonal focus for ethnographies of illness experience. *Qualitative Health Research, 2*(2), 127-134.

Knafl, K., Breitmayer, B., Gallo, A., & Zoeler, L. (1996). Family response to childhood chronic illness: Description of management styles. *Journal of Pediatric Nursing, 112*(5), 315-326.

Koocher, G. P., McGrath, M. L., & Gudas, L. J. (1990). Typologies of nonadherence in cystic fibrosis. *Journal of Developmental and Behavioral Pediatrics, 11*(6), 353-358.

Kushner, C., & Rachlis, M. (1997). Consumer involvement in health policy development. In National Forum on Health (Ed.), *Health and health care issues: Summaries of papers commissioned by the National Forum on Health.* Ottawa, ON. Retrieved January 15, 2000 from the World Wide Web: www.nfh.hc-sc.gc.ca/publicat/issuesum/kushner.htm.

Lather, P. (1991). *Getting smart: Feminist research and pedagogy with/in the postmodern.* New York: Routledge.

Lather, P. (1993). Fertile obsession: Validity after poststructuralism. *Sociological Quarterly, 34*(4), 673-693.

Lazarus, R. S., & Folkman, S. (1984). *Stress, appraisal, and coping.* New York: Springer.

LeFort, S. M. (1993). The statistical versus clinical significance debate. *IMAGE: Journal of Nursing Scholarship, 25,* 57-62.

Longino, H. E. (1990). *Science as social knowledge: Values and objectivity in scientific inquiry.* Princeton, NJ: Princeton University Press.

Lynn, M. R. (1989). Meta-analysis: Appropriate tool for the integration of nursing research? *Nursing Research, 38,* 302-305.

Maas, M. L., Johnson, M., & Moorhead, S. (1996). Classifying nursing-sensitive patient outcomes. *IMAGE: Journal of Nursing Scholarship, 28*(4), 295-301.

Martin, K. S., & Scheet, N. J. (1995). The Omaha System: Nursing diagnoses, interventions, and client outcomes. In N. M. Lang (Ed.), *Nursing data systems: The emerging framework* (pp. 105-113). Washington, DC: American Nurses Publishing.

McAllister, W. (1994). Concrete fictions and hegemonic methodologies: Doing policy research in government. *Journal of Health Politics, Policy and Law, 19*(1), 91-106.

McKeever, P. (1996). The family: Long-term care research and policy formation. *Nursing Inquiry, 3*(4), 200-206.

Melhado, E. M. (1998). Economist, public provision, and the market: Changing values in policy debate. *Journal of Health Politics, Policy and Law, 23*(2), 215-263.

Micek, W., Berry, L., Gilski, D., Kallenbach, A., Link, D., & Scharer, K. (1996). The link between nursing diagnosis and interventions. *Journal of Nursing Administration, 26*(11), 29-35.

Mitchell, P. H., Ferketich, S., Jennings, B. M., & American Academy of Nursing Expert Panel on Quality Health Care. (1998). Quality health outcomes model. *IMAGE: Journal of Nursing Scholarship, 30*(1), 43-46.

Mitchell, P. H., Heinrich, J., Moritz, P., & Hinshaw, A. S. (1997). Outcome measures and care delivery systems: Introduction and purpose of the conference. *Medical Care, 35*(11), NS1-NS5.

Moritz, P. (1995, May). *Outcomes research: Examining clinical effectiveness.* Paper presented at the Communicating Nursing Research, San Diego, CA.

Morse, J. M., & Carter, B. (1996). The essence of enduring and expressions of suffering: The reformulation of self. *Scholarly Inquiry for Nursing Practice, 10*(1), 43-74.

National Center for Nursing Research. (1991). *Patient outcomes research: Examining the effectiveness of nursing practice.* Rockville, MD.

Navarro, V. (1984). The political economy of medical care: An explanation of the composition, nature, and functions of the present health sector of the United States. In P. R. Lee, C. L. Estes, & N. B. Ramsay (Eds.), *The nation's health* (2nd ed., pp. 338-354). San Francisco: Boyd and Fraser.

Newacheck, P. W., Stoddard, J. J., & McManus, M. (1993). Ethnoculutral variations in the prevalence and impact of childhood chronic conditions. *Pediatrics, 91*(5S), 1031-1047.

Patterson, J. M., & Blum, R. W. (1993). A conference on culture and chronic illness in childhood: Conference summary. *Pediatrics, 91*(5S), 1025-1030.

Perrin, E. C., Newacheck, P., Pless, I. B., Drotar, D., Gortmaker, S. L., Leventhal, J., Perrin, J. M., Stein, R. E. K., Walker, D. K., & Weitzman, M. (1993). Issues involved in the definition and classification of chronic health conditions. *Pediatrics, 91*(4), 787-793.

Pierce, D., & Frank, G. (1992). A mother's work: Two levels of feminist analysis of family-centered care. *American Journal of Occupational Therapy, 46*(11), 972-980.

Playle, J. F., & Keeley, P. (1998). Non-compliance and professional power. *Journal of Advanced Nursing, 27,* 304-311.

Reynolds, N. R., Timmerman, J. A., & Stevenson, J. S. (1992). Meta-analysis for descriptive research. *Research in Nursing and Health, 15,* 467-475.

Richardson, L. (1991). Postmodern social theory: Representational practices. *Sociological Theory, 9,* 173-179.

Robinson, C. A. (1993). Managing life with a chronic condition: The story of normalization. *Qualitative Health Research, 3*(1), 6-28.

Rodgers, B. L. (1989). Concepts, analysis, and the development of nursing knowledge: The evolutionary cycle. *Journal of Advanced Nursing, 14,* 330-335.

Rosnow, R. L., & Rosenthal, R. (1989). Statistical procedures and the justification of knowledge in psychological science. *American Psychologist, 44*(10), 1276-1284.

Ryan, P., & Delaney, C. (1995). Nursing minimum data set. In J. Fitzpatrick, R. Taunton, & A. Jacox (Eds.), *Annual Review of Nursing Research* (Vol. 14, pp. 169-194). New York: Springer.

Sandelowski, M. (1996). Using qualitative methods in intervention studies. *Research in Nursing and Health, 19,* 359-364.

Scott, C. B., & Moneyham, L. (1995). Perceptions of senior residents about a community-based nursing center. *IMAGE: Journal of Nursing Scholarship, 27*(3), 181-186.

Seidman, S. (Ed.). (1994). *The postmodern turn: New perspectives on social theory.* Cambridge: Cambridge University Press.

Slakter, M. J., Wu, Y.-W. B., & Suzuki-Slakter, N. S. (1991). *, **, and ***; Statistical nonsense at the .00000 level. *Nursing Research, 40*(4), 248-249.

Smith, D. E. (1990). *The conceptual practices of power: A feminist sociology of knowledge.* Boston: Northeastern University Press.

Smith, K. (1983). Tests of significance: Some frequent misunderstandings. *American Journal of Orthopsychiatry, 53*(2), 315-321.

Smith, S. (1997). Deepening participatory action-research. In S. Smith, D. Willms, & N. Johnson, *Nurtured by Knowledge* (pp. 173-263). New York: Apex Press.

Stetler, C. B. (1994). Refinement of the Stetler/Marram model for application of research findings to practice. *Nursing Outlook, 42*(1), 15-25.

Sullivan, M. D. (1993). Placebo controls and epistemic control in orthodox medicine. *Journal of Medicine and Philosophy, 18,* 213-231.

Tanenbaum, S. J. (1994). Knowing and acting in medical practice: The epistemological politics of outcomes research. *Journal of Health Politics, Policy and Law, 19*(1), 27-44.

Tanenbaum, S. J. (1996). "Medical effectiveness" in Canadian and U.S. health policy: The comparative politics of inferential ambiguity. *HSR: Health Services Research, 31*(5), 517-532.

Thorne, S. E. (1990). Constructive noncompliance in chronic illness. *Holistic Nursing Practice, 5,* 62-69.

Toulmin, S. (1972). *Human understanding.* Princeton, NJ: Princeton University Press.

VanSciver, M. M., D'Angelo, E. J., Rappaport, L., & Woolf, A. D. (1995). Pediatric compliance and the roles of distinct treatment characteristics, treatment attitudes, and family stress: A preliminary report. *Developmental and Behavioral Pediatrics, 16*(5), 350-358.

Walker, L., & Avant, K. (1988). *Strategies for theory construction in nursing.* Norwalk, CT: Appleton & Lange.

Ware, J. E. (1995). What information do consumers want and how will they use it? *Medical Care, 33*(1), JS25-JS30.

Wuest, J. (1993). Removing the shackles: A feminist critique of noncompliance. *Nursing Outlook, 41,* 217-224.

Wuest, J. (1994). A feminist approach to concept analysis. *Western Journal of Nursing Research, 16*(5), 577-586.

Wuest, J. (1997). Illuminating environmental influences on women's caring. *Journal of Advanced Nursing, 26,* 49-58.

Dialogue:

The Form of Data

SWANSON: All that qualitative data has to come out of our mouths, or our response to the questionnaires, or physiological tests, or from the environment, or something. I mean, the fact that people write all around the questionnaires—I do it all the time, and nobody can capture my experience by writing questions. I see it all the time. Take physiological tests. Besides the fact that these tests often do not have good sensitivity, are they valid? There is a new study that came out that says there is a "white coat blood pressure phenomenon," and they found out that all these pregnant women's blood pressure would go up sky high only when they were in a clinic setting, around a white coat, and someone was taking their blood pressure. The rest of the time it was okay; for 24 hours they would be fine. They found out that the doctors were treating them, and they should not be treating them. So even the physiological stuff is questionable. They are in as bad a shape as we are.

ESTABROOKS: Even worse, in fact, for policy makers, the data are not collected from people. They are collected from records and banks, and secondary sources. But that is the form in which policy makers have become used to receiving their research information. In that context, there is this qualitative movement going on . . .

SWANSON: The first nurse we had on the legislature in California was, I think, in the 1960s, and that nurse was the sole source of information regarding health issues for the guys. Before that, the only information was from a vet who was a legislator. And everything was in terms of counts. COUNTS! It's incredible!

KUZEL: We just have to focus on what we have to offer in terms of working on practical problems for policy makers and clinicians. We just have to focus on what we can do for you. . . . Maybe we can help.

4

Questions in Use

JANICE M. SWANSON

In this chapter, I address issues about questions in the use of qualitative evidence. Although it is a commonly held tenet that the research question is the primary question in an investigation, there are additional questions of a different nature that are of considerable importance to each study. I take the position that

- the types and nature of questions asked are essential in the use of qualitative evidence;
- the types of questions found in research include formal research questions, data collection questions, and analytic questions asked about the data;
- the nature of these questions differs in quantitative and qualitative investigations;
- the nature of these questions also differs in common qualitative research approaches;
- how you get from the research question to what you ask people participating in the study is a vital yet often neglected or unreported aspect of the study; and
- the nature of the question varies depending upon who asks the question: the clinician, the participant, or the decision maker.

This position is supported through the examination of current research approaches, comparison of these approaches, and through my own experience. I propose that the nature of the questions and how they are asked are key to the use of questions that may be answered through qualitative inquiry in order to generate qualitative evidence.

The Nature of the Question and How It Is Important

The nature of the question asked in an investigation leads to variation in questions asked throughout the study, which leads to the eventual generation and use of qualitative evidence to guide practice and set policy. Many types of questions are asked during an investigation, the most important being (a) research questions, (b) questions asked about the data in the analysis, and (c) analytic questions.

Research Questions

Research questions in qualitative investigations tend to be general, because they cannot yet name the major concepts that will be discovered during the research process. They will, however, usually name the population to be studied. The qualitative research question will usually note the area of study and the nature of the outcomes, such as the questions asked in a grounded theory study (Chenitz & Swanson, 1986; Strauss & Corbin, 1990): "What is the social-psychological process engaged in by young adults living with multiple sclerosis (MS)?" Additional, more specific questions might ask, "Under what conditions do young adults live with MS?" "What strategies are used by young adults living with MS?" and "With what consequences do young adults live with MS?" To answer the research question in a qualitative study, questions that elicit spontaneous answers are asked of each participant at one time or during successive periods of time. In addition, observations of behavior and the environment may be made and recorded as well. Other data, such as videotapes, journals, and printed materials, may also be used. The narrative and other data produced are analyzed using a process of coding and concept or category building.

Types of questions used in data analysis, however, are distinct and based on whether the study is a quantitative or a qualitative study.[1] Research questions in quantitative investigations name the two or more variables to be investigated and the population in which the variables will be investigated. The variables must be measurable, and valid and reliable instruments must be available for data collection. Also, the population must be described. For example (Swanson, Dibble, & Chapman, 2000): "In young adults with genital herpes, does a group psycho-educational intervention led by nurses decrease sexual health risk and improve psychosocial adaptation?" (p. 246). To answer the research question in a quantitative study, instruments such as questionnaires may be given to each participant at specific periods of time. Each questionnaire contains uniform questions and answers that are quantified for the process of statistical analysis. In this study, valid and reliable instruments were used to measure sexual health risk and psychosocial adaptation in order to allow the investigators to answer the research question.

Formal research questions, as those above, are important to the design of the study and the type of study. Questions that are asked during the data collection process and analytic questions asked during the process of analysis are also important to the design and purpose of the study.

Data Collection Questions

To elicit data in a research study, subjects or informants may be asked questions, or, for example, questions may be used to guide the observations of a setting, which will be recorded in field notes. Questions then often guide the process of data collection. Types of questions used in data collection are distinct from formal research questions and questions used in the analysis of data.

The sets of questions asked by the investigators during data collection in a qualitative investigation will very likely change as the work progresses. Different questions might be asked of different participants. As the questions themselves are different, there is no set order for asking the questions. The questions will most likely be asked in an interview format with open-ended questions. Or the data will consist of observations made by the investigators or members of the research team and noted as field notes either by audiotape, videotape, word processing, or handwritten notes. The hypotheses or hunches that arise from the data change as the work progresses. The purpose of data collection questions in a qualitative study is to contribute to theory development. In other words, different questions, which change over time, are asked of the participants so that through the analysis of concepts, categories will emerge that will generate theory, such as in the development of grounded theory, ethnography, or phenomenology.

It is important to note that the nature of the questions asked in a qualitative investigation may vary. Kidder and Fine (1987) have noted a distinction between qualitative data collection that gives insights into the interpretation of findings in a quantitative study and qualitative data collection that generates categories and concepts that lead to theory generation. Insightful questions may, for example, be sets of uniform questions that are semistructured or open-ended and are asked as a part of a quantitative study to enrich the interpretation of the questions asked to test the hypotheses. Answers to these questions may shed light on the interpretation of prestated hypotheses from pre-selected theoretical concepts chosen to guide the study. The use of insightful questions only hinders theory development, whereas the use of the theory-generating questions promotes theory development. As stated by Judd (1987), "Theoretical knowledge about social behavior and the social factors that are responsible for those behaviors" (p. 26) is needed. Theoretical knowledge is generated from qualitative studies that ask theory-generating questions and is not generated from quantitative studies that insert a set of uniform questions that limit findings to insights.

Glaser (1992) warns that in a grounded theory, for example, the investigator must trust in the discovery of a problem; this core problem will emerge if one is true to what presents in the data. Therefore, the investigator should not be forced to preconceive a problem or to limit questions in data collection until the core problem emerges. Although the core problem will be "delimited" (Glaser, 1992, p. 24), depending on constraints such as the investigator's training, the nature of the sample, and the source of funding, the study of abstract problems and the processes that informants are engaged in to resolve those problems are very different from unit analysis. The problem to be studied must come from the informants themselves; only they can articulate what is relevant to them. Thus, questions must be open-ended, practical, and must not introduce preconceived problems or topics to the informant.

The following are examples of questions asked in data collection interviews of informants in a grounded theory study of young adults' experience of living with genital herpes (Swanson & Chenitz, 1993; from the files of the author, J. M. Swanson):

> Tell me what it was like when you first started having symptoms.
> Tell me about getting a diagnosis.
> In what ways has having this disease affected your life?
> How do you bring up the topic of having this disease with a partner?

Follow-up questions include probes such as "when," "where," and "under what conditions do you bring up the topic?" Other questions may pertain to other parts of the research such as deciding when data collection will occur, deciding the composition of the sample, noting who will be interviewed, where interviews will take place, who will carry out the interviews, where participant-observation or observation will take place, what media will be used to make the observations, duration of observations, variation in observations, and so forth.

In a quantitative investigation, however, the investigators ask the participants the same data collection questions. Furthermore, they may well ask the questions in the same order, or they may purposely vary the order in which questions are asked. Participants are asked a question, or a set of uniform questions, so that some light can be shed on the interpretation of prestated hypotheses from preselected theoretical concepts chosen to guide the study. The questions are likely closed-ended but may elicit some spontaneous responses that then are usually coded into measurable quantities. The following are examples of statements used to collect data in a quantitative study testing the effects of nurse-facilitated psychoeducational group interventions on sexual health risks and psychosocial adaptation in young adults with genital herpes (Swanson, Dibble, & Chapman, 1999):

I know of precautions I could take to reduce my risk of giving genital herpes.

I would rather risk taking my chances on giving my partner herpes than try and make changes in my sex life.

Before I had sex with a new partner, I would discuss herpes protection with him or her.

Participants rated their responses to these statements, and others, noting how true each statement was for themselves in the prevention of genital herpes, on a 4-point Likert-type scale (Swanson et al., 1999, pp. 844-845). The scale ranged from (1) "not at all true of me" to (4) "completely true of me."

Analytic Questions of Data

To analyze data in a research study, questions are asked of the data. The nature of the questions, then, often guides the process of data analysis. Types of questions used in data analysis are also distinct, as noted in this section.

In a qualitative investigation, the sets of questions asked by the investigator(s) in concert with a study team and/or consultants analyzing the data will also very likely change as the work progresses. Here also, different questions may be asked, depending on the findings as the analysis progresses. The order for asking questions depends largely on the theoretical framework selected at the initiation of the study and on the research questions or hypotheses.

Glaser (1992) states that questions asked during analysis must be "totally neutral to get at relevance" (p. 51). He suggests that this applies to the first step, called *open coding*. In open coding, each phrase of the transcript of an interview or field notes of observations or other qualitative data is coded line by line using exact words of the informants themselves or a term or phrase that connotes those words. Glaser (1992) stresses that questions to guide analysis should be neutral, such as "What is this data a study of?" (p. 51). Constant comparisons are made of the data at several levels, beginning with comparisons of incidents. The investigator may ask questions such as "Why does this action occur in this incident and not in a similar incident?"

The following are some sample questions from the qualitative study described earlier on the process of living with genital herpes in young adults (Swanson & Chenitz, 1993). The investigators observed that some informants always told their partners about their disease before initiating sexual contact with them; others did not. Line-by-line data were then coded, and similar codes were grouped into the category, or concept, "telling a partner." An analytic question at this point asked, "Under what conditions does telling a partner of one's diagnosis with the disease occur?" Conditions under which a partner tells or withholds telling about his or her diagnosis with the disease were then coded. Additional categories or concepts were then formed. Practical conditions were coded and included conditions such as "during an outbreak" or "only a one-night stand." Personal conditions were also coded, and included conditions such as "a bit of a conflict" and "feeling inferior." The concept "valued self" was then generated in the described manner, and another analytic question was asked of the data: "What hypotheses can be asked of the data at this point?" One hypothesis that was formed and used to question the data was that "the higher the value of self, the more likely one would tell a partner they had herpes before initiating sex." Then, as the investigators continued to code and compare the concepts to more incidents, another analytic question was asked: "Are there recurring patterns in the data, and if so, what are they?" One of the major recurring patterns is described in the following quote (Swanson & Chenitz, 1993):

> The major strategy for preserving oneself was to adopt a management style that allowed control of information about self.... Informants adopted one of three styles of controlling information about their disease: revealing, accommodating, and avoiding. Regardless of the style adopted, it enabled respondents to live with herpes over time. (p. 289)

Some informants reported the pattern of always revealing they had genital herpes to potential sexual partners. Some reported the pattern of accommodating, that is, telling a partner they had the disease only under certain conditions, such as during an outbreak of the disease or if they were in an ongoing relationship. Other informants reported the pattern of always avoiding telling their sexual partner they had the disease, including informants who were married and had a child. The three patterns reflected the variations used by informants in their quest to preserve a sense of self at all costs.

Thus, the analytic questions vary as the process of analysis progresses in a qualitative study. Types of research questions, data collection questions, and analytic questions presented here as examples were drawn from grounded theory studies. These types of questions will vary depending on the type of qualitative research methodology chosen for the study. Other influences inevitably affect the process, such as the particular interests of the investigators, prior experience, and varying perspectives, all of which must be recorded in field notes and utilized in the process of analysis and interpretation.

In a quantitative investigation, the sets of questions asked by the investigator(s) in consort with statisticians analyzing the data will also very likely change as the work progresses. Different questions may be asked depending on the findings as the analysis progresses. The order for asking questions depends largely on the theoretical framework selected at the initiation of the study and the research questions or hypotheses. The following are some sample questions asked during analysis of a quantitative study on the gender differences in the predictors of depression in young adults with genital herpes (Dibble & Swanson, 2000; from the files of the author, J. M. Swanson):

What are the descriptive statistics (such as demographics) related to sample characteristics?

What are the descriptive statistics (such as demographics) related to the other variables of interest?

Because differences by gender were of particular interest in this analysis, appropriate analytical steps were taken (Dibble & Swanson, 2000):

> To analyze the research questions, multiple regression techniques, including graphic residual analyses (Ferketich & Verran, 1984) for both model testing and building procedures, were performed. In this technique the initial model, based on significant univariate correlations, is tested and then the residual is compared graphically with other variables collected in the study but not necessarily contained in the initial model. This iterative technique is one of the ways to ensure that the assumptions underlying the regression procedure are met. (p. 190)

Further specific questions asked in this analysis and further statistical procedures are found in the literature, such as in the Ferketich and Verran (1984) article.

How Does the Nature of the Research Question Asked Differ in Major Qualitative Research Approaches?

Morse (1994) makes a very clear statement about the similarities and differences between three qualitative research approaches: phenomenology, ethnography, and grounded theory. She distinguishes between the type of research questions asked in each research approach. In addition, she emphasizes that the type of research questions stem from the paradigm underlying each research approach. The following examples are given.

Phenomenology

The type of research questions asked in a phenomenological study are meaning questions designed to elicit the essence of experiences

(Morse & Field, 1995). This is done through direct inquiry using in-depth conversations. Constant questioning provides insights into one's lived experience. The paradigm is philosophy. An example is MacIntyre's (1999) monograph, *Mortal Men*, which presents the lived experience of HIV-positive gay men as they juggle sex, the use of illicit drugs, and their T-cell levels. When the men found that their T-cell levels were low, they curtailed risky sexual encounters and the use of illicit drugs, but when they found that their T-cell levels were high, they felt safer and resumed these behaviors. As is true of a phenomenological study, no preconceived theories or frameworks guide the collection and analyses of data. In this study, the experience or life-worlds of the gay men are described and are open to interpretation by the reader. Theories, models, or explanations are not generated from the analysis. Gay men's experiences of increasing or decreasing their sexual practices and use of illicit drugs based on their T-cell levels are described.

Ethnography

The type of research questions asked in an ethnographic study are descriptive questions that describe the values, beliefs, and the practices of a cultural group (Morse & Field, 1995). An ethnography describes a cultural group or a phenomenon associated with such a group. The paradigm is ethnography. An example is Lipson and Omidian's (1997) examination of the health beliefs of Afghan refugees. The investigators used data collected primarily via open-ended interviews and participant observation over approximately a 10-year period from the largest Afghan immigrant community in the United States, in northern California. The authors reported the social context in which Afghan refugees find themselves as they confront interactions with U.S. citizens and health and social service providers. The report particularly related to information needs and cultural differences and misunderstandings, as the refugees coped with life in their host country while maintaining an Islamic identity across generations. Thus, this ethnography allows the reader to understand behavior related to health and illness in the context in which that behavior occurs. An ethnography allows us to understand the topic of study from the view of the participants; it allows the "emic" or natives' point of view.

Grounded Theory

The type of research questions asked in a grounded theory study are process questions that elicit experience and change over time (Morse & Field, 1995). Grounded theory questions change and may have stages and phases. The paradigm of grounded theory is sociology, originating from symbolic interactionism (Blumer, 1969; Mead, 1934). As they interact with others, people construct their own realities through the creation of symbols. Thus, individuals are involved in creating meaning in a situation. Grounded theory generates explanatory theories of human behavior. Participants are selected through a process called theoretical sampling (Glaser & Strauss, 1967) that is based on their experience with the topic and the needs of the theory as it develops. Observation, unstructured interviews, and other forms of fieldwork are used in data collection. Analysis occurs jointly with data collection and involves constant comparison of one piece of data with another as well as the generation of a process (through coding and memo writing) that describes change over time, usually in stages or phases that participants go through to solve a social-psychological problem that they have identified. An example of grounded theory is the study just presented, which describes the process of regaining a valued sense of self following a diagnosis of genital herpes in young adults living in the San Francisco Bay Area in California (Swanson & Chenitz, 1993). Data consisted of interviews conducted as semi-open discussions that pursued concerns introduced by the participants. The process of adaptation to living with genital herpes occurs in three stages: (1) a stage of *protecting oneself* from a devalued sense of self following the stigmatization that they connected with the disease; (2) a stage of *renewing oneself* by reaching out and attempting to balance their lives; and (3) a stage of *preserving oneself* by adopting a style of management that allows them to preserve their sense of self, be it always revealing to a potential sexual partner that they have the disease, accommodating by telling some potential partners conditionally, or avoiding telling a potential partner. As a grounded theory study, the process, in addition to having distinct stages, also describes the contexts in which it occurs and the major conditions for change. The process of adapting to living with a chronic sexually transmitted disease occurred within the following contexts: (a) that of a social world marked by instability and change; (b) self-imposed privacy and isolation due to the stigma attached to the disease; and (c) varied lifestyles, often including the use of illicit drugs, common in young adults. The conditions under which the process could change included the stability of the relationship and the course of the disease. For example, little change occurred under the condition of a supportive partner and stable disease course. However, a new partner, a new infection site, or an increase in the frequency of recurrences of the disease could force the participants to go back and repeat earlier stages of the process.

Others

It is important to remember that there are many other qualitative research approaches; each approach has its own distinctive way of stating research questions. Some of these approaches include the following: feminist research, action research, participatory research, critical research, and historical research (for an overview, see Burns & Grove, 1999).

How Do You Get From the Research Questions to What You Ask People?

Essentially, the research questions vary depending on whether you are conducting an insightful, small qualitative study or a larger theory-generating study. It is important to distinguish between these types of qualitative studies; in so doing, it is important to note that the qualitative worldview makes the following assumptions (Burns & Grove, 1999):

- There is no single reality,
- Reality is based on perceptions,
- Reality is different for each person,
- Reality changes over time, and
- What we know has meaning only within a given situation or context. (p. 339)

Examples

Insightful Study: Breast Cancer

Qualitative methods that use an insightful approach as an adjunct to a quantitative study are found frequently in the literature. Use of an insightful approach is often appropriate, depending on the purposes of the study. One example of the use of an insightful approach is a study by Hatch and her colleagues (1999) in which they used qualitative social science methods and applied them to a research question in chronic disease epidemiology: breast cancer research. Concerned with the dual problems of the cultural relevance of standardized questionnaires and memory decay and recall bias in retrospective epidemiological studies, they conducted a pilot study. To aid in instrument development, the authors used qualitative research data collection and analysis techniques to elicit information in the words of the participants themselves regarding important events, body development, and types of physical activity engaged in during their peripubertal period of development (between 9 and 16 years of age). Data collected from Hispanic, Caucasian, and African American breast cancer patients were analyzed using category development to discover the differences in recall of peripubertal exposures and experiences based on cultural differences. The authors have used the data to construct questionnaire modules that provide familiar phrasing and memory cues and that embed questions from the study within sets of context questions using the cues and phrasing that generate descriptions of culturally sensitive past events more accurately than direct, cold questions have in the past, such as age at menarche.

In this primarily quantitative study, the authors have turned to the use of qualitative data in a secondary way, to act as a supplement to the quantitative study. Questions were asked in this study to assist the investigators in constructing questionnaire modules that provided familiar phrasing, memory cues, and questions that will elicit better responses and will provide insight into the interpretation of findings of the quantitative study. This use of qualitative data, secondarily, is limited to providing insight into a quantitative study; such use stands in contrast to the use of qualitative data as the primary source of data in a qualitative study that generates theory and is useful in addressing an unresolved health problem. The latter is illustrated in the next section, in a report of an anthropological study (Vecchiato, 1997) carried out using qualitative methodology to investigate the sociocultural aspects of tuberculosis (TB) control in a rural community in the mountains of Ethiopia, where a number of biomedical efforts based on quantitative epidemiological research had produced no change in the epidemiological situation related to TB (Styblo & Rouillon, 1991).

A Call for the Use of a Theory-Generating Study: TB

An example of a study that calls for the use of a theory-generating method was carried out by Vecchiato (1997). Vecchiato's ethnographic research contributed to theory by supporting Garro's (1988) rendition of a "prototypical cultural model of illness" (p. 194). Hodes and Azbite (1993) had previously described the national TB programs in Ethiopia, using the current focus of Western medicine, as "virtually non-functional" (p. 280) and having little influence on the extent of the disease in the country. TB was a major cause of death in hospitals in the country despite a research focus on clinical, epidemiological, and bacteriological aspects of the disease. The authors cited problems arising from funding, reporting of cases, the organization and staffing of medical services, the supply of medications, and the monitoring of patients and facilities. These authors recommended that TB services be incorporated into the primary health care model to affect the delivery of TB programs. The outcomes of the TB program whose measurable entities were reported by the Ethiopian Ministry of Health (MOH, 1991), such as prevalent rates of diagnosis of TB compared to other top diseases and ranking by cause of hospital deaths, attested to the persistence of pulmonary TB as a major health problem in Ethiopia. TB was the main cause of hospital deaths, ranking third in males (6.1%) and sixth in females (3.2%) in diseases diagnosed in the years 1988 and 1989. Research had focused on traditional clinical, bacteriological, and epidemiological dimensions of the disease (Gebre et al., 1995; Hodes & Kloos, 1988; Zerihun & Esscher, 1984). One study (Demissie & Kebede, 1994) pointed to various sociocultural factors underlying the lack of compliance to treatment such as lack of education, little knowledge, a feeling of improvement despite underlying existence of the disease, and negative attitudes toward care providers in the TB center. In addition, an early monograph (Schaller & Kuls, 1972) based on research in the 1960s suggested disease-transmitting behaviors existed, for example, communal water pipe smoking and sharing drinking vessels at community gatherings such as funerals. The World Health Organization sponsored measures of national control using three long-term strategies: (1) improving socioeconomic conditions in the country; (2) BCG vaccination; and (3) case-finding and treatment. Yet, these biomedical efforts had produced no change in the epidemiological situation related to TB (Styblo & Rouillon, 1991).

In contrast to the biomedical approach, Vecchiato (1997) designed an anthropological study to investigate the sociocultural aspects of TB control in a rural community in the mountains of Ethiopia. The author employed qualitative methods, including fieldwork, which consisted of structured, open-ended interviews with traditional medical specialists, patients and informants, and participant observation, as well as a quantitative survey of illness concepts and behavior.

Vecchiato (1997) observed that the Sidama lived in windowless, single-room, thatched-roof huts and used wood fires in the huts, employed common drinking vessels, smoked common water pipes, and drank raw milk. He reported that "a normative, culturally transmitted body of knowledge and practices concerning this infectious disease" exists among the Sidama (p. 195). This work documented an ethnomedical approach to TB that is evidenced in ethnomedical etiology and ethnobotanical remedies, summarized in the following:

Ethnomedical Etiology With no knowledge of the germ theory of disease and elementary knowledge of TB, the ethnomedical etiology of the disease as perceived by the participants was described. The cause of TB was seen as debilitation due to excessive work, excessive exposure to the sun, carrying heavy loads, and malnutrition.

Ethnobotanical Remedies Because the Sidama conceptualized TB as having multiple causes, they described multiple ethnobotanical remedies, for example: nutritious food; drinking animal blood; cautery, which was carried out by a traditional medical specialist burning the chest with a red hot-rod; and the use of various herbal remedies, including emetics to rid the body of bad blood. Lack of compliance to Western medical treatment was explained by the fact that the Western treatment, using the pharmaceuticals isoniazid, rifampin, and streptomycin, lacked an emetic effect, required by the cultural belief to cleanse the body.

The conclusions drawn by Vecchiato (1997) were that the "management of actual illness episodes is shaped not solely by culturally transmitted ethnomedical axioms, but also by practical, financial, social, structural, and geographic considerations" (p. 195). He recommended that intervention programs should accept the *convergence* of the ethnomedical approach to TB practiced by the Sidama with that of Western medicine by, for example, building communication regarding symptom recognition and the importance of diet and nutrition. He also recommended that such programs work on *divergence* between these two approaches to the control of TB by, for example, addressing factors such as beliefs in etiology and treatment of the disease. Approaches to these recommendations, according to the author, must include sensitivity to the importance of communal and community factors and use of socially relevant means, such as enlisting full community involvement in case finding and treatment. Yet, the author, on the basis of his findings, warns that "active community participation in TB control programs will not be successfully elicited in Ethiopia or other developing countries without knowledge of the 'health culture' of patients and their support groups" (p. 195).

Vecchiato's study produced more than mere insight. A free-standing qualitative anthropological study, Vecchiato's study calls for a theory-supported approach to disease control based on a cultural model of illness shared by community members. He suggests that documenting cultural gaps and understanding and integrating alternative indigenous approaches into the delivery of care are critical. Questions that elicit the health culture of a people are critical questions. Anthropological studies such as this, as well as other qualitative research studies, can produce theoretically useful findings that will enhance biomedical outcomes in the future. Further research that incorporates the health culture into Western approaches to disease control and that examines the impact of the integrated approach upon Western biomedical outcomes, such as the incidence or prevalence of a disease, is needed.

Whose Question Is It? How Should It Be Asked? How May It Be Answered Through Qualitative Inquiry or Through Going From Experience to Theory-Generating Research?

Questions From Experience

Questions from experience must be recognized. It is important to ask whose question it is, how should it be asked, and how may it be answered through qualitative inquiry. I raised the following questions in the process of recognizing questions from both clinical and research experience that resulted in research that progressed eventually to theory-generating research.

What Is the Nature of the Clinician's Question?

The clinician's question is derived from practice. It may be a question posed by a patient, or it may be a question that is distilled over time by the clinician in response to repeated questions from patients, or it may be a group of similar questions from various dimensions of one's practice.

An example of the clinician's question is drawn from my early clinical experience. Clinical questions arise early in one's practice experience. Without benefit of graduate courses, a graduate degree, a course in research, or even a baccalaureate degree, I was faced with a challenge in practice that still exists today, a quarter of a century later. While practicing as a campus nurse in a small, 10-bed infirmary at a small, private college on the West Coast of the United States, I was routinely challenged by such occurrences as a student who fell from a 75-foot fir tree and another student, high on peyote, who walked through a second-story plate glass window in a dormitory. These challenges were met in stride as appropriate emergency procedures were carried out, allowing students to return to their normal lives. I was also faced with another challenge. Many times during the year, I received telephone calls from young women students at the airport. The young women would state that they had just returned on a flight from someplace like Tijuana, Mexico, or Seattle, Washington, where they had undergone an illegal abortion, and were "running a high fever. . . . Please come get me." A book of standing orders, established long before the terms "primary care" or "nurse practitioner" were in use, directed me on an immediate course of action. Following an examination by the college health physician who was called to the infirmary, the young woman was admitted into the infirmary and started on a course of antibiotics. The following morning, I would enter the young woman's room, sit on the edge of her bed, and say something like "It must be hard to go through something like this." The young woman would, without hesitation, usually reply with something like "I don't understand how this could have happened to me. After all, he didn't put it in all the way!"

The question posed by the client challenged me. After all, there were two intelligent young people in this scenario: a young woman and a young man. The young woman was receiving aftercare, but the young man, well, the staff were just glad that he showed up and closed the door to her room while he visited with her. His needs were not addressed further. I, however, was troubled. The young woman's question stirred something in my "clinical gut," where my practice concerns were taken into a meditative state. I went to the ivy-covered campus library and found, in among the leather-bound editions of Dante, proper texts on human anatomy and physiology. However, these texts were not, in my estimation, readily accessible or understandable to my clients. I found that little was published about birth control in the early 1960s because giving clients information about birth control was illegal at that time.

Through the years of clinical practice that followed, in settings as varied as the Harvard University Health Services in Cambridge, Massachusetts, a small Athabascan Indian village in a northern corner of Alaska, a public health nursing district in the inner city in Detroit, Michigan, shortly before the riots in the 1960s, and a segregated hospital in southern Mississippi, I learned through experience that information and intelligence were not necessarily clear determinants of behavior. The client's question from that first clinical experience resonated as it gained momentum from similar experiences of other clients in my practice.

Whence the Participant's Question(s)?

Graduate school, at last, gave me some tools and a venue for investigating this clinical question. Reviewing the literature, I found many studies that addressed family planning. However, these studies were almost entirely focused on women. I could not forget the young man, the partner of the client who had endured an illegal abortion. I conceptualized a study, a survey of men and contraceptive use. Unable to locate an appropriate instrument, I adopted a tool used with women that was developed by a major research and policy-making organization worldwide, The Population Council (1972). After adjusting selected questions and pretesting, I used the tool to survey married men. Upon collecting the questionnaires from the men, I was struck by their comments, which were given in hushed tones and included questions such as "And what should she do if she forgets to take the pill for 3 days in a row? And how long should she leave the diaphragm in after we have sex? Would you go over to the high school and talk to my son? He's a senior and needs this information, but I'm uncomfortable talking to him about it." Again, I was deluged with questions that did not fit into the research design of a survey. When examining the questionnaires themselves, I found that many men had written their comments and questions around the borders of the questionnaire. How often, I thought, have I done the same thing, or have been tempted to do the same thing, regardless of the questionnaire's topic. Obviously, the questionnaire failed to capture the men's experience with contraception and to anticipate their questions. However, these data, I thought, are important data. Yet, there was no place for these data to go. These data did not answer the preconceived survey research questions, and thus, they were not included in the analysis. These rich data had no place to go except into my clinical gut, along with the experiences of the young women.

Shortly thereafter and still early in my academic career, I had the experience of hearing the late Dr. Anselm Strauss present his work using a qualitative research method called grounded theory. He stated that this method of qualitative research was appropriate to use when there was no research in an area and when there was research but the findings were not of value to the clinician in practice. The comment rang true to my experience related to men and family planning. However, there was almost nothing in the literature that addressed this problem. Although literature existed that addressed family planning and women's experiences, the majority of this work was carried out by demographers and described the relationships between the use of contraception in women and many demographic variables such as age, income, marital status, race/ethnicity, and the like. Unfortunately, very little existed to actually assist the clinician in dealing with clinical questions such as I had faced in practice. I shared my experience and concern with Dr. Strauss and, upon his invitation, eventually became the first federally funded institutional postdoctoral fellow in nursing in the United States.

I began my postdoctoral program of research in a newly opened, federally funded pilot program in San Francisco, which provided reproductive health services, including family planning, to men. While learning qualitative research methodology from Dr. Strauss, I engaged in observation, participant-observation, and both formal and informal interviewing at this site. After a period of fieldwork, which included formal interviews with 30 young men, I was beset again by a request from one of the potential participants. He stated that his female partner wanted to be interviewed with him and asked if this would be possible. Concerned that this would affect my study of men and family planning, I sought advice from Dr. Strauss, expressing my initial fears that having partners in the study would somehow contaminate the sample. Anselm asked me, "What is the natural unit here? Men or the couple?" I replied that men were the target population for the study, but that the behavior of the couple was of interest because there would be no need for contraception if the couple were not involved. Anselm again asked, "Would they be seen as a unit in the clinic?" I again replied that they probably would not, as staff members were not generally comfortable seeing couples together but were accustomed to working with women. Anselm replied that the behavior I was interested in—the couple's interaction around contraceptive choices and use—could not be observed. Thus, it would be necessary for me to interview the couple as a unit, and that would be as close to "between the covers" behavior as I, as a researcher, could get.

I then started interviewing couples as a unit, and the entire focus of the study changed. In fact, I published a study of the original 30 men (Swanson, 1980) and then went on to complete a second study on couple interaction around contraception (Swanson, 1988).

Throughout this evolution, the nature of the question changed. First, there was the clinician's question, which was based on my experience with clients and their questions. These clinicians' questions are important because they provide the basis for research questions that will address the needs of practitioners, thus providing evidence on which to base practice. Problems for practice professions arise, however, when the roles of the researchers take them out of practice or limit their contact with people in practice.

What Is the Nature of the Decision Maker's Question?

The nature of the decision maker's question is particularly important because it determines the shape of the outcome(s). For example, upon completion of the described research project, I published a paper describing the process of the couples' experiences finding contraceptive options (Swanson, 1988). The work described a social-psychological process with several phases. The process and subprocesses explained the "why" regarding couples' interaction regarding contraception and its use. It was one of the first studies to document patterns of both simultaneous and sequential use of multiple methods of contraception by individual couples. Until that time, when examining demographic reports of contraceptive use, the pattern was to gather data from women only. The question asked, from The Population Council's questionnaire, was "What method of contraception do you use?" When I, unsure of myself in my initial interviews with men in the men's reproductive health clinic, asked them, "What method of contraception do you use?" the men replied something like this:

> It depends . . . do you mean at night or in the morning? During the week or on weekends? At her safe time of the month or during other times of the month? You see, we use the diaphragm on weeknights so she can take it out and wash it in the morning before going to work, and she doesn't have to wear it to work, then risk washing it in a public restroom. Then in the morning, we use foam and condoms, and she wears a pad so she doesn't drip. When she is in her safe period we may use nothing, but when she is most fertile, we will use four methods at one time.

Indeed, it was the use of multiple methods that may have saved these couples from the experience of an unwanted pregnancy and the decision whether or not to have an abortion.

When examining the demographers' published periodic surveys of contraceptive use by married women in the United States (Westoff, 1972), I noted that the pill was the most popular method at that time, and male methods, such as condoms, withdrawal, and vasectomy, were among the least popular methods. The use of multiple methods was not acknowledged in the body of the article. Upon closer examination, however, I noted that the report of multiple methods used was footnoted.

It was stated by the demographer that he accounted for multiple methods use by choosing to report only one method used by each participant, that method being the "most effective method" named by the woman. The most effective method was determined in separate studies that examined the efficacy of individual methods of contraception. Thus, these studies did not account for the joint use of multiple methods. In addition, the context was also stripped away, as only the central variable, contraceptive use, was reported.

Answering the Question:
Contexualization Versus Decontextualization

As seen in the preceding section, the participants present their constructions of reality (i.e., use of contraception) in broad contexts that are rich with descriptions of the social, psychological, and even environmental milieus. The contexts explain the choices made and the clear rationale used by the actors on the various scenes for making such choices. Thus, the accounts in the empirical world are heavily contextualized. The way in which the research question is asked, however, may capture the rich contexts as in qualitative research. Or another research question of a different genus may decontextualize or strip away the context in which the action has meaning to the actors, such as "What method of contraception do you use?" The answer cannot be contained in one word but is embedded in a story that contains rich details about a process engaged in by the storyteller.

Issues for Consideration in Use

Questions in Use of Evidence

Important issues exist that must be considered when using research findings. They include the process of applying findings in the everyday real world, such as to practice or to changing policy (see Chapters 11 & 12). One approach to examining the questions in use is to address questions that arise in the use of evidence. Questions arise in attempts to apply both quantitative and qualitative evidence.

The reader who attempts to apply quantitative research findings in support of a particular theory usually finds that the theory is too narrow or is insufficiently broad enough to account for the wide range in diversity experienced by the reader in the ever changing daily world of reality. The quantitative study may support or fail to support a preconceived theory. This study is based on precisely measured, validated facts. Facts, however, tend to change quickly, leaving the researcher with a theory that may have applied at one point in time or may have applied partially but does not have sufficiently diverse concepts to account for the fast-changing scene in the world of practice. The few variables in the quantitatively derived theory may be well known, but they might account for only a portion of the picture (Glaser & Strauss, 1967). The readers who must apply the rigid theory might interpret the theory to mean that if the facts are correct, then so is the theory, thus leaving them with little chance of applying it in a complex work world.

Thus, a major problem faced by researchers who seek to publish their findings is that of conveying the credibility of their work. Whether the work rests on quantitative or qualitative data, the reader of the work, when thinking about or using the work, enters what Glaser and Strauss (1967) term "the discounting process" (p. 231).

The Discounting Process

According to Glaser and Strauss (1967), the discounting process takes several forms. The theory may be: (a) corrected, (b) adjusted, (c) invalidated, and/or (d) deemed inapplicable. The theory that is presented by the researcher in his or her work is corrected due to the design, as in a study of health care professionals that fails to include data collected from administrators. Here, the reader would correct the theory to allow for the one-sided design. The theory may be adjusted to allow for other structural conditions not addressed by the researcher as well, such as new models of care delivery not yet in practice when the theory was tested. The theory may even be "invalidated for other structures through the reader's experience or knowledge" (p. 232), such as the reader's prior practice experience, which the reader may compare to the theory and consider the theory to be invalid. The theory may be labeled as inapplicable to other structures such as social worlds or social structures other than the one(s) used to test the theory.

Questions in Use of Qualitative Evidence

Because the reader makes these necessary adjustments when thinking about or using a researcher's theory, the researcher has the task of making the theory credible to the reader. As the researcher cannot address every qualification that would be brought up by the myriad of readers, his or her task is twofold: (1) presenting the theory so that readers can understand it and (2) describing the data vividly so that the reader can see and hear the people. However, the description must always be "in relation to the theory" (Glaser & Strauss, 1967, p. 228). Thus, descriptions must be complex and real yet not too cumbersome so as to interfere with the flow of ideas. According to Glaser and Strauss (1967), both the researcher and the reader must take responsibility. The researcher must present the theory and the data clearly, paying particular attention to areas that might be deemed dubious by the reader. The reader must expect and insist on an explicit rendering of the theory and its description, because when this falls short, the reader is left to make judgments based on what *is* provided in the report, which may be limiting.

Issues of Application

To practically apply qualitative research, judgments must be made about the nature of the theory. Using grounded theory as an example, Glaser and Strauss (1967) state that four properties of the theory must exist: (1) fit, (2) understanding, (3) generality, and (4) control (also see Chapter 5).

Fit The theory must fit the substantive area to which the reader may apply the theory. That is, the substantive theory must fit the data. Without a fit between theory and data, the data must be forced and distorted to attempt a fit. Furthermore, data that have been collected in the research study that do not fit must be left out of the analysis. Lack of fit becomes problematic when the reader must try to match the theory with everyday reality as it is lived, which is ever changing. To ensure fit between the theory and the substantive area, the researcher must be diligent in inducing the theory from diverse data drawn from the everyday realities of the substantive area. Only if this occurs will the theory assist the reader in dealing with the everyday realities faced by the reader in the substantive area.

Understanding The theory must also make sense to the people who are working in the substantive area and be understandable to them. A theory cannot be applied by the reader without understanding. The theoretical concepts in a substantive theory provide a bridge between the theoretical thinking of the researcher and the thinking of the people who work in the substantive area. The bridge is a necessity because it allows the researcher to be in touch with the everyday practical world, yet at the same time, it allows the reader to understand and manage or use the theory. The concepts that make up the substantive theory allow the reader to take them into the everyday world and test them out, against their own hypotheses, to see if they hold up or must be adjusted in some way. The concepts assist the reader, in effect, to see and hear the people in everyday situations, but they do so in relation to the theory (Glaser & Strauss, 1967). In application of the theory, the reader may see and hear other conditions, other alternatives, or other consequences that might have gone unheeded before being armed with the theory, thus allowing the reader to adjust his or her practice in ways not accessible to the reader before reading the theory.

Generality The theoretical concepts, or categories, as they are called in grounded theory, should not be so abstract that they lose their ability to sensitize the reader to the concept. They should, however, be sufficiently abstract to allow the reader to apply them to multiple conditions in ever changing daily situations. Thus, the reader should be able to bend or adjust the flexible theory or, if necessary, quickly reformulate it as it is applied on the spot, so to speak, in order to improve the reader's "situational realities" (Glaser & Strauss, 1967, p. 242): "The person who applies theory becomes, in effect, a generator of theory, and in this instance the theory is clearly seen as process: an ever-developing entity" (p. 242).

The theory should also be sufficiently general to apply to the scene as a whole. If the theoretical concepts account for a wide range of diversity, rather than for a narrow range of facts, the concepts or categories that would be subject to qualification will be general enough to withstand shifts in direction and magnitude by sets of new conditions encountered in the constantly changing everyday world of practice. The application of the theory further tests and validates the theory by correcting, for example, inaccuracies in observation and reintegrating them into the theory (Glaser & Strauss, 1967).

Control The theory must give the reader sufficient control in everyday situations to be able to apply the theory and to make the alterations in application that are necessary. The reader must have at least partial control of the structure in a situation and, in addition, have at least partial control of the process that is ongoing and changing in the situation over time. Besides control, the reader needs access to the situation in order to practice the application of theory. In the use of grounded theory, a substantive or grounded theory will specify contexts, conditions, strategies or goals, and a range of consequences. These will give the user "the means by which to predict and thereby control for desired outcomes" (Corbin & Strauss, 1992, p. 15). Because the theory is a general theory, the details of each new case encountered by the reader in practice must be worked out. As this occurs and theory is applied, "the more control for desired outcomes will increase" (p. 15).

Types of Questions in Qualitative Research and Their Use

The Political Nature of Research All research findings are a challenge to the status quo: that is, they challenge what is known and accepted in the field. If they did not, there would be no reason to conduct the research in the first place. Therefore, it is important to recognize the political nature of research. For example, Krieger (1999) notes that often epidemiologists and others argue that "all decisions about science, from the choice of topics to the methods and interpretation of research, are . . . political and moral decisions" (p. 1151). In contrast, Savitz et al. (1999) feel strongly that scientists should do science and not appeal to emotion or morality, and they should leave policy making to the policy makers who take on an advocacy role selectively drawing on both research and other arenas of influence, such as economics, culture, and ethics. Although the latter issue has yet to be decided upon, there is a general agreement about the political nature of research.

In a recent paper on the importance of combining political activity and public health, McKinlay and Marceau (2000) present the following alternative courses of action that John Snow, the father of epidemiology, could have taken when faced with the findings of his field observations about the cholera mortality rates in homes that used different sources of water supplies:

1. He could have *embarked on a health education campaign*—to dissuade those at risk from ever using the contaminated well;
2. He could have *presented his evidence to the profit-driven water company,* with recommendations that it take immediate action to correct a life-threatening practice;

3. He could have *presented his results to professional colleagues at prestigious scientific meetings* (e.g., the Royal Society) or could have published them in a leading medical journal. (pp. 49-50)

Instead, he took the evidence-based socially responsible action based on his research findings and removed the handle from the contaminated Broad Street water pump, which was effective, as the cholera mortality rates quickly dropped in the homes of those previously using water from this source. McKinlay and Marceau (2000) conclude:

> If the health of a population is socially determined, then public health must take place in the social policy arena. Hence, public health is inescapably a political activity. . . . To disregard these sociopolitical determinants of the health of society is to relegate public health solely to the prevention and promotion of individual risk behaviors—which are mere epiphenomena. (p. 51)

Thus, there is a political nature to research. The use of research, whether to set policy or to change practice, often occurs in a political arena.

Types of Questions in Qualitative Research Use must be circumscribed by the nature of the questions that are asked. Different kinds of knowing must be linked with the types of questions asked. Examples of different types of questions used in qualitative research include the following: (a) questions asked in the process of conducting qualitative research and developing theory, (b) questions asked in the use of an area of focus in qualitative research in the everyday world of practice, (c) questions asked in the process of using qualitative research to inform us about treatment that will change practice, and (d) questions asked in the process of generating qualitative research to change policy.

Questions Asked in the Process of Conducting Qualitative Research and Developing Theory: Death and Dying

In the early 1960s, Glaser and Strauss (1965, 1968) and Quint-Benoliel (1967) of the University of California at San Francisco initiated a study of the process of dying. The study was born of two of Strauss's personal death experiences, which, although quite different from each other (one was sudden and the other was "lingering"), raised important questions that led not only to the research project but also to the birth of a qualitative research method, grounded theory (Glaser & Strauss, 1967). The approach used to address the problem of dying by these authors and the complexity of the processes involved, including contexts, is revealed in the following personal communication during a graduate seminar in grounded theory analysis that I attended as a postdoctoral fellow at the University of California at San Francisco, recorded in class notes on April 17, 1980:

> I came here in 1960 shortly after two personal death experiences (mother and 36-year-old colleague); I hired a nurse, Jeanne Quint, and Barney, and I spent 6 months on a hospital ward; I did the work, and Glaser listened and coined the words for what I was doing, such as *theoretical sampling.*
>
> Of the two personal death experiences, one was sudden, and the other occurred over a long period of time; I knew dying takes *time,* and there is lots of flim-flam which occurs over it. I went first to the premature nursery, where there would be no awareness by the infant of impending death. I found that some died right away without names, even, and some died later, after several days or weeks. Internal comparisons were built in. Nurses felt bad if an infant lived 5 days and then died; led to development of *"social loss."* Developed variations around this category.
>
> Next, I went to a neurosurgical ward, where patients were unconscious, with no awareness, conscious, with awareness, and where some became unconscious while they were there, while others got better, went home, and came back to the hospital again at a later date. Took variation and went back to the premature nursery with more questions.
>
> Then, I went to the intensive care unit (ICU), where lots of people were dying, and where quick dying occurred, as with the infants; saw new features. Here new nurses were coming and going, and as many as four people would die in quick order. A cancer unit was the next ward, chosen on *theoretical* grounds. Here some patients were aware they were dying, and some were not; some were aware they had cancer and some were not. Some people did not die here; some went home; some people came back to die here. Began to think *comparatively.* Also became more aware of organizational features.
>
> Became very interested in *duration* and *awareness,* then in *expected* and *unexpected;* we picked the place where we worked by the *dimensions* of each

of these, then looked for *variations*. You *generate dimensions* as you go. When you come in with a lot of preconceived ideas, look for all the *opposites*. For example, I sent a nurse to observe on a cancer ward, and she came back and wrote an article about how depersonalized, inhumane, etc., it was. I was outraged; I immediately sent her back to look for all the opposites, how personalized, humane it was.

Looked for maximized, minimized, variant. Our work is a mixture of inductive and deductive method, really. You start with the data, downplay theories, check some ideas out, and generate others. For example, a group of scientists were looking at the amount of wax (not fat) in sea organisms; they theorized that the wax provided some protection against the temperature. They theoretically sampled at different depths, in different climates and sea temperatures all over the world. They found more wax in the organisms that lived further down, in colder climates, the world over.

You are *verifying* as you go; it is built into the method. We were halfway through the *Discovery* (1967) book before Barney (from Columbia University, steeped in quantitative methodology) gave up the idea that you need to check out a theory quantitatively when you complete the qualitative piece. Read the literature *selectively* after you do your work, depending on where you are going.

Anyone can collect good data and write good descriptive pieces; you need to move off the concrete to the abstract level. The key to good research is to ask the right question, a *generative question*. For example:

> What difference does it make that people die?
> What difference does it make that people know they will die, or don't know?
> What difference does it make that people die in an organizational context?

If you are a good researcher and know where you are going, you will ask better questions.... A generative research question demands a cluster of other questions. Must look for what is salient and what is not salient; cannot give one answer, have to give many answers; look for density, complex interrelationships. World is terribly complex; it is the researcher's job to catch some of that complexity; people may disagree with you but they can at least say where, how they differ. For example, in Italy we found wards with 150 people together, some of which were dying quite visibly; here in the U.S. people die usually in the presence of only 3 or 4; this did not negate our theory; new conditions modify it. Find out from people when they disagree with you, all about the disagreement, and modify your theory to account for those conditions also.

Proceeding from the research, two monographs that deal with time (Glaser & Strauss, 1965) and awareness (Glaser & Strauss, 1968) of this largely unpredictable event were published.

Questions About Illness Used in Practice: Chronic Illness Trajectory

Corbin and Strauss's (1992) chronic illness trajectory framework is an example of the use of qualitative research in a focused area of practice that has been widely used in the everyday world of practice. The framework is built on decades of research that was initiated by the major study of death and dying in the 1960s by Glaser and Strauss (1965, 1968) and Quint-Benoliel (1967). They decided to use the term *trajectory* to conceptualize their insight that dying takes time, and many strategies can be used by professionals and family alike to manage and shape the dying course. Later work by the authors and their graduate students amassed a body of grounded theory studies on people with chronic illness.

That chronic illnesses have a course and can be shaped through management was introduced as a framework to help people in practice and research in the text *Chronic Illness and the Quality of Life* (Strauss & Glaser, 1975). The book was eventually revised, based on a much greater body of research about chronic illness; this latter text used the term *trajectory* as the central organizing concept/conceptual framework of the management of chronic illness (Strauss et al., 1984). The model has implications for practice and policy making. The model provides general guidelines about living with chronicity for application to practice by health professionals working with patients with chronic illness. The practitioners must work out the details by asking informal questions about how the model can be used to its full advantage in their practice. For example, some of the initial types of questions that could guide the use of this focal area of research in the everyday world of practice include the following:

What is the course of this chronic illness?
How does the course of chronic illness vary for this disease?

How is the course of this chronic illness affected by management?
In this patient or group of patients?
At this time and over time?

The implications for policy making include the necessary need for a shift from reimbursement of nurses and other health professionals for largely technical task performance to other vitally necessary functions such as teaching, counseling, making referrals, advocating, and meeting emotional needs (Corbin & Strauss, 1992). Corbin and Strauss presented their chronic illness trajectory framework in a special issue of the journal *Scholarly Inquiry for Nursing Practice* (which was later reprinted in a book: Woog, 1992). The presentation was followed by reactions to the framework by six expert nurses working with patients with various chronic diseases. Corbin and Strauss then responded to these experts, noting their comments. The model contributes to the conceptualization of the course of a chronic illness and enables the practitioner to conduct research to enhance understanding and, with the understanding, to "give better care" and to "create better policy" (Woog, 1992, p. 5).

Questions About Treatment Used in Practice: Adherence to Antituberculosis Treatment

The work of Judy Dick (Dick & Lombard, 1997) in Cape Town, South Africa, is an example of how the need for information about treatment through the use of qualitative methodology can change practice. Despite many efforts, practitioners failed to reduce high rates (approximately 40%) of lack of adherence to antituberculosis treatment in patients in Cape Town Local Authority health clinics (Dick & Lombard, 1997). Nurses delivered litanies of instructions about the needed treatment, such as the necessity of receiving the tablets at the clinic each day and the need to screen close contacts of the patient. Treatment behavior is complex and poorly understood, yet adherence to treatment in a well-managed TB control program could decrease the incidence of TB by 50% (World Health Organization, 1990). Research of health education strategies to improve adherence indicate that a combination of educational and behavioral strategies achieve greater success than the use of educational strategies alone. The authors tested a combined strategy of a patient-centered interview and a specially developed educational booklet on adherence to prescribed treatment in TB patients in two adjacent Cape Town Local Authority health clinics: Clinic A was the intervention clinic, and Clinic B was the control clinic. The intervention was based on prior qualitative research undertaken by Dick (1995) during her dissertation work at the University of Cape Town, Cape Town.

Previous qualitative research conducted in the Cape Town TB clinics explored ways to improve the clinic nurses' interaction with patients newly diagnosed with TB (Steyn, van der Merwe, Dick, Borcherds, & Wilding, 1997). Video recordings of nurse-patient interviews were transcribed and analyzed. Results indicated that the interviews were nurse-centered and that patients were poorly received, rarely confirmed, and were not equally in control. Following communication skill training, a shift occurred in the interactions; they were more patient centered and mutually satisfying to both the patient and the nurse. A second qualitative research project involved the clinic nurses in the process of "exploring how tuberculosis patients experience their disease" (Dick, Van der Walt, Hoogendoorn, & Tobias, 1996, p. 173). From this project, a photonovel was developed, Waar daar 'n wil is . . . (Where there is a will . . .), that incorporated not only the TB patients' experience of their disease but also the informational needs of newly diagnosed patients and a calendar to assist them in monitoring their progress during treatment. In the booklet, technical information plus motivational support are given. A role model, portrayed by the heroine, confronts obstacles to adherence such as the stigma of having TB, depression, and side effects of the medication. The mean adherence rate of Clinic A over the course of a year during the intervention was 72.4%; the rate in the subset who received the intervention (the first 60 consecutive patients with pulmonary TB) was 95%, a statistically significant improvement (t test $p < .0001$). The mean adherence rate of Clinic B was 77%. The subset (the first 60 consecutive patients with pulmonary TB) achieved a mean adherence rate of 83%, an improvement that was not statistically significant (t test $p < .0902$). Thus, qualitative research provided the basis for the intervention that made a difference in outcomes in the first test in South Africa of the effects of a health education approach to improving adherence rates to medication regimens in patients with active pulmonary TB. Questions about interventions such as "Why are we getting this outcome when we want another?" may lead to questions such as "What is happening here?" and qualitative methodology that will yield answers that then can be tested in a clinical trial.

Questions That Will Change Policy: Infant Mortality in Indonesia

The work of Terry Hull and his colleagues (Hull, Djohan, & Rusman, 1998) in Lombok, Indonesia, is an example of the use of information, gained via qualitative methodology, that will lead to findings that can change policy. Despite multiple efforts, Lombok continues to have the highest recorded rate of infant and child mortality in modern Indonesia (Hull et al., 1998). A qualitative research study was undertaken in three villages by three investigators who all had training in anthropology; two had advanced degrees in demography, which involved research using anthropological field methodology. In the course of the study, the investigators also reviewed demographic methods for making estimates of infant mortality in Indonesia. They documented many problems, such as inadequate survey and census data that led to errors stemming from, for example, mothers who may give "more or less" accurate answers about infants born to them, interviewers who may record their responses in "more or less" accurate detail (Hull et al., 1998, p. 23), or the use of biased model life tables used to convert child death rates to the infant mortality rate.

The study team commenced fieldwork in the three villages, training indigenous interviewers and interviewing themselves. Just obtaining a list of infant deaths yielded insights into infant mortality in the villages. People at the district, subdistrict, and village levels, including clinics, birthing centers, traditional midwives, health personnel, and religious leaders, all gave different numbers and conflicting information about the time, age, and circumstances of the death. For example, religious leaders who must bathe corpses as a part of their duties reported 4 or 5 times the numbers of deaths reported by officials. Accurate information came from those closest to the family experiencing the death. Thus, third parties who relied on hearsay may have entered errors into village or clinic records: for example, often the name of the infant and/or the parents would be incorrect, deleted, or a nickname would be used, creating problems in verification.

The investigators used the Rashomon Technique (Akutagawa, 1952; Hull et al., 1998) of qualitative research, which uses traditional field methods to record the stories of each person's perceptions of the same tragic event, the death of an infant or child. The technique is based on a Japanese story and film in which people who witnessed a rape all gave very different descriptions of the same event. In the technique's application to social science methodology, the various accounts of truth become useful for explanation and also for policy advice as they are applied to the various contradictions stemming from the social realities. Various people who played different roles in trying to save the lives of the infants, such as parents, neighbors, religious leaders, traditional healers, and personnel from the health center, often reported conflicting roles when the infant became ill. Behaviors and beliefs that influenced the treatment of the ill infant, whether the attempts succeeded or failed, were gleaned by recording each person's story and analyzing both similarities and differences in the accounts: "The task of the interviewer is to fully and faithfully record the story of the . . . death or crisis, from the personal viewpoint, and in the precise words of the witness" (Hull et al., 1998, p. 35). The types of questions that may be asked include "What is this person's account of their experience of this event?" and "How does this person relate the details of their experience of this event, such as time, duration, people involved, and outcome?" In a process of analysis of a myriad of truths from the various witnesses, along with supporting information from a wide variety of sources, the research team identified major themes that reflected common perceptions, experiences of the witnesses, or problems encountered. Based on the findings, realistic yet complex sets of policy recommendations were then made that include actions necessary to resolve contradictions and develop beneficial care practices in the case of these preventable deaths. Thus, findings were used in decision making in setting policy that would prevent the preventable deaths and hasten the decrease of infant mortality rates.

Conclusions

In this chapter, I have discussed issues about questions in the use of qualitative evidence, their nature and their significance, focusing on formal research questions, data collection questions, and analytic questions. The nature of each type of question differs in qualitative investigations from questions in quantitative investigations, as well as across major qualitative research approaches. I describe how the researcher gets from the research questions in a qualitative investigation to what is asked of people participating in the study. Differences between the nature of the clinician's question, the participant's question, and the decision maker's question are drawn from my own experience.

The nature of the questions asked are key to the use of questions to generate qualitative evidence that will challenge the status quo, both in practice and in setting policy.

Note

1. While it may no longer be popular to make quantitative versus qualitative comparisons, in this context, it is useful.

References

Akutagawa, R. (1952). *Rashomon and other stories* (T. Kojima, Trans.). Tokyo: Charles E. Tuttle.
Blumer, H. (1969). *Symbolic interaction: Perspective and method.* Englewood Cliffs, NJ: Prentice Hall.
Burns, N., & Grove, S. (1999). *Understanding nursing research* (2nd ed.). Philadelphia: W. B. Saunders.
Chenitz, W. C., & Swanson, J. M. (1986). *From practice to grounded theory: Qualitative research in nursing.* Menlo Park, CA: Addison-Wesley.
Corbin, J. M., & Strauss, A. (1992). A nursing model for chronic illness management based upon the trajectory framework. In P. Woog (Ed.), *The chronic illness trajectory framework: The Corbin and Strauss nursing model* (pp. 9-28). New York: Springer.
Demissie, M., & Kebede, D. (1994). Defaulting from tuberculosis treatment at the Addis Ababa Tuberculosis Centre and factors associated with it. *Ethiopian Medical Journal, 32,* 97-106.
Dibble, S. L., & Swanson, J. M. (2000). Gender differences for the predictors of depression in young adults with genital herpes. *Public Health Nursing, 17*(3), 187-194.
Dick, J. (1995). *Adherence to anti-tuberculosis treatment in Cape Town.* Unpublished doctoral dissertation, University of Cape Town, Cape Town, South Africa.
Dick, J., & Lombard, C. (1997). Shared vision—a health education project designed to enhance adherence to anti-tuberculosis treatment. *International Journal of Tuberculosis and Lung Disease, 1*(2), 181-186.
Dick, J., Van der Walt, H., Hoogendoorn, L., & Tobias, B. (1996). Development of a health education booklet to enhance adherence to tuberculosis treatment. *Tuberculosis and Lung Diseases, 77*(2), 173-177.
Ferketich, S. L., & Verran, J. A. (1984). Residual analyses for causal model assumptions. *Western Journal of Nursing Research, 6,* 41-60.
Garro, L. C. (1988). Explaining high blood pressure: Variation in knowledge about illness. *American Ethnologist, 15,* 98-119.
Gebre, N., Karlsson, U., Jonsson, G., Macaden, R., Wolde, A., Assefa, A., & Miorner, H. (1995). Improved microscopial diagnosis of pulmonary tuberculosis in developing

countries. *Transactions of the Royal Society of Tropical Medicine and Hygiene, 89,* 191-193.

Glaser, B. G. (1992). *Basics of grounded theory analysis: Emergence vs. forcing.* Mill Valley, CA: Sociology Press.

Glaser, B., & Strauss, A. (1965). *Awareness of dying.* Chicago: Aldine.

Glaser, B., & Strauss, A. (1967). *The discovery of grounded theory: Strategies for qualitative research.* Chicago: Aldine.

Glaser, B., & Strauss, A. (1968). *Time for dying.* Chicago: Aldine.

Hatch, M., von Ehrenstein, O., Wolff, M., Meier, K., Geduld, A., & Einhorn, F. (1999). Using qualitative methods to elicit recall of a critical time period. *Journal of Women's Health, 8*(2), 269-277.

Hodes, R. M., & Azbite, M. (1993). Tuberculosis. In H. Kloos & Z. A. Zein (Eds.), *The ecology of health and disease in Ethiopia* (pp. 265-284). Boulder, CO: Westview.

Hodes, R. M., & Kloos, H. (1988). Health and medical care in Ethiopia. *The New England Journal of Medicine, 31,* 918-924.

Hull, T. H., Djohan, E., & Rusman, R. (1998). *They simply die: Searching for the causes of high infant mortality in Lombok.* Canberra: Demography Program, Research School of Social Sciences, Australian National University.

Judd, C. M. (1987). Combining process and outcome evaluation. In M. M. Mark & R. L. Shotland (Eds.), *Multiple methods in program evaluation* (pp. 23-41). San Francisco: Jossey-Bass.

Kidder, L., & Fine, M. (1987). Qualitative and quantitative methods: When stories converge. In M. Mark & R. Shotland (Eds.), *Multiple methods in program evaluation* (pp. 57-75). San Francisco: Jossey-Bass.

Krieger, N. (1999). Questioning epidemiology: Objectivity, advocacy, and socially responsible science. *American Journal of Public Health, 89*(8), 1151-1153.

Lipson, J., & Omidian, P. (1997). Afghan refugee issues in the U. S. social environment. *Western Journal of Nursing Research, 19,* 110-126.

MacIntyre, R. (1999). *Mortal men.* Rutgers, NJ: Rutgers University Press.

McKinlay, J. B., & Marceau, L. D. (2000). Upstream healthy public policy: Lessons from the battle of tobacco. *International Journal of Health Services, 30,* 49-69.

Mead, G. H. (1934). *Mind, self and society.* Chicago: University of Chicago Press.

Ministry of Health (MOH). (1991). *Comprehensive health service directory: Selective information. 1981 E.C. (1988/89 G.C.).* Addis Ababa, Ethiopia: Planning and Programming Department, Ministry of Health (MOH).

Morse, J. M. (1994). Designing funded qualitative research. In N. Denzin & Y. Lincoln (Eds.), *Handbook of qualitative research* (pp. 220-235). Thousand Oaks, CA: Sage.

Morse, J. M., & Field, P. A. (1995). *Qualitative research methods for health professionals* (2nd ed.). Thousand Oaks, CA: Sage.

The Population Council. (1972). *A manual for surveys of fertility and family planning: Knowledge, attitudes, and practice.* New York: The Population Council.

Quint-Benoliel, J. (1967). *The nurse and the dying patient.* New York: Macmillan.

Savitz, D. A., Poole, C., & Miller, W. C. (1999). Reassessing the role of epidemiology in public health. *American Journal of Public Health, 89*(8), 1158-1161.

Schaller, K. F., & Kuls, W. (1972). *Ethiopia: Geomedical monograph series.* New York/ Heidelberg: Springer-Verlag.

Steyn, M., van der Merwe, N., Dick, J., Borcherds, R., & Wilding, R. J. (1997). Communication with TB patients: A neglected dimension of effective treatment? *Curationis, 20*(1), 53-56.

Strauss, A., & Corbin, J. (1990). *Basics of qualitative research.* Newbury Park, CA: Sage.

Strauss, A., Corbin, J., Fagerhaugh, S., Glaser, B., Maines, D., Suzeck, B., & Wiener, C. (1984). *Chronic illness and the quality of life* (2nd ed.). St. Louis, MO: Mosby.

Strauss, A., & Glaser, B. (1975). *Chronic illness and the quality of life.* St. Louis, MO: Mosby.

Styblo, K., & Rouillon, A. (1991). Tuberculosis. *Health Policy and Planning, 6,* 391-397.

Swanson, J. M. (1980). Knowledge, knowledge, who's got the knowledge? The male contraceptive career. *Journal of Sex Education and Therapy, 6*(2), 51-57.

Swanson, J. M. (1988). The process of finding contraceptive options. *Western Journal of Nursing Research, 10*(4), 492-503.

Swanson, J. M., & Chenitz, W. C. (1993). Regaining a valued self: The process of adaptation to living with genital herpes. *Qualitative Health Research, 3,* 270-297.

Swanson, J. M., Dibble, S. L., & Chapman, L. (1999). Effects of psycho-educational interventions on sexual health risks and psycho-social adaptation in young adults with genital herpes. *Journal of Advanced Nursing, 29,* 840-851.

Swanson, J. M., Dibble, S. L., & Chapman, L. (2000). A psychoeducational program increased knowledge and decreased sexual risk behaviors in young adults with genital herpes. *Western Journal of Medicine, 172,* 246.

Vecchiato, N. L. (1997). Sociocultural aspects of tuberculosis control in Ethiopia. *Medical Anthropology Quarterly, 11*(2), 183-201.

Westoff, C. (1972). The modernization of U.S. contraceptive practice. *Family Planning Perspectives, 4,* 9-12.

Woog, P. (1992). *The chronic illness trajectory framework: The Corbin and Strauss nursing model.* New York: Springer.

World Health Organization. (1990). *Tuberculosis control and research strategy for the 1990s. Report and recommendations of a WHO meeting.* Geneva: World Health Organization.

Zerihun, G., & Esscher, E. (1984). Ten years' experience of tuberculosis meningitis in children. *Ethiopian Medical Journal, 22,* 49-54.

III

The Nature of Standards

Dialogue:

Developing a Perspective
Developing a Chapter

KUZEL: I was talking with Ben Crabtree about this book, and Ben said to me, "You know, Tony, you've been thinking about this 'standards' stuff for years, and you've written a couple of times on it. If you're going to do this general chapter, just don't do the same thing you've done before. Do something different with it."

   I had to take that challenge to heart. And so I was toying with the idea of "pragmatism" as a concept and trying to understand. . . . You know, people talk about that all the time, but do I personally understand what that really means? I was successful in getting John Engel, one of my mentors, to be involved in writing this chapter, and he said, "Well, let me tell you about some books that might be useful."

   I was thinking, in writing it, that our book is going to start with philosophical perspectives. Maybe I could take on pragmatic philosophy and try to summarize some of the important ideas that come out of that tradition, and then try to make the case for how they relate to the issue of standards and how they are actually very harmonious with the work of clinicians.

BUT LATER, A CAUTION . . .

MADJAR: I think that the message . . . is that we can use pragmatism in order to understand what's going on here, but it doesn't necessarily mean that we ought to live by it. There is more to life, there is more to philosophy, there is more to a whole lot of things.

AND REFLECTIONS ON OTHERS' WORK . . .

KUZEL: I'm personally comfortable with where Sally Thorne came from in her chapter, saying that, "Well, of course the disciplines have an enormous impact on what gets done and how it is judged. But let's get more reflective about it, about how they are having an impact." To me, that's very consistent with this framework of pragmatism. There's no conflict here at all.

AND QUESTIONS . . .

MORSE: Why are these [criteria] particular to qualitative research?

KUZEL: They are not.

MORSE: Do they need to be?

KUZEL: I sort of discovered, as I went through this process, that they had a broader application.

MADJAR: I think it's regrettable that we don't communicate that somehow one evaluates qualitative research in such a different way from how one might evaluate quantitative research . . . that the two have nothing in common. . . . In a sense, the standards are of *inquiry*, and the *systematic nature* of that inquiry. . .

5

Some Pragmatic Thoughts About Evaluating Qualitative Health Research

ANTON J. KUZEL
JOHN D. ENGEL

Faced with multiple perspectives, competing purposes, and limited resources, providers, policy makers, and patients must make decisions about what needs are most important and what actions yield the greatest benefit. The authors of the earlier chapters have made a compelling case for acknowledging and embracing the role of qualitative evidence in planning, delivering, and evaluating health care. The growing popularity and use of qualitative inquiry allows for a richer, experienced-based dialogue about the quality of such work. Public and private agencies that want to fund health-related research are looking for guidance on how to evaluate qualitative research (Devers, 1999). In this chapter, we offer some general ideas about how stakeholders may make judgments about research proposals and completed works that follow qualitative traditions and methods. We begin with basic considerations, move (in the spirit of the first chapter) to a discussion about a relevant philosophy, and close with some principles for evaluating qualitative research proposals and completed work. In the next chapter, Sally Thorne considers how academic traditions shape the practice of qualitative research design and evaluation. The third chapter of this section, by Nancy Gibson and colleagues, looks at an increasingly popular model of qualitative research—participatory inquiry—and proposes a model for planning and critique.

General Considerations

Those readers schooled in clinical epidemiology undoubtedly are sometimes confused by the language and the myriad of traditions that are used in qualitative health research. A second difficulty, for those more familiar with prevailing biomedical research, is that qualitative work is inherently interpretive and subjective and necessarily resists efforts to define a hierarchy of evidence: There is no qualitative analogy to the gold standard of clinical epidemiology: the randomized control trial. Indeed, radical (in the sense of antifoundational) proponents of qualitative inquiry (e.g., Derrida, 1976; Fish, 1989; Rosenau, 1992) insist that all knowledge claims can only be understood as the idiosyncratic views of individuals in a particular time and place. For those holding this view, consensus is an illusion and generalizations are folly. Such a perspective can be terribly frustrating for clinical epidemiologists, who have been raised in another research tradition. This reaction is illustrated in the rhetorical question from Poses and Isen's (1998) critique of qualitative clinical research: "How can one evaluate the claims of people who deny the existence of truth?" (p. 32). Although understandable from their position, it is at the same time a statement that suggests intolerance, hegemony, and caricature.

Even though we understand the historical context of the postmodern position and will have more to say about it later in this chapter, we believe that a search for plausible explanations and expectations is a reasonable goal. In thinking about the evaluation of qualitative work, we suggest a pragmatic focus: that is, a consideration of whether rationality and action are useful for the practical concerns of patients, providers, and policy makers. Pragmatism is one of several virtues that thought and action can have; others include aesthetics and ethics. We believe that health professionals—a principal audience for this book—are concerned with all of these in their daily work. We will focus our discussion on the implications of pragmatism for the evaluation of qualitative health research, but we in no way imply that other considerations are less important.

Health professions define themselves as being in the *service* of individuals and communities. Researchers in these professions are more likely to think of themselves as *applied* rather than basic scientists. There are even those outside the health professions who see them more like *trades* than professions and point to guildlike organizational structures and apprenticeships that are the final requirement before one can be considered a prepared *practitioner* (Freidson, 1970). The nature of the work of the health professions is focused on practical ends: "The ends of medicine are ultimately the restoration or improvement of health and, more proximately, to heal, that is, to cure illness and disease or, when this is not possible, to care for and help the patient to live with residual pain, discomfort, or disability" (Pellegrino & Thomasma, 1993, pp. 52-53).

This pragmatic purpose and meaning is consecrated in the solemn promises required of newly initiated members. In the United Kingdom, each registered nurse, midwife, and health visitor is held to a code of professional conduct that emphasizes competence in the service of client interests:

> You are personally accountable for your practice, and, in the exercise of your professional accountability, must:
>
> 1. Act always in such a manner as to promote and safeguard the interests and well-being of patients and clients;
> 2. Ensure that no action or omission on your part, or within your sphere of responsibility, is detrimental to the interests, condition or safety of patients and clients; and
> 3. Maintain and improve your professional knowledge and competence. (United Kingdom Central Council, 1992)

Medicine's Oath of Hippocrates includes these words: "I will follow that system of regimen which, according to my ability and judgment, I consider for the benefit of my patients, and abstain from whatever is deleterious and mischievous. . . . Into whatever houses I enter, I will go into them for the benefit of the sick" (full text on multiple Web sites, e.g., emory/edu/WHSC/MED/HTN/Andrew/hippocrates.html). Returning to Pellegrino and Thomasma (1993), we highlight their claim that phronesis, or practical wisdom, is an indispensable virtue of clinical practice:

> Phronesis . . . practical wisdom, the capacity for moral insight, the capacity, in a given set of circumstances, to discern what moral choices or course of action is most conducive to the good of the agent or the activity in which the agent is engaged. Phronesis is the intellectual virtue that disposes us habitually to *attain truth for the sake of action,* as opposed to truth for its own sake. (p. 84)

We suggest, therefore, that it is consistent with the nature of the health professions to evaluate qualitative inquiry with attention to how well it informs practice. A focus on pragmatism does not mean that one should not be concerned with theory: Being practical is not at odds with being theoretical. "That's fine in theory, but not in practice" makes no sense to us; we prefer Kurt Lewin's (1948) view that there is nothing so practical as a good theory. It is worth looking at the philosophical tradition of pragmatism to understand the relationship of theory and practice, to examine proponents' views regarding reality and knowledge, and to discern some guidelines to the evaluation of qualitative inquiry.

Pragmatist Philosophy

We will provide only a brief review of some of the pertinent ideas from pragmatist philosophy. For a more in-depth discussion about pragmatism, we refer interested readers to the works of John Dewey (1938), Charles Peirce (1934), William James (1907), George Mead (1934), and Kurt Lewin (1948). Although commonly identified with turn-of-the-century American philosophers, pragmatist thinking has roots that can be traced back to ancient Greek philosophers (Rescher, 1977). Some recent reviews and contributions come from Hammersley (1989), Putnam (1995), and Rescher (1992), and it is from these authors that we draw our summary.

Putnam (1995) suggests that pragmatists see the inescapable linkage and mutual shaping between facts on the one hand and theories, values, and interpretations on the other. For them, the question of "which came first, the fact or the theory" is a chicken-egg worry that can only be resolved by allowing one to make certain prior assumptions. Rescher (1992) agrees, stating that "presumptions . . . play a crucial role in the cognitive sphere. For we cannot pursue the epistemic project—the quest for information about the world—without granting certain initial presumptions" (p. 17). Rescher goes on to suggest that the claims that are presumptively justified would be (a) based on ordinary sensory data or on memory, (b) useful to explain circumstances, (c) analogous with what has worked in other contexts, and (d) coherent with other accepted theses.

Prior assumptions not only allow inquiry to happen, they also condition it, because inquiry is driven by what does not fit with what we take for granted. Hammersley (1989) says that for pragmatist philosopher Charles Peirce, this means that doubt is the starting point of inquiry, and "inquiry is directed towards fixing belief: towards finding a stable resolution to the doubt that stimulated it" (p. 49). Peirce probably saw "fixing belief " as important for confident, effective action, but Hammersley says that George Mead, a pragmatist who followed Peirce, makes this explicit:

> Much action is subconscious. Reflective consciousness arises when an act is checked, where contact experiences do not match our expectations. Where a problem emerges the individual sets about resolving it by evaluating the initial expectations and the contact experiences to find some way of bringing them into harmony, to find a course of action that will consummate the act. (pp. 59-60)

How do pragmatists suggest that we go about reestablishing harmony and finding the best course of action? Clearly, they expect us to modify our expectations, which we take to mean the assumptions and theories that structure the way we describe, explain, or predict. But since there are many ways in which we might modify our expectations, are there any principles that can guide our choice? Rescher (1992) suggests that we should generate several conflict-resolving options, often by employing inductive reasoning. Rather than inferring conclusions from given premises, it is sometimes necessary to

> "jump to conclusions," albeit in the safest way relative to all we know. . . .
> Induction aims to the best manageable balance between the unknown leap required to get answers to our questions and the safety net of an optimal linkage to what we can already substantiate. (p. 131)[1]

Having generated multiple options, we must then choose the one that best accounts for the data, is linked in some way with prior theory, and is the most simple, as judged by the "community of inquiry." This collaboration is fundamental to the inquiry process, and Putnam (1995) states that the pragmatists, particularly Dewey, had very specific ideas about how it should proceed:

It is not only that, on Dewey's conception, good science requires respect for autonomy, symmetric reciprocity, and discourse ethics—that could be true even if scientific theories and hypotheses were, in the end, to be tested by the application of an algorithm—but . . . the very *interpretation* of the *non*-algorithmic standards by which scientific hypotheses are judged depends on cooperation and discussion structured by the same norms. Both for its full development and for its full application to human problems, science requires the *democratization of inquiry.* (pp. 72-73)

The corollary to this assertion is that social structures and processes powerfully shape the circumstances that become identified as problems, the way those problems are engaged, and which of the multiple options is judged the best solution. This corollary is a major focus for the kinds of inquiry that have an emancipatory thrust (Thorne, 1997), and we will have more to say about this later as preamble to Gibson et al.'s fuller treatment in Chapter 7.

There is one more criterion by which pragmatists suggest we may choose from among various conflict-resolving options: the extent to which our choice is *generally* helpful. Hammersley (1989) summarizes William James's position as follows: "This is not a matter of believing what serves our purposes on a particular occasion. Rather, we accept as true those ideas that work for us in a broad sense and in the long run. For James, truth is what it has proved to be generally expedient to believe" (p. 51). This directly asserts the desirability of generalizations, but with the understanding that such claims are inevitably shaped by culture and history: "Truth claims are always fallible, even when universal consent seems to have been attained. This is because future cultures might find reasons to discard the truths of today" (Carspecken, 1996, p. 84). There is, of course, considerable danger in generalizing: It can lead to gross simplifications of complex systems in an effort to find one size that fits all. Yet, inquiry is still driven to generalize because of two forces: the need for instruction and the need for validation, both of which are present in those directly involved in the research and in the audience for the research. Even research for oneself is more attractive if the results are instructive, that is, if it is helpful in other contexts. If the research is also for others, then clearly its value (as judged by others) will largely rest upon how well it provides lessons, the moral of the story of the inquiry. This value in the eyes of others becomes a mirror in which we see ourselves (Carspecken, 1996); hence, validation is the second driver for generalizability.

Experience may eventually show that our prior assumptions, subsequent interpretations, generalizations, and choices of action were not justified, but Rescher (1992) argues that such risks are acceptable and manageable:

> To be sure, the risk of deception and error is present throughout our inquiries: our cognitive instruments, like all other instruments, are never fail proof. Still, a general policy of judicious trust in certain presumptions is eminently cost effective. In inquiring, we cannot investigate everything; we have to start somewhere and invest credence in something...
>
> In trusting our senses, in relying on other people, *and even in being rational,* we always run a risk. Whenever in life we place our faith in something, we run a risk of being let down and disappointed. Nevertheless, it seems perfectly reasonable to bet on the general trustworthiness of the senses, the general reliability of our fellow human beings, and the general utility of reason...
>
> We proceed in cognitive matters in much the same way that banks proceed in financial matters. We extend credit to our informative sources and resources, doing so at first to only a relatively modest extent. When and if they comport themselves in a manner that shows that this credit was well deserved and warranted, we proceed to give them more credit and extend their credit limit, as it were. (pp. 29-30)

Expanding on the issue of risk, Rescher (1992) talks about "misfortunes of the first kind," in which one rejects something that, in retrospect, should have been accepted and thereby suffers a loss. "Misfortunes of the second kind" are just the opposite, in which the gamble is taken but does not pay off.[2] Those who seek risk experience many misfortunes of the second kind and relatively few of the first. For risk avoiders, it is the other way around. Rescher (1992) suggests that a middle ground in which risk is accepted but with caution and calculation might result in the greatest benefit and the fewest losses (whether of opportunities or resources).

All these ideas and guides to action depend on a vigorous discourse:

> The problem of subjectivity and intersubjectivity was in the minds of the pragmatists from the beginning—not as a metaphysical worry about whether we have access to a world at all, but as a real problem in human life. They

insisted that when one human being in isolation tries to interpret even the best maxims for himself and does not allow others to criticize the way in which he or she interprets those maxims, or the way in which he or she applies them, then the kind of "certainty" that results is *in practice* fatally tainted with subjectivity. . . . The introduction of new ideas for testing likewise depends on cooperation, for any human being who rejects inputs from other human beings runs out of ideas sooner rather than later, and begins to consider only ideas which in one way or another reflect the prejudices he or she has formed. Cooperation is necessary both for the formation of ideas and for their rational testing. (Putnam, 1995, pp. 71-72)

In pragmatist philosophy, several key elements can inform the evaluation of qualitative proposals and completed work: the interrelatedness of facts, values, theories, and interpretations; the necessity of granting presumptions; the judicious approach to risk through trust tempered by experience; and the essential role of a community of inquiry guided by democratic values. With these ideas in mind, we now review the suggestions that other health professionals (members of our inquiry community) have made about assessing the value of qualitative inquiry.

Published Suggestions for Evaluating Qualitative Health Research

In 1994, we collaborated with psychologist Richard Addison and sociologist Stephen Bogdewic on a review of "desirable features of qualitative research." We grouped these as values, characteristics, techniques, and outcomes:

values which guide inquiry
Empathy (for research participants)
Collaboration (with participants, and with colleagues and critics)
Service (in the sense of shared power)
Moral sensitivity (having a notion of a greater good)

characteristics of the inquiry and report
Clarity
Assumptions—explicitly stated

Purpose—explicitly stated
Language—avoidance of jargon
Coherence
Internal—effectively interprets the context; fit between purpose and
     style of investigation
External—relates the context to bigger picture

techniques of inquiry
Dialogue among participants
Triangulation of sources and investigators
Sampling which looks for confirming and disconfirming evidence
Immersion in the context of inquiry

outcomes
For participants—new knowledge and behavior that is useful
For readers—vicarious experience and learning (Kuzel, Engel,
     Addison, & Bogdewic, 1994, p. 376)

Nurse researcher Sally Thorne (1997) recently discussed "the art
(and science) of critiquing qualitative research" (p. 117). She organizes
her suggestions in two groups, the first of which describes criteria for
evaluating qualitative inquiry:

Epistemological integrity: "There is a defensible line of reasoning from the
assumptions made about the nature of knowledge through to the methodological rules by which decisions about the research process are explained"
(p. 120); representative credibility: "The theoretical claims they purport to
make are consistent with the manner in which the phenomenon under
study was sampled" (p. 120); analytic logic: "Makes explicit the reasoning of
the researcher from the inevitable forestructure through to the interpretations and knowledge claims made on the basis of what was learned in the
research" (p. 121); and interpretive authority: "Assurance that a researcher's
interpretations are trustworthy, that they fairly illustrate or reveal some
truth external to his or her own bias or experience." (p. 121)

Moving "beyond evaluation," Thorne (1997) also suggests principles
of critique that "call upon qualitative researchers to account for the

ways in which their findings should or should not contribute to disciplinary knowledge" (p. 122). These normative standards are:

Moral defensibility: "Convincing claims about why we need the knowledge that we are extracting from people, what will be the purpose in having such knowledge once we obtain it" (pp. 122-123); disciplinary relevance: "Whether or not the knowledge is appropriate to the development of the disciplinary science" (p. 123); pragmatic obligation: "Researchers in this field are obliged to consider their findings 'as if' they might indeed be applied in practice" (p. 124); and probable truth: Research seeks to "create meaning, to construct images from which people's 'fallible and tentative views of the world can be altered, rejected, or made more secure.' " (p. 125, quoting Eisner, 1981)

Medical sociologist Jennie Popay is the principal coordinator of the qualitative inquiry section of the Cochrane Collaboration. She and her colleagues (1998), sociologists Anne Rogers and Gareth Williams, assert that "interpretation of subjective meaning, description of social context, and attention to lay knowledge" are "the foundation of good qualitative health research" (p. 341). They specifically suggest that the following questions should guide the evaluation of published reports:

Does the research, as reported, illuminate the subjective meaning, actions, and context of those researched?

Is there evidence of the adaptation and responsiveness of the research design to the circumstances and issues of real-life social settings met during the course of study?

Does the sample produce the type of knowledge necessary to understand the structures and processes within which the individuals or situations are located?

Is the description provided detailed enough to allow the researcher or reader to interpret the meaning and context of what is being researched?

How are different sources of knowledge about the same issue compared and contrasted?

Are subjective perceptions and experiences treated as knowledge in their own right?

How does the research move from a description of the data, through quotation or examples, to an analysis and interpretation of the meaning and significance of it?

What claims are being made for the generalizability of the findings to either
other bodies of knowledge or to other populations or groups? (pp. 346-348)

In addition, they state that "in the context of HSR [health services re-
search], qualitative research should have some clear implications for
policy and practice" (p. 349).

Psychologist Richard Frankel (1999) reflects on 30 years of doing
qualitative research and reading about other people's work, and suggests that great qualitative work is that which represents a breakthrough,
exhibits particular creativity or parsimony, or deals with problems of
core clinical significance. Frankel (1999) also acknowledges the framework for evaluating published qualitative work developed by family
physician William Miller and medical anthropologist Benjamin Crabtree. Miller and Crabtree (Frankel, 1999) propose several questions
that can help a practitioner-reader determine relevance:

> Did the authors study an outcome that patients would care about?
> Is the problem common to your practice, and is the intervention feasible?
> Will the information, if true, require you to change your practice?

Miller and Crabtree (Frankel, 1999) suggest several more questions
that can help determine validity:

> Was the appropriate method used to answer the question?
> Was appropriate and adequate sampling used to get the best information?
> Was an iterative process of collecting and analyzing data used and data
> saturation achieved?
> Was a thorough analysis presented?
> Are the background, training, and preconceptions of the investigators
> described? (p. 341)

In concluding his review, Frankel (1999) confesses that "much earlier
in my career, I was a 'methodological imperialist,' asserting that the
only 'proper' approach to research was a single theory and a single
method. In late midcareer, I have become much more pragmatic and, in
fact, much more interested in what works and generates new knowledge" (p. 345).

When we look at these four expositions, we are struck by the fact that
none of them (including our own!) explicitly referenced any of the

pragmatic philosophers whose thinking we reviewed earlier, yet it seems to us that all are consistent with that tradition. We now understand our 1994 synthesis as a call for democratic values among a community of inquirers, with a hint at power issues. The characteristics of the inquiry and report we suggested involve stating prior assumptions (although we did not state that one *must* grant this in order to get started) and seeking parsimonious language ("avoidance of jargon"). Our "coherence" ideals acknowledge the importance of context, hint at clarity of logic, and call for linkage to existing theory. We imply the value of generalizability of results, but we were not brave enough to say that. The outcomes to which we ascribe importance are the basic imperatives of a pragmatic system of thought and action.

Thorne's (1997) construction seems to be quite consistent with a pragmatist philosophy. She calls for attention to the nature of knowledge, its derivation, and assessment of truth claims, all of which are included in the pragmatist system of thought. Her advice to only make claims for that which you have sufficient evidence is appropriate, but it seems to be a corollary to the notion of community and its consent to truth claims (Carspecken, 1996). We understand the criterion of "analytic logic" to be identical to the pragmatist's "plausibility criteria" of explicit presumptions and logical linkage between new and existing knowledge. Thorne's "interpretive authority" depends once again on evidence (implicit or explicit) of the consent of the community of inquiry, while "moral defensibility" acknowledges the pragmatist's linkage of values, facts, interpretations, and theories, and hints at emancipatory inquiry. She draws a distinction between "disciplinary relevance" and "pragmatic obligation," which seems to make a distinction between theory and action, something pragmatists would not do. However, both of these qualities speak to the generalizability of the inquiry results. Finally, the criterion of "probable truth" appears to directly address the plausibility of findings with language that makes explicit their "fallible and tentative" (p. 125) nature. This is surely harmonious with pragmatist philosophy, and such a system of thinking clarifies the basis for community judgments of plausibility.

Popay and colleagues (1998) emphasize democratic values ("attention to lay knowledge") and the impact of social structures and processes ("description of social context"). They also speak about the "interpretation of subjective meaning," which we take to mean that subjective data has validity and importance.[3] Their specific suggestions emphasize that change is wrought by issues that arise in a meaningful, active, social context. They reemphasize an accounting of the role of social structures and processes and again call for a democratization of inquiry. "How does the research move . . ." reminds us of Thorne's (1997) representative credibility and analytic logic criteria. Two of their questions directly call for the generalizability of findings, and they close with an emphasis on "clear implications for policy and practice" (Thorne, 1997, p. 349). Surely we are once again on solid pragmatist ground.

Finally, Frankel's (1999) characteristics of "great" qualitative work are easily understood from the same philosophical perspective. "Breakthrough" studies may represent brilliant inductive reasoning, or they might create doubt where there was complacency. When Frankel speaks about "creative" inquiry, he seems to mean "novel" or "challenging and improving the conventional wisdom." The creativity results in new knowledge that is useful. His fondness for parsimony needs no elaboration. As for studies that have "core significance" and get "to the heart or essence of the research question" (p. 338), it seems again that these qualities will depend on consensual validation and analysis that makes explicit linkages between presumptions, facts, values, interpretations, and theories. Miller and Crabtree's (Frankel, 1999) first two questions presume a community of inquiry, and the third question recognizes that without "shared doubt," the reader is not engaged by the report. After several questions that emphasize technique,[4] the closing question asks if the study provides not only description but also interpretation such that "something new is learned" (Frankel, 1999, p. 341). Clearly, Miller and Crabtree believe that learning is for the sake of patients and the goal of improved practice. The final question highlights the importance of prior assumptions, that is, "background, training, and preconceptions of the investigators" (Frankel, 1999, p. 341), and Frankel's closing confession drives our point home.

So it seems to us that many of the most widely read and acknowledged treatments of standards for qualitative health research are fundamentally based in a pragmatist philosophy. This is not surprising, given that the authors whose works we reviewed are all practitioners as well as researchers. It also seems to bear out our earlier characterization of the health professions as essentially pragmatist in their values and everyday work. But is there any other significance to this exercise, beyond a demonstration of an unacknowledged philosophical basis for how we judge our inquiry? We have two additional purposes: (1) to offer another framework with which to approach the task of judging research proposals and completed work that can be applied to both purely qualitative and mixed method research, and (2) to provide a clear link to the increasingly emancipatory nature of our work (Macaulay et al., 1999; Thesen & Kuzel, 1999; Thorne, 1997; Wuest & Merritt-Gray, 1997).

As to our first purpose, we offer the following list of questions that a practitioner grounded in pragmatist philosophy might put to a research proposal or completed work:

Do the investigators state the presumptions that are the context of doubt?

Do the investigators demonstrate a sensitivity to the linkage between presumptions, facts, values, interpretations, and theories?

Do the investigators demonstrate an understanding of the consequences of their choices of methods for data gathering, analysis, and representation?

Does new theory meet basic criteria for plausibility, namely, connection with past theory, explicit and clear logic, parsimony, and utility?

Does the inquiry involve a community of inquirers? Are they guided by democratic values? Do they account for the impact of social structures and processes?

Does the study make an effort to allow for generalizing results over contexts or time?

These questions represent the next iteration in how we think about the issue of standards. We do not mean to imply that they are superior to those suggested by Thorne, Popay et al., or Frankel and Crabtree and Miller—many readers might find their language more engaging, their logic more lucid, and their suggestions more useful. Rather, we believe our suggestions are *consistent* with all of their frameworks and make explicit some of the ideas that we see implied in their language. We prefer this synthesis to our own earlier version and provide another option for those that review and judge qualitative health research. It is a response to the concern raised by Miller and Fredericks (1995): "How does a qualitative researcher know when and how a claim can be put forth as being credible?" (p. 62). It is consistent with Morse's contention in Chapter 9 (this volume) that qualitative research is verified against the phenomenon itself, tested by implementation, and further checked by comparison with others' work. It acknowledges Upshur's contention in Chapter 1 (this volume) that evidence is provisional, emergent, and incomplete.

In addition, our current synthesis seems applicable to either qualitative studies or those that employ mixed methods, which are increasingly popular and whose review poses unique challenges (Devers, 1999). We are not the first to recognize the natural fit between pragmatist philosophy and studies that use counting and statistics as well as observations, interviews, and interpretations. Authors such as Howe (1988), Cherryholmes (1992), and Tashakkori and Teddlie (1998) assert that pragmatism allows for the rapprochement of the qualitative and quantitative camps. Tashakkori and Teddlie, in fact, see it as a paradigm and contrast it with positivism, postpositivism, and constructivism (p. 23). Whether labeled a paradigm or a philosophical tradition, there seems to be an increasing recognition that pragmatism provides an appropriate basis from which to design, implement, and evaluate mixed method studies. It offers a model of evidence that accommodates qualitative and quantitative modalities (see Chapter 1, this volume).

In fact, multimethod studies mirror the work of the clinic, where professionals and patients must consider beliefs that derive from both clinical epidemiology ("Studies have shown that women who get mammograms find breast cancer at an earlier stage and are more likely to have good outcomes") and personal or family experience ("My mother and aunts are old and none of them have had breast cancer; the only time I had a mammogram it was quite painful") to derive a decision for action that is guided by moral principles. Greenhalgh (1998) states that health professionals *must* attend to these multiple bases for thinking and action:

> Health professionals, perhaps especially those in primary care, frequently experience frustration when trying to apply "evidence-based" research findings to real-life case scenarios. I would suggest that this occurs most commonly when they abandon the interpretive framework and attempt to get by on "evidence" alone. . . . The irrevocably case based (i.e., narrative based) nature of clinical wisdom is precisely what enables us to contextualize and individualize the problem before us. (pp. 262-263)

Stated differently, a pragmatist will employ values, beliefs, and methods that seem likely to result in desired consequences. Adhering to a narrow set of options reduces the possibilities for positive action (Kuzel, 1986).

Not only do we see our framework for evaluation as applicable to both purely qualitative and mixed method (qualitative and quantitative) studies, but we also believe they are relevant for inquiry that is ostensibly focused only on description and interpretation. For example, some proponents of interpretive qualitative traditions such as phenomenology argue that this work is or should be atheoretical. For them, a focus on the use and development of theory in the context of phenomenology is inappropriate because it constrains or distorts interpretation (e.g., Van Manen, 1996). We, however, believe that it is impossible to derive an interpretation without some reference to assumed facts, values, and theories; this *stock of knowledge* is what brings meaning to experience (Schutz, 1967). Even granting the assertion that phenomenology is atheoretical is an act that is theory- and value-laden.

We also do not believe that description and interpretation can be so neatly separated from action. Whether as direct participants in or as members of an audience for the work, qualitative inquiry that describes and interprets changes our stock of knowledge about the world, and this inevitably will affect our future actions. We agree with Morse (1997) that all qualitative inquiry is properly concerned with the production of theory, and note that most of her criteria for assessing qualitatively derived theory—clarity, logical structure and coherence, generalizability, and pragmatic utility—are entirely consistent with our current framework.

We stated earlier that our criteria for evaluating qualitative inquiry may be applied to both proposals and completed work, but evaluating proposals deserves more discussion. There are now many places where qualitative inquiry may be presented or published, but it is our impression that agencies that fund health research are still more skeptical of qualitative work than are journal editors or program committees for professional meetings. We believe our criteria might help address this problem because they seem to have both a rational and an emotional appeal, and as Morse (1994a) points out, proposals are about selling an idea. The criteria challenge the investigator to describe the context of the problem, not merely by giving a picture of the setting and the phenomenon of interest but also by making explicit the facts, values, and theories that have also helped create the problem. We also ask for clear statements about the logic of inquiry—the basis for the plausibility of any derived theory—as well as attention to methods. Both of these criteria have a strong rational appeal. Our emphasis on practical implications seems to be part of the fabric of clinical work as well as the standards that others have proposed. The democratic involvement of participants is consistent with values that are deeply held by many social groups and provides a second appeal to the emotion of reviewers. This is in no way a manipulation of the reviewer by the author of the proposal, but rather, it is a practical strategy that aligns the values and beliefs of the stakeholders in the grant process.

Critical Perspectives

Pragmatist philosophy's emphasis on democratic social values and attention to the role of social structures and processes in the production of knowledge and action provide an important conceptual basis for more recent inquiry models, including emancipatory and critical inquiry. These labels state the emphases in these models: goals of empowerment that are achieved by uncovering and challenging the false consciousness that perpetuates unequal social power relations (e.g., Freire, 1970). Many vigorous research strands have grown from this vision of social justice and come under the labels of "action research," "participatory action research," "feminist" inquiry, and "critical" versions of anthropology and sociology. Practitioners using these models typically cite the pragmatists (particularly Dewey) as the source of the intellectual framework from which they work. They are explicit about the logical and practical need to attend to power issues. Carspecken (1996) articulates how these values are inextricably linked to truth claims:

> Unequal power distorts truth claims [since consent is coerced]. Critical epistemology will have to be precise about the many ways, a good number of them highly subtle, in which power corrupts knowledge. This matter goes to the very heart of critical epistemology, and it allows fundamental value orientations (for democracy, equality, and human empowerment beyond the merely democratic) to fuse with epistemological imperatives. (p. 21)

Carspecken (1996) further states that this "critical epistemology" (theory of knowledge) acknowledges the existence of an "objective realm" to which we all have access, and contrasts this with a "subjective realm" and "normative realm":

> *The objective realm* [is] characterized by the principle of multiple access. Objective validity claims are associated with assertions about the world; about what is, about what took place, and about what sorts of events regularly precede other sorts of events.
> *The subjective realm* [is] characterized by the principle of privileged access. Subjective validity claims are associated with assertions about your, her, or my world: about feelings, intentions, and states of awareness.
> *The normative/evaluative realm* . . . is implicated in position-taking. Position-taking with others necessarily carries claims and assumptions about what is "proper" that soon expand into cultural understandings about what is right, wrong, good, or bad. The normative/evaluative realm has to do with our world, as it is or should be. (pp. 84-85)

Carspecken (1996) describes five stages of critical qualitative inquiry:

Stage One: Completing the primary record (observations);
Stage Two: Preliminary reconstructive analysis (articulating those cultural themes and system factors that are not observable and that are usually unarticulated by the actors themselves);
Stage Three: Dialogical data generation (interviews);
Stage Four: Discovering system relations: looking for relationships between a specific social site of study and other social sites; and
Stage Five: System relations as explanations of findings (connecting reconstructive analyses with social theories). (p. 7)

The objective realm is observed in Stage One and tentatively interpreted in Stage Two. Interviews provide some insight into the subjective realm: The espoused theory presented by informants (reasons people give for their actions) can be compared to the theory-in-use inferred by the outside observer (Argyris & Schön, 1978). The notion of emic versus etic perspectives applies here (Taylor & Bogdan, 1984). The normative realm, first uncovered in Stages One through Three, is the particular focus of Stages Four and Five. Not all qualitative or mixed method inquiries will follow this sequence or incorporate all of these steps—they clearly flow from anthropology's tradition of ethnography—but we believe it is a useful guide for pragmatist research. Those qualitative studies that are more narrowly focused or that use a single method (e.g., focus group interviews) would still benefit from considering context, social structures, and social processes.

Carspecken (1996) also suggests specific techniques to promote validity claims, including multiple data sources, multiple observers, thick description, prolonged engagement, peer debriefing, and member checks. Some authors (e.g., Janesick 1994) argue that reliance on technique to produce valid results is misguided. We agree that technique alone is an inadequate basis for validity claims, but those advocated by Carspecken are appealing to us for at least two reasons: First, they are consistent with a pragmatist (albeit critical) framework and thus are linked to the values and knowledge theories of that system; and second, they have widespread and enduring support among qualitative investigators from many traditions (Creswell, 1998) and therefore represent practical advice from a diverse research community.[5] Rather than being slaves to method (what Janesick, 1994, has called "methodolatry"), we see the considered use of some of these techniques as "methodological awareness," an understanding of the "consequences of particular methodological decisions during a research study, whether they relate to the production of data or the choice of writing style" (Seale, 1999, p. 33). We, therefore, have included this as one of our current criteria for evaluation of qualitative inquiry.[6]

Postmodern Critiques

As reviewed by Denzin and Lincoln (1994), Vidich and Lyman (1994), and Seale (1999), postmodernism is a rejoinder to those (like us!) who would systematize qualitative inquiry. Postmodernists see such systems as merely another version of academic oppression that imposes conformity to the wishes of the ruling elite. Even a fallabilistic construction (Seale, 1999), such as the one we offer, strikes these critics as a forced consensus, ignoring the idiosyncratic and ultimately unknowable nature of human existence (Derrida, 1976; Fish, 1989; Rosenau, 1992). Furthermore, Lincoln and Denzin (1994) describe a "crisis of representation" (p. 577); referring to the work of feminist Judith Stacey (1988), they point to the

> difficulties involved in representing the experiences of the Other about whom texts are written. . . . A major contradiction exists in this project, despite the desire to engage in egalitarian research characterized by authenticity, reciprocity, and trust. This is so because actual differences in power, knowledge, and structural mobility still exist in the researcher-subject relationship. The subject is always at grave risk of manipulation and betrayal by the ethnographer. In addition, there is the crucial fact that the final product is too often that of the researcher, no matter how much it has been modified or influenced by the subject. (Lincoln & Denzin, 1994, p. 577)

They also speak about the "crisis of legitimation" as a circular logic in which the text validates itself, that is, when the author represents adherence to principles and methods as evidence of the strength of truth claims, the source of the text's power. Referring to this as "epistemological validity" (p. 579), Lincoln and Denzin (1994) point out that postmodern critics offer alternative constructs, most notably Patti Lather's (1986) suggestions for validities that emphasize self-doubt, multiple voices and positions, and opposition to dominant perspectives.

Some have taken these critiques to a logical extreme, portraying them as radically relativistic and ultimately nihilistic: "Anything goes; nothing matters; everything matters; and so forth." We think such a reaction is simplistic, unfair, and misses the contribution made by postmodernism to the debate (Seale, 1999). We believe these ideas have great value in sensitizing researchers to questions such as "What warrant do I have for this work? How can I avoid imposing my agendas and yet not have to forgo them entirely? Who are the members of the 'community' with whom I work? Who owns the data? Who owns the results? Who decides where and how results are represented, and for what purpose?" Action-oriented health researchers who work with communities have taken on these questions directly (e.g., Greenwood & Levin, 1998; Macaulay et al., 1999; Thesen & Kuzel, 1999; Wuest & Merritt-Gray, 1997). As we see health professionals work collaboratively with communities in projects aimed at personal and collective development, we point to one more set of ideals with which the academics in such endeavors may guide their efforts.

   Family physicians Ann Macaulay, William Freeman, and Peter
Twohig, human ecologist Nancy Gibson, and community advocates
Laura Commanda and Carolyn Robbins recently published their experiences with a community-based and directed diabetes prevention
project (Macaulay et al., 1999). Continuing a line of such work among
Canadian investigators (Green et al., 1994; Herbert, 1996; Macaulay
et al., 1997) and citing several other examples of participatory research
(Lindqvist, Timpka, & Schelp, 1996; Matsunaga et al., 1996; Plough &
Olafson, 1994; Rispel, Doherty, Makiwane, & Webb, 1996), Macaulay
and colleagues proposed a code of ethics for research with communities that was recently adopted as a policy statement by the North American Primary Care Research Group (Macaulay et al., 1998). Speaking
from their own and others' experiences, they suggest that researchers
and communities should clearly specify and negotiate agreement on
the following issues:

> Research goals and objectives
> Methods and duration of the project
> Terms of the community-researcher partnership
> Degree and types of confidentiality
> Strategy and content of the evaluation
> Where the data are filed, current interpretation of data, and future
> control and use of data and human biological material
> Methods of resolving disagreements with the collaborators
> Incorporation of new collaborators into the research team
> Joint dissemination of results in lay and scientific terms to communi-
> ties, clinicians, administrators, scientists, and funding agencies.
> (Macaulay et al., 1999, p. 778)

Nancy and Ginger Gibson and Ann Macaulay build on this framework
in Chapter 7 (this volume), in which they suggest strategies for evaluating participatory inquiry.
   Pragmatist philosophy points the way to such collaborative models
of inquiry, and critical epistemologies like those espoused by
Carspecken (1996) or Greenwood and Levin (1998) sensitize privileged participants (like health professionals) to hidden power and the
value of diversity. This same sensitivity is appropriate for those of us
who participate in judgments about one another's work in the form of
proposals or publications. We are in a privileged position and will do

well to reflect on and make public the values, theories, and purposes we serve in making those judgments. In the spirit of encouraging dialogue and debate (Devers, 1999), this chapter offers several perspectives on this challenge.[7]

Notes

1. What Rescher calls "inductive" reasoning is what Charles Peirce called "abductive" reasoning: to make sense of an observation requires a change in the assumptions or premises. Peirce would then have tested this "leap of logic" with an experiment, which he called "inductive reasoning." The terminology becomes confusing, and we prefer to focus on the process involved: the restructuring of prior assumptions to resolve a puzzle, predicament, or paradox. See also Chapter 1 for more on deduction, induction, and abduction.

2. These are also commonly called "type I" and "type II" errors.

3. We have not yet directly addressed pragmatist beliefs about reality (ontology); we will come back to this when we review emancipatory forms of inquiry. Our discussion will include a consideration of objective, subjective, and normative "ontological categories" (Carspecken, 1996, p. 20).

4. We will also speak later about the place of techniques as quality indicators.

5. Some of these techniques are part of the several criteria for qualitative research we summarized earlier. For a more detailed analysis and critique of these and other techniques, see Clive Seale's (1999) excellent review.

6. In this chapter, we have not included any explicit discussion of qualitative analysis, although much is implied in our suggested framework of evaluation. Interested readers may wish to consult Strauss and Corbin (1990), Silverman (1993), Miles and Huberman (1994), Morse (1994b), or Crabtree and Miller (1999) for examples of guides to qualitative analysis.

7. We hope readers will share their experiences, suggestions, and criticisms with us at akuzel@hsc.vcu.edu and jengel@neoucom.edu.

References

Argyris, C., & Schön, D. (1978). *Organizational learning.* Reading, MA: Addison-Wesley.

Carspecken, P. F. (1996). *Critical ethnography in educational research: A theoretical and practical guide.* New York: Routledge.

Cherryholmes, C. C. (1992). Notes on pragmatism and scientific realism. *Educational Researcher, 21,* 13-17.

Crabtree, B. F., & Miller, W. L. (Eds.). (1999). *Doing qualitative research* (2nd ed.). Thousand Oaks, CA: Sage.

Creswell, J. W. (1998). *Qualitative inquiry and research design: Choosing among five traditions.* Thousand Oaks, CA: Sage.

Denzin, N. K., & Lincoln, Y. S. (1994). *Handbook of qualitative research.* Thousand Oaks, CA: Sage.

Derrida, J. (1976). *Of grammatology.* Baltimore: Johns Hopkins Press.

Devers, K. J. (1999). How will we know "good" qualitative research when we see it? Beginning the dialogue in health services research. *Health Services Research, 34,* 1153-1188.

Dewey, J. (1938). *Logic: The theory of inquiry.* New York: Henry Holt.

Eisner, E. (1981). On the difference between scientific and artistic approaches to qualitative research. *Educational Researcher, 10*(3), 5-9.

Fish, S. (1989). *Doing what comes naturally.* Durham, NC: Duke University Press.

Frankel, R. M. (1999). Standards of qualitative research. In B. F. Crabtree & W. L. Miller (Eds.), *Doing qualitative research* (2nd ed., pp. 333-346). Thousand Oaks, CA: Sage.

Freidson, E. (1970). *Profession of medicine: A study of the sociology of applied knowledge.* New York: Dodd, Mead.

Freire, P. (1970). *Pedagogy of the oppressed.* New York: Herder & Herder.

Green, L. W., George, M. A., Daniel, M., Frankish, C. J., Herbert, C. J., Bowie, W. R., O'Neall, M. (1994). *Study of Participatory Research in Health Promotion.* Ottawa: Royal Society of Canada.

Greenhalgh, T. (1998). Narrative based medicine in an evidence based world. In T. Greenhalgh & B. Hurwitz (Eds.), *Narrative based medicine* (pp. 247-265). London: BMJ Books.

Greenwood, D. J., & Levin, M. (1998). *Introduction to action research: Social research for social change.* Thousand Oaks, CA: Sage.

Hammersley, M. (1989). *The dilemma of qualitative method: Herbert Blumer and the Chicago tradition.* London: Routledge.

Herbert, C. P. (1996). Community-based research as a tool for empowerment: The Haida Gwaii diabetes project example. *Canadian Journal of Public Health, 87,* 109-112.

Howe, K. R. (1988). Against the quantitative-qualitative incompatibility thesis, or dogmas die hard. *Educational Researcher, 17*(8), 10-16.

James, W. (1907). *Pragmatism: A new name for some old ways of thinking.* New York: Longmans, Green.

Janesick, V. J. (1994). The dance of qualitative research design: Metaphor, methodolatry, and meaning. In N. K. Denzin & Y. S. Lincoln (Eds.), *Handbook of qualitative research* (pp. 209-219). Thousand Oaks, CA: Sage.

Kuzel, A. J. (1986). Naturalistic inquiry: An appropriate model for family medicine. *Family Medicine, 18*(6), 369-374.

Kuzel, A. J., Engel, J. D., Addison, R. B., & Bogdewic, S. P. (1994). Desirable features of qualitative research. *Family Practice Research Journal, 14*(4), 369-378.

Lather, P. (1986). Issues of validity in openly ideological research: Between a rock and a soft place. *Interchange, 17,* 63-84.

Lewin, K. (1948). *Resolving social conflicts.* New York: Harper.

Lincoln, Y. S., & Denzin, N. K. (1994). The fifth moment. In N. K. Denzin & Y. S. Lincoln (Eds.), *Handbook of qualitative research* (pp. 575-586). Thousand Oaks, CA: Sage.

Lindqvist, K., Timpka, T., & Schelp, L. (1996). Ten years of experiences from a participatory community-based injury prevention program in Motala, Sweden. *Public Health, 110,* 339-346.

Macaulay, A. C., Commanda, L. E., Freeman, W. L., Gibson, N., McCabe, M. L., Robbins, C. M., & Twohig, P. L. (1998). *Responsible research with communities: Participatory research in primary care.* Policy statement of the North American

Primary Care Research Group. Retrieved July 1, 1999, from the World Wide Web: http://views.vcu.edu/napcrg/napcrg98/exec.html.

Macaulay, A. C., Commanda, L. E., Freeman, W. L., Gibson, N., McCabe, M. L., Robbins, C. M., & Twohig, P. L. (1999). Participatory research maximizes community and lay involvement. *British Medical Journal, 319*, 774-778.

Macaulay, A. C., Paradis, G., Potvin, L., Cross, E. J., Saad-Haddad, C., McComber, A. M., Desrosiers, S., Kirby, R., Montour, L.T., Lamping, D. L., Ledvc, N., & Rivard, M. (1997). The Kahnawake Schools diabetes prevention project: Intervention, evaluation and baseline results of a diabetes primary prevention program with a Native community in Canada. *Preventive Medicine, 26*, 779-790.

Matsunaga, D. S., Enos, R., Gotay, C. C., Banner, R. O., DeCambra, H., Hammond, O. W., Hedlund, N., Ilaban, E. E., Issell, B. F., & Tsark, J. A. (1996). Participatory research in a native Hawaiian community: The Wai'anae Cancer Research Project. *Cancer, 78*, 1582-1586.

Mead, G. H. (1934). *Mind, self, and society.* Chicago: University of Chicago Press.

Miles, M. B., & Huberman, A. M. (1994). *Qualitative data analysis* (2nd ed.). Thousand Oaks, CA: Sage.

Miller, S. I., & Fredericks, M. (1995). Can there be "rules" for qualitative inquiry? *Journal of Thought, 30*, 61-71.

Morse, J. M. (1994a). Designing funded qualitative research. In N. K. Denzin & Y. S. Lincoln (Eds.), *Handbook of qualitative research* (pp. 220-235).Thousand Oaks, CA: Sage.

Morse, J. M. (1994b). "Emerging from the data": The cognitive processes of analysis in qualitative inquiry. In J. M. Morse (Ed.), *Critical issues in qualitative research methods* (pp. 23-43). Thousand Oaks, CA: Sage.

Morse, J. M. (1997). Considering theory derived from qualitative research. In J. M. Morse (Ed.), *Completing a qualitative project: Details and dialogue* (pp. 163-188). Thousand Oaks, CA: Sage.

Peirce, C. S. (1934). *Collected papers: Vol. 5. Pragmatism and pragmaticism.* C. Hartshorne and P. Weiss (Eds.). Cambridge, MA: Harvard University Press.

Pellegrino, E. D., & Thomasma, D. C. (1993). *The virtues in medical practice.* New York: Oxford University Press.

Plough, A., & Olafson, F. (1994). Implementing the Boston Health Start Initiative: A case study of community empowerment and public health. *Health Education Quarterly, 21*, 221-234.

Popay, J., Rogers, A., & Williams, G. (1998). Rationale and standards for the systematic review of qualitative literature in health services research. *Qualitative Health Research, 8*(3), 341-351.

Poses, R. M., & Isen, A. M. (1998). Qualitative research in medicine and health care: Questions and controversy. *Journal of General Internal Medicine, 13*, 32-38.

Putnam, H. (1995). *Pragmatism: An open question.* Oxford: Blackwell.

Rescher, N. (1977). *Methodological pragmatism: A systems-theoretic approach to the theory of knowledge.* New York: New York University Press.

Rescher, N. (1992). *A system of pragmatic idealism: Vol. 1. Human knowledge in idealistic perspective.* Princeton, NJ: Princeton University Press.

Rispel, L., Doherty, J., Makiwane, F., & Webb, N. (1996). Developing a plan for primary health care facilities in Soweto, South Africa: Part 1. Guiding principles and methods. *Health Policy Planning, 11,* 385-393.

Rosenau, P. (1992). *Post-modernism and the social sciences: Insights, inroads, and intrusions.* Princeton, NJ: Princeton University Press

Schutz, A. (1967). *The phenomenology of the social world.* Evanston, IL: Northwestern University Press.

Seale, C. (1999). *The quality of qualitative research.* London: Sage.

Silverman, D. (1993). *Interpreting qualitative data: Methods for analysing talk, text, and interaction.* London: Sage.

Stacey, J. (1988). Can there be a feminist ethnography? *Women's Studies International Forum, 11,* 21-27.

Strauss, A., & Corbin, J. (1990). *Basics of qualitative research: Grounded theory procedures and techniques.* Newbury Park, CA: Sage.

Tashakkori, A., & Teddlie, C. (1998). *Combining Qualitative and Quantitative Approaches.* Thousand Oaks, CA: Sage.

Taylor, S. J., & Bogdan, R. (1984). *Introduction to qualitative research methods: The search for meanings.* New York: John Wiley.

Thesen, J., & Kuzel, A. J. (1999). Participatory inquiry. In B. F. Crabtree & W. L. Miller (Eds.), *Doing qualitative research* (2nd ed., pp. 269-292). Thousand Oaks, CA: Sage.

Thorne, S. (1997). The art (and science) of critiquing qualitative research. In J. M. Morse (Ed.), *Completing a qualitative project: Details and dialogue* (pp. 117-132) Thousand Oaks, CA: Sage.

United Kingdom Central Council for Nursing, Midwifery and Health Visiting (1992). *Code of Professional Conduct.* 23 Portland Place, London, England W1N 4JT.

Van Manen, M. (1996). Phenomenological pedagogy and the question of meaning. In D. Vandenberg (Ed.), *Phenomenology and educational discourse* (pp. 39-64). Durban, South Africa: Heinemann.

Vidich, A. J., & Lyman, S. M. (1994). Qualitative methods: Their history in sociology and anthropology. In N. K. Denzin & Y. S. Lincoln (Eds.), *Handbook of qualitative research* (pp. 23-59). Thousand Oaks, CA: Sage.

Wuest, J., & Merritt-Gray, M. (1997). Participatory action research: Practical dilemmas and emancipatory possibilities. In J. M. Morse (Ed.), *Completing a qualitative project: Details and dialogue* (pp. 283-306). Thousand Oaks, CA: Sage.

Dialogue:

The Constraints of Publishing

MEADOWS: Well, certainly one of the challenges in qualitative research—and it may not be limited to the type of research but more to the disciplines in which we work—is the publication expectations that we grapple with in our academic environments. For instance, I hear over and over that in order for my research to be well represented, I need to publish my ongoing work as at least a monograph or maybe as a chapter in a book that provides a context for my work in women's health. But when I go up for merit at the end of the year, I get zero—that is, no salary increment for publishing in that domain.

MORSE: Well, maybe that is part of the education process in which we need to engage and start taking a stand. As the coeditor of a book, I could write letters to the authors' department heads or chairs explaining that the chapters are reviewed and rigorous. For instance, this book is all about the nature and rigor of evidence, and it would be ironic if this authorship wasn't properly credited.

THORNE: Of course, another part of the difference between good, developing, and rich qualitative research and smaller projects or studies is that evidence builds, theories develop, samples are expanded, and so on. And although often in bench research or some other environments one publishes every time a new solution is used or a cell divides, we are trying to look at a holistic environment and develop theories so our productivity may appear to be lower or take longer.

MADJAR: Perhaps we need to take a couple of positions or courses of action. If we can encourage and guide our graduate students to situate their smaller and less mature studies in the context from which they grow, they may be more publishable and contribute to the literature in a complementary way. But we must work with them, guide their first author attempts, and be willing to have our names there and be part of the evaluative process—then we are responsible as well. And for our own work, we may need to either ask journals to publish longer articles or to accept that as we publish a series of articles from our research establishing our concepts, theories, methods, etc., the articles will be of the usual length but have a lot of cross-referencing—or citations—from our earlier publications.

MEADOWS: So then we get it out, the count rises, our careers are enhanced, our research merited as it deserves, and, in addition, we foster and encourage the careers of our students at all levels while doing the secondary educational task of working with our peers who don't do or aren't familiar with standards of qualitative work.

KUZEL: It's the same in any field, with any method. When the field is young, there is variation in quality as folks learn the skills and try things out. Then after a number of years, the field stabilizes, standards become implicitly and explicitly agreed upon, and the field settles down. Until the next person comes along to stir things up again!

6

The Implications of Disciplinary Agenda on Quality Criteria for Qualitative Research

SALLY E. THORNE

Although attention to credibility traditions within discrete disciplines has been a hallmark of excellent scholarship, recent shifts toward breaking down academic disciplinary boundaries and working within interdisciplinary inquiry teams have begun to erode some aspects of quality criteria. As an inherently interdisciplinary exercise, qualitative health research has evolved as a direct challenge to the research traditions within most of the disciplines in which it has flourished and has moved toward embracing its own emerging set of standards and criteria. Because the work of qualitative health researchers places them somewhat outside their own disciplinary traditions and naturally aligns them with researchers representing a range of other academic disciplines, it has become popular in qualitative research circles to ignore or discount the implications that the various disciplines and their traditions have upon the nature, structure, and quality of the research product.

In this chapter, I will problematize the implications of disciplinary traditions and argue that they have influenced and will continue to influence the scope, direction, and style of our inquiry. I will do this by considering the epistemological and historical traditions of some of the more prominent disciplinary perspectives that have been active in contributing to the qualitative health research enterprise and by examining the implications of the various theoretical and practical sciences to the research undertaking. From this foundation, I will critically examine the degree to which disciplinary perspective influences the style and substance of research and, therefore, shapes the nature of knowledge that derives from inquiry. Considering the objectives of a disciplinary tradition as distinct from the objectives of an inherently

interdisciplinary qualitative health research enterprise, I will speculate
that various and distinct quality criteria may in fact obstruct the process of developing coherent knowledge on the basis of diverse bodies of
qualitative health research. In so doing, I hope to stimulate dialogue
about the inherently disciplinary grounding that much of our research
reveals and to suggest preliminary strategies for determining the basis
on which we can decide whether or not our diverse studies contribute
to coherent knowledge. On this basis, I will propose ways in which we
can become more fully informed about the implications of disciplinary
tradition upon the form, structure, substance, and quality of our qualitative health research initiatives.

Major Disciplinary Traditions

The history of qualitative health research reveals its roots in a
number of distinct but related disciplinary traditions. Specifically, the
major methods in use today include such approaches as phenomenology (adapted by psychology from philosophy), grounded theory
(from sociology), and ethnography (from anthropology), as well as a
wide range of variations on each theme (Thorne, 1991). These three
social sciences have long traditions in academic circles, and the specific
qualitative methodologies that have survived in them represent only a
subset of the methodological strategies developed for the purposes of
each discipline. More recently, that is, in the last two decades of the 20th
century, the health science disciplines have adopted and adapted the
qualitative methods developed within the social sciences and elsewhere
and have applied them to a range of practical and theoretical problems
within health care. While many health disciplines are currently represented within the community of qualitative health researchers, nursing
and medicine (especially psychiatry) have taken the lead and continue
to represent the strongest methodological voices. For this reason, my
analysis will focus on the disciplinary traditions of psychology, sociology, and anthropology within the social sciences, and medicine and
nursing within the health sciences, with apologies to those many disciplines whose involvement in our enterprise has also been important
(among these are education, social work, speech sciences, counseling,
nutritional sciences, dentistry, pharmacy, and rehabilitation).

For our purposes in this analysis, the most important distinction between the social sciences and the health sciences is the nature of their disciplinary projects. Psychology seeks to understand the workings of the human mind, sociology works out the patterns of social behavior inherent in human nature, and anthropology directs its inquiry to the question of variations and universals within human behavior and experience. Despite the recent emergence of "applied" subspecialties, each of these disciplines traces its origin to human philosophical curiosity and remains to a considerable degree grounded in theoretical challenges rather than practical problems (Reason, 1996). In contrast, medicine and nursing (as well as the other health sciences) trace their roots to social problem solving rather than theoretical inquiry. Their very nature is the development of applied knowledge toward a socially recognized activity, and their theoretical work is inherently secondary to that mandate (Chenail, 1992). Although it is well recognized that many social scientists conduct their work in applied contexts and that many health scientists make important contributions to theory, I believe that the underlying foundations of the disciplines can be shown to have a sustaining influence on the disciplinary traditions with regard to what counts as good science. Because of this, the theoretical and applied traditions of the disciplines warrant consideration for their influence upon our understanding of quality criteria.

Influence of the Disciplinary Traditions

While none of the disciplines involved in this discussion represent unitary monoliths, each does have a tradition of scholarship that influences a number of variables; these variables will determine what distinguishes adequate methodological applications from inadequate ones. These distinctions emerge in every aspect of the inquiry process, from the questions that are asked and the theoretical framework within which they are located, to the design, sample selection, sorting, and analysis of data and interpretation of implications. Within each discipline, a tradition exists of scholarship that privileges certain methodological decisions over others by virtue of many factors, including the following: (a) their fit with the extant theory upon which the research is justified; (b) their familiarity to those persons who fund and review scholarly work within the discipline; and (c) the patterns of socialization and mentorship that neophyte researchers will obtain within the field.

Until recent years, many educators, scholars, and theorists exhibited a distinct disdain for work beyond the boundaries of their discipline. Beyond the obvious advantages for building elite scholarly communities, it is arguable that such attitudes reflected an adherence to the trappings of "normal science," the paradigmatic consensus by which regulations are entrenched (Crotty, 1998) for the purpose of credibility within academic and scientific communities. Certainly, until recent years, the social sciences were often referred to as the "soft" sciences, and the health sciences were often considered to be markets for the application of science rather than disciplines in which science itself could be generated (Schwandt, 1997). Paradoxically, the upsurge of enthusiasm for qualitative research helped create the academic climate within which interdisciplinarity gained credence as legitimate scholarship. To establish scientific legitimacy, early qualitative researchers had to frame the foundational assumptions underlying their work as an intentional challenge to the inherent limitations of knowledge gained from traditional scientific methods alone. This challenge, coinciding with social trends that demanded multiple methods and novel strategies, broke down the traditional supremacy of logical positivism as an inquiry method and diminished the social authority of its adherents. Within a span of two decades, we have shifted the culture of academic scholarship to the point where it has become almost politically incorrect to acknowledge disciplinary traditions.

I have had several years of experience as part of a meta-study group comprised of six researchers attempting to unravel the knowledge that could be extracted from the existing qualitative research on living with chronic illness.[1] On the basis of this experience, I have become convinced that aspects of our disciplinary culture are almost hardwired into our research methods, regardless of our enthusiasm for collaborating and crossing interdisciplinary boundaries. Although I had read much of the research for other purposes over the years, the exhaustive systematic analysis of a recent meta-study project served as a lens through which previously invisible patterns within the available literature emerged with a sharpened focus. Among the most fascinating insights was the growing awareness that the author's (or lead author's) discipline was almost always apparent in the nuances of design, strategy, and interpretation, regardless of any explicit mention. In other words, where I had previously understood the body of literature to be an evolving source of knowledge about a common phenomenon, now my colleagues and I had the opportunity to see the literature as a series of competing arguments with regard to which disciplinary orientation ought to achieve prominence as the most viable theoretical frame within the field. What I discovered was that researchers were almost inevitably speaking to the assumptions inherent in their own discipline, even when they were drawing (often uncritically) upon the knowledge developed across disciplines. Thus, the insider's subjective perspective of a phenomenon like chronic illness was systematically skewed by the conceptualizations and motivations of the discipline and embedded in the academic culture within which the researcher was socialized.

An example may be instructive to illustrate this claim. Within qualitative health research, the methodology of grounded theory or variations upon it have become popular over recent years. Because it is well recognized that human health and illness experiences are complex matters influenced by a range of competing variables or factors, most grounded theorists advocate some form of theoretical sampling to ensure that their findings are reasonably representative of the anticipated range of the phenomenon of interest. However, their selection of variables that might express maximal variation frequently betrays their disciplinary orientation. In research about breast cancer, for example, the sociologist conducting a qualitative study might sample for high versus low socioeconomic status, the anthropologist for ethnicity, the psychologist for the presence or absence of depressive symptomatology, the physician for pre- and postmenopausal status, and the nurse for the presence or absence of dependent children at home. Each has drawn upon the theoretical frame of his or her own discipline to identify the primary feature upon which the sample is presumed to vary. Each recognizes that it might prove difficult to establish the credibility of the final research project with colleagues in the discipline, if these specific variables are not given primary consideration. Due to the complexity of qualitative data analysis and the appropriate sample size for each study, it would not be appropriate to insist that each researcher recruit a sample that is sufficiently representative of an unlimited number of such variables. However, the ones we select, and the way they reveal the assumptions our discipline has taught us would matter in the world of academic credibility, make it exceedingly difficult to build knowledge on the basis of such various inquiries.

Another example, perhaps even closer to the heart of the issue, is the kinds of questions that will be asked within the context of each discipline. To illustrate, I refer to the heated debate that flared up within nursing circles and was documented in letters to the editor when a research report on career women with tattoos was published in a respected peer-reviewed nursing journal (Armstrong, 1991). Had the same paper appeared in a journal directed toward sociologists, anthropologists, or psychologists, the audience would almost certainly have responded with an immediate recognition of the theoretical claims upon which the author had built. Such findings would have been considered an appropriate contribution to a rather obscure but mildly interesting social, cultural, or psychological phenomenon of our times. Had the paper been directed toward an audience of physicians, the focus might have been on the documentation of infection rates or requests for surgical reversal. Perhaps, in health care venues oriented toward public health, an audience might have presumed that the relevance had to do with the implications of body piercing as a potentially high-risk behavior, a predictor of impulse control, or an indicator of peer pressure. For nurses, however, the publication of this paper violated a sense of what constitutes knowledge for professional practice, since the findings were in no way linked to any useful clinical application. They angrily took the journal to task for its abandonment of relevance as a quality criterion for scholarly research in the field (Anonymous, 1992; Moyer, 1992; Winton, 1992).

Thus, it appears that disciplinary perspectives may play a considerably larger role in the articulation of explicit and implicit quality criteria in qualitative health research than we typically acknowledge (Thorne, 1997; Thorne, Reimer Kirkham, & MacDonald-Emes, 1997). Not only do the studies that derive from various disciplinary perspectives bear the brand of disciplinary orientation, but our ideas about what constitutes good and bad science are indelibly stamped with the hallmarks of these distinct traditions. Because our analytic discussions typically categorize us by methodological allegiance, we tend to assume that our quality criteria are a logical extension of the methodological theory rather than an application of principles within a range of diverse contexts. We assume, for example, that ethnographies are all more or less alike, and that our anthropological colleagues will be better authorities on issues associated with quality criteria because it is their discipline that invented the approach. Similarly, we afford sociologists authority over grounded theory, despite the fact that it is probably used more often by health researchers than by sociologists in the current academic climate. And we assume that psychologists will be the experts when it comes to resolving problems inherent in phenomenological and hermeneutic approaches because their discipline's explicit objective is to unravel the mysteries of the human psyche.

However, I would argue that a much more useful and meaningful categorization we might consider is that of the applied versus the theoretical disciplines. Although I appreciate that individual members of each tribe may play a variety of roles, the inherent nature of the disciplinary groups is quite distinct. Psychology, anthropology, and sociology exist to generate theoretical understanding about some aspect of the human condition (Durrenberger & Thu, 1999; Porter & Ryan, 1996). In contrast, the health sciences are solidly grounded in the social mandate to do something about specific problems and challenges within that human condition (Chenail, 1992). This essential distinction must influence decisions about what constitutes good science as well as relevant knowledge.

To illustrate, nurses in my community of Vancouver, Canada, are studying the prenatal concerns of Asian immigrant women. Their qualitative inquiries are based on the entirely functional belief that sensitive and effective health care is dependent upon some critical aspects of understanding this population that are currently missing from the existing literature. From their perspective, a defensible theoretical sampling appropriate to such a study might include attention to such dimensions as whether or not the women speak English, whether or not their mother has also immigrated to Canada, or whether this is a first or subsequent child. However, from the perspective of an anthropologist, it would be highly problematic to consider Asian immigrant women as a homogenous group. Sensitivity to the subtle and not-so-subtle nuances of culture would require the researcher to take into consideration whether they were recent or established immigrants, whether they were from mainland China or some other country, from rural or urban areas, from what particular province, and so on. Furthermore, a researcher would have to pay serious attention to the implications of the specific linguistic group involved, as well as to whether their cultural allegiance was to traditional Confucian philosophy and Chinese medicine, to Western biomedical traditions, or some combination of the two. Thus, a study that might seem credible and quite relevant from the perspective of an applied discipline might have significant flaws from the perspective of a more theoretical discipline.

Just as knowledge that is credibly added to the repertoire of the applied disciplines cannot always be accepted as credible in the theoretical social sciences, the qualitatively derived knowledge that is obtained in psychology, anthropology, and sociology is not always accessible for the applied disciplines. For example, a sociological inquiry that is grounded in a particular claim about how human social behavior is determined and structured may use qualitative methods to test or extend that claim with a particular population, such as ill people or health care consumers. However, because the findings of that study will be grounded primarily in that claim, they cannot be used for knowledge about that population from an applied perspective. For example, sociologists have often studied such diseases as epilepsy as prototypical cases for uncovering knowledge about stigma and disclosure (Scambler & Hopkins, 1990; Schneider & Conrad, 1980). However, health care professionals would be remiss in their clinical practice if they understood this body of evidence as confirmation that epilepsy is the chronic condition for which disclosure issues are inherently the most problematic. Thus, I suggest that what is considered good and bad science can be strongly linked to the disciplinary perspectivism of our judgments, and to address the problem, we must acknowledge the importance of discipline.

Implications of the Knowledge Derived From Various Disciplinary Traditions

Beyond the recognition of the fact that the form, style, and scope of knowledge derived from the qualitative inquiries of various disciplines may shape the findings that are reported and the quality criteria with which we judge the science, my experience with qualitative metasynthesis has convinced me that to fully comprehend the knowledge that emerges from the science of various disciplines, we must appreciate that discipline's essential nature. By *essential nature,* I refer to its philosophical tradition, its social and historical positioning within the domain of empirical science, and its interpretation of its own social mandate, its raison d'etre. Taking into consideration the core philosophical traditions that underlie our own disciplines as well as those of the authors whose works we read and interpret plays a critical role in our ability to determine when we ought to accept research findings at their face value and when we ought to regard them with skepticism. Without this consideration, we run the risk of inadequately evaluating each other's contributions to knowledge and trying to build knowledge upon a very insecure foundation.

Even within the most theoretical strands of social science, it must be recognized that knowledge development has a purpose, and that purpose extends beyond political expediency. Each of our disciplines has a recognized social mandate, whether it is solving social problems or simply theorizing. As we engage in increasingly interdisciplinary projects, we may take on additional purposes, but we typically do so only to the extent that they do not compromise our understanding of our own discipline's contribution in the larger sense.

One arena in which some of these troubling issues of a disciplinary nature will inevitably emerge is the philosophical positioning we take as we approach our qualitative inquiries. Although many early qualitative researchers in the health field distinguished their science from logical positivism because it was ontologically idealist in orientation, it is now well recognized that qualitative inquiries have application within the full spectrum, including realism (Engel & Kuzel, 1992). For example, many of the phenomenological inquiries directed toward uncovering the essential structure of what is assumed to be foundational human experience—such as pain, loneliness, and grief—reflect a decidedly realist philosophical stance. Although our understanding of the phenomenon may be accessible only through the lens of subjective consciousness, the use of these methodological approaches presupposes that these phenomena do have a nature of their own, independent of subjective interpretation or social construction. In contrast, studies from various postmodern perspectives reveal a fundamental assumption that because there is no relevant social reality apart from what is subjectively experienced, consideration of objective realities becomes irrelevant. Thus, pain, loneliness, and grief become whatever the sufferer claims them to be. Over recent years, within the qualitative health research field, there has been a considerable trend toward various postmodernisms, and ideas such as *co-construction of knowl-edge* have gained credibility within various scholarly communities as well as within the sociopolitical domain.

It becomes important, then, to consider each discipline's theoretical relationship to the idea of how subjectively and objectively derived knowledge contributes to good science. Traditional empiricism repre-sented an attempt to circumvent the inherent problems associated with reason alone, and the various forms of logical positivism that emerged as the gold standard for science developed intricate strategies for ensuring that subjectivities did not contaminate scientific processes and their products. While the social and health sciences developed in the context of a culture that privileged reductionist objectivity in its "normal science" (Berkwits, 1998; Flick, 1998), each sought to develop scientific approaches that were both credible and consistent with disciplinary philosophical foundations. Thus, anthropologists created intricate taxonomies for human behaviors and physicians developed extensive protocols for randomized clinical trials (RCTs). Although leaders within our various disciplines continued to struggle with the relevance of normal science for their larger social mandates, it was not until Thomas Kuhn's (1962) writings on the philosophy of science became widely accessible that a way to articulate alternative definitions of science became socially viable. Qualitative research in the health field capitalized heavily on the paradigm debate, polarizing traditional (quantitative) science as inherently realist in ontology and reductionist in epistemology and making room for an alternative form of science that captured subjectivity and violated many of the accepted standards of what constituted good science. Thus, this historical location of qual-itative health research has shaped much of what we now understand it to represent.

For the health sciences, the qualitative research thrust provided an opportunity to enter into the study of human health and illness experi-ence that included people's minds and souls as well as their physiology and biochemistry. For the social sciences, this "revolution" created a credible platform upon which to rethink the theoretical advances that had been made in the name of understanding human behavior. Despite our newly found affinity for subjectively derived knowledge, we also recognize the unavoidable degree to which subjective knowledge is inherently bounded. Although we may have made great advances in technology, the mind still cannot operate outside temporal, contextual, and embodied constraints. These constraints have demonstrable implications, and to some extent, we have attempted to resolve these. Historical analysis, for example, can help us deconstruct the temporal influence of subjective knowledge, just as cross-situational analysis can help us understand social and political context. However, we have no viable alternatives to embodiment. Subjective knowledge, therefore, is inherently dependent on fragile biochemical influences upon the body and the brain. Given specific biochemical changes, even the most disciplined mind will have predictable logical, perceptual, and conceptual shifts, and the extent to which these systematically limit our ability to know our world itself is unknowable.

Thus, truths in the subjective domain are always a different species of truths than those in the objective domain, which strive toward answering general questions to do with those fixed aspects of the human condition, what makes human beings uniquely human, and so on. They are, therefore, an inherently different form of science, and their truths are a different sort of truths (Heshusius, 1994; Kvale, 1995; Silverman, 1998). They are often more appropriately understood as grounded philosophies, using the mental processes of many people rather than the reasoning prowess of a single philosopher and basing some sense of truth on what might be common patterns in thinking and reasoning. Because we know from historical analysis of social trends and dominant values that group behavior can powerfully influence individual thought, it becomes difficult to argue that there is any relationship between what people think and a truth outside the context of shared thinking as it shifts over time and situation.

No matter how comfortably we collaborators from various disciplines work within the language, and indeed rhetoric, of subjectively derived knowledge, psychology exists to decode the mechanisms within the human mind, anthropology exists to seek answers to the questions of human universals, and sociology exists to understand how our inherently collective nature shapes our existence. Nursing, medicine, and other health sciences must regularly attend to subjectivities within the individual cases they confront, and can benefit considerably from learning how to do that better. However, they are also bound to acknowledge that their very existence is dependent upon the acceptance of some objective realities as fundamental. If human health, for example, is not independent of our current social constructions, then there is no goal toward which science in these disciplines can reasonably aspire.

Knowledge becomes a kind of parlor game, a matter of infinite variation and intellectual curiosity, rather than an inherent component of a
socially relevant and mandated professional activity (Silverman, 1998).

Therefore, it seems that by engaging in the development of the
science of subjectivity, we create an opportunity to rediscover our
foundational disciplinary truths, and in so doing, we must acknowledge how essentially different those truths can be. Because of this, the
evaluation rules for our science must be necessarily different (Engel &
Kuzel, 1992). Beyond the dialogue in the domain of samples, data sources,
analytic strategies, and credibility measures, it is time to engage in a
more philosophical discussion of what it is that our disciplinary
perspectives inherently mean for the way we theorize, the way we define
what constitutes reality, and the way we make sense of our various
observations in the study of human health and illness experience.

Discipline-Specific Quality Criteria

If, as I claim, there are sufficient differences in the essential nature of
the various health and social science disciplines to warrant a reexamination of the criteria that we use to determine the quality of our scientific products, then a discussion of how this applies in the practice of
research becomes important. Not only do we currently collaborate
together on multidisciplinary teams, but we also review each other's
grant proposals and manuscript submissions, consult with each other
on the proper application of methodological principles, and even
participate in the education of each other's neophyte researchers. Thus,
we will have to grapple with the issue of discipline-specific criteria in
order to make transparent our assumptions and guiding values and to
create a climate in which qualitative health research as a legitimate
social and health science enterprise can maintain some credibility in
the academic as well as in the health practice and policy domains.

To begin, I propose that we reconsider one of the classic issues that
arises when qualitative researchers from various perspectives evaluate
each other's research—the theoretical framework. Inherent in the assumptions underlying the social sciences is the enduring requirement
that any qualitative inquiry be anchored substantively (in addition to
methodologically) within a particular theoretical interpretation that
applies in some way to the phenomenon being studied (Strauss, 1995).

This assumption is both a cultural tradition within the social sciences and a remnant of traditional empirical science guidelines. The reason for this rigid policy is that individual studies in and of themselves are never entirely relevant; what makes them relevant is their contribution to the theoretical challenge that is central to the discipline. In other words, the purpose of research in these traditions is to develop, challenge, or extend existing theory. Therefore, failure to articulate precisely what theory and in what manner a new piece of research directs itself toward renders that research meaningless. When the applied health science researchers began to draw on the methods of the social sciences to answer their own research questions, they brought forward some of the same theoretical baggage. Thus, a generation of qualitative health researchers in nursing, medicine, social work, and other professions have been trained to look for a theoretical foundation and theoretical significance as a hallmark of quality. However, a theoretical framework undeniably shapes the questions that are asked, the way the research design is framed, and the researcher's freedom to interpret findings (Mitchell & Cody, 1993). Thus, many health science researchers have borrowed rather extensively from the least restrictive (that is, most neutral) social science theories. Furthermore, although they locate their research in these theoretical frameworks, they do so in such a manner that they can claim some theoretical significance without unduly interfering with their rather atheoretical descriptions of the clinical problems or phenomena under study. I would therefore argue that we need to rethink the standard that all qualitative health research requires not only a methodological strategy but also a direction from an explicit substantive theoretical framework. Instead, researchers from various disciplines should be challenged to articulate the logic of their inquiries in accordance with their disciplinary motivations. Thus, a nursing study of smoking cessation behavior, for example, would not be expected to contribute significantly to a specific self-efficacy theory; instead, it would be understood as an opportunity to test out the usefulness of some clinical hunches about smoking cessation within a study population. By freeing such an inquiry from its theoretical boundaries, the researcher may be better positioned to explore the field in a more clinically relevant manner (Reason, 1996) and ask questions like "Why do these two people differ so dramatically in their belief that they can succeed? How do they interpret the risks of trying to quit smoking?"

Another core distinction that we ought to make relates to our understanding of sample size. While it has been common in qualitative health research to judge appropriate sample sizes on the basis of balancing depth with breadth and determining what volume of data it is humanly possible to analyze inductively, we rarely link sample size decisions to our larger disciplinary projects. I believe that this failure to critically examine sample size determinations places qualitative health researchers at risk for legitimate skepticism within our scientific communities. For example, while exhaustive case analysis might be an entirely appropriate method for a psychologist trying to untangle the complexities of how the human mind handles a particular situation or context, it would be entirely inappropriate as a foundation for a health science inquiry whose explicit intent is to challenge a particular health policy. On the other hand, although qualitative studies involving large numbers of participants may inherently survey the phenomenon in a rather superficial manner, smaller studies designed to access depth may systematically exclude important aspects of the phenomenon that only become visible when a wider cross-section of the phenomenon is considered. Therefore, the disciplinary purposes of research ought to inherently influence our understanding of sample size in quite different ways. An anthropologist whose intent is to understand the foundations of human kinship behavior may require much larger sample populations than a physician studying parental anxiety following acute childhood illness. Similarly, a psychologist studying human denial mechanisms might use considerably different approaches than a nurse seeking to develop supportive interventions to families that are in conflict about acknowledging a medical diagnosis.

The third issue that warrants considerable reexamination is the matter of data collection strategies. Many qualitative health inquiries rely heavily on data consisting of verbatim transcriptions of face-to-face interviews between individuals who have experience with the phenomenon under question and researchers trained to loosely guide an open-ended conversation (Silverman, 1998). Documentary analysis, participant and nonparticipant observation, and various other data collection strategies are often used as an adjunct to the subjectively co-constructed data that are gleaned from such interviews. However, depending on the essential nature of the disciplinary knowledge toward which the study is directed, reliance on interview data may or may not be justifiable. For example, because we know how much of social behavior is inaccessible to consciousness, we would not expect to find evidence of basic social processes in interview data alone. To understand why people ignore certain bodily cues that have critical meaning for their health behaviors, we might find observation of patterns across large samples with diverse populations a necessary part of our inquiry. Similarly, because we recognize that many human experiences are exceedingly difficult to articulate within the constraints inherent in language, we would have more confidence in findings about such phenomena if they drew upon data that extend beyond what people can tell us in words. For instance, we find certain aspects of alienation and grief to be more accessible in art and music than they might be in verbal material. However, in the applied health sciences, there is an infinite number of clinical problems for which the kinds of knowledge that can be gained from interview data are entirely appropriate and sufficient. For example, while an observational survey might tell us how many questions were asked in a medical consultation and how much information was provided, it will be the accounts of the recipients that will tell us whether the patient left feeling informed, understood, and satisfied with the options provided.

Where interview data are a significant element of the research, the tradition of verbatim transcription and line-by-line coding represents another opportunity for disciplinary variations. Much of the analytic tradition that has dominated qualitative health research derives from the intricate methodologies developed by anthropology to detect subtle nuances in language use, nonverbal cues such as pauses, and wordless utterances. Within the health sciences, this tradition has been uncritically borrowed, so that researchers typically assume significant transcription costs to document each encouraging sound ("mm," "hmm" from the researcher, and "um, um, um . . ." from the subject) that is audible on audiotape. Typically, facial expression, body posture, and other expressions of encouragement, hesitation, or connection are systematically ignored. Thus, in many such instances, verbatim transcriptions reveal an obsessive attention to a single dimension of communications information that is typically irrelevant to the analytic process and edited out in the final report. In contrast, hermeneutic textual analysis might require careful and systematic attention to all accessible details of terminology, syntax, and flow of ideas in order to detect subtle meanings within the structure of the language (Allen, 1995; Clavarino, Najman, & Silverman, 1995). For example, a sociologist seeking to uncover power relations between physicians and their pa-tients by examining narrative recordings in medical charts might find it absolutely necessary to decode and interpret language at the most minute level. Thus, it seems possible to argue that our disciplinary tradi-tions may have important differences to contend with not only in the material that we will consider worthy as data but also in the processes by which we render those data into credible research findings.

The final issue I will raise here deals with disciplinary variations in what constitutes rigor within our approaches and credibility within our findings. Specifically, I believe that there are significant variations be-tween the social and health sciences with regard to the conditions that must be met before practical application of the findings becomes de-fensible and ethical. For example, when a sociologist proposes a theory about human behavior that is of interest to health care professionals, it would normally be quite problematic to alter professional practice on that basis without investigating the implications of the claim in a criti-cal manner. Although a team of social scientists revealed that women who were unmarried were more likely to reach the five-year survival milestone after diagnosis with breast cancer (Waxler-Morrison, Hislop, Mears, & Kan, 1991), no applied health researcher would consider that an appropriate basis upon which to intervene in their patients' marital status in order to help them live longer. However, there have been numerous qualitative studies by health science researchers whose find-ings are immediately understood as applicable within the clinical con-text. For example, when a team of nurse researchers discovered that practicing nurses seriously underestimated the rate of dyspnea among terminally ill cancer patients at home because the symptom was ren-dered invisible by coping strategies (Roberts, Thorne, & Pearson, 1993), a protocol to standardize assessment beyond overt patient complaints of such symptoms was implemented immediately. To me, these exam-ples emphasize the fundamental difference between knowledge that is developed for a social science and may, with translation, eventually have a practical application, and knowledge whose very nature demands its application to practice.

Thus, in relation to many aspects of our research enterprise, it can be argued that we ought to strive for quality standards that are not only consistent with the philosophical traditions of our qualitative research methods but are also true to our disciplinary mandates. On this basis, consensus about methodological adequacy, rigor, and credibility will inevitably require that we reduce our dependence on the rules and regulations advanced by those who originally developed the specific methods, and that we continue to develop and refine variations of those methods to best suit the problems each discipline faces and the kinds of knowledge that it seeks to generate.

Conclusions

Because credibility criteria, design decisions, and ideas about the very nature of truth vary considerably among diverse disciplinary traditions, I believe that an ongoing dialogue about disciplinary standards will be an enlightening and informative one. For example, as we begin to understand quality standards in nursing research and how such standards ought to be distinct from high-quality sociological inquiry, I think we will be better able to guide our collaborations with a sense of our unique contributions that transcend methodological and design traditions. When we read and draw upon each other's work, it will become possible to appreciate the implications of interpreting knowledge through a decidedly disciplinary lens; we will begin to make transparent our various embedded assumptions about what matters and why it matters. When we review each other's grant proposals and manuscript submissions, we will need to attend not only to the strengths of our own particular disciplinary orientation but also to its limitations. Of course, one possible effect of this reflective process might be that we decide not to work together at all, and to increasingly regard other disciplinary research with suspicion. However, I am convinced that by understanding ourselves not only as individual researchers involved in a reflective inductive process but also as embodiments of discrete academic disciplinary traditions, we ought to be able to tolerate complexity, to respect our differences, and to eventually gain sufficient self-confidence to clearly articulate the linkages between our various knowledge traditions. I believe that distinct disciplinary standards are a fundamental requirement for qualitative health research to survive as a credible inquiry tradition. Thus, as we continue to embrace an interdisciplinary ideal, we must not forget to honor and celebrate our differences.

Note

1. The Chronic Illness Meta-Study Group is led by principal investigator Barbara Paterson; additional coinvestigators include Carol Jillings, Connie Canam, Gloria Joachim, and Sonia Acorn. It has been funded by the Canadian Nurses Foundation as well as other sources and operates out of the University of British Columbia School of Nursing.

References

Allen, D. (1995). Hermeneutics: Philosophical traditions and nursing practice research. *Nursing Science Quarterly, 8,* 174-182.
Anonymous. (1992). Letter to the Editor. *IMAGE: Journal of Nursing Scholarship, 24*(1), 80.
Armstrong, M. L. (1991). Career-oriented women with tattoos. *IMAGE: Journal of Nursing Scholarship, 23,* 215-220.
Berkwits, M. (1998). From practice to research: The case for criticism in an age of evidence. *Social Science & Medicine, 47,* 1539-1545.
Chenail, R. J. (1992). A case for clinical qualitative research. *The Qualitative Report, 1*(4), 1-11. Retrieved August 10, 1999, from the World Wide Web: www.nova.edu/ssss/QR/QR1-4/clinqual.html.
Clavarino, A. M., Najman, J. M., & Silverman, D. (1995). The quality of qualitative data: Two strategies for analyzing medical interviews. *Qualitative Inquiry, 1,* 223-242.
Crotty, M. (1998). *The foundations of social research: Meaning and perspective in the research process.* London: Sage.
Durrenberger, P. E., & Thu, K. M. (1999). Why we're worried about cultural anthropology. *Society for Applied Anthropology Newsletter, 10*(3), 3-5.
Engel, J. D., & Kuzel, A. J. (1992). On the idea of what constitutes good qualitative inquiry. *Qualitative Health Research, 2,* 504-510.
Flick, U. (1998). *An introduction to qualitative research.* London: Sage.
Heshusius, L. (1994). Freeing ourselves from objectivity: Managing subjectivity or turning toward a participatory mode of consciousness. *Educational Researcher, 23*(3), 15-22.
Kuhn, T. S. (1962). *The structure of scientific revolutions.* Chicago: University of Chicago Press.
Kvale, S. (1995). The social construction of validity. *Qualitative Inquiry, 1,* 19-40.
Mitchell, G. J., & Cody, W. K. (1993). The role of theory in qualitative research. *Nursing Science Quarterly, 6,* 170-178.
Moyer, N. (1992). Letter to the Editor. *IMAGE: Journal of Nursing Scholarship, 24*(1), 80.
Porter, S., & Ryan, S. (1996). Breaking the boundaries between nursing and sociology: A critical realist ethnography of the theory-practice gap. *Journal of Advanced Nursing, 24,* 413-420.
Reason, P. (1996). Reflections on the purposes of human inquiry. *Qualitative Inquiry, 2,* 15-28.
Roberts, D., Thorne, S. E., & Pearson, C. (1993). The experience of dyspnea in terminal cancer: Patients' and nurses' perspectives. *Cancer Nursing, 16*(4), 310-320.

Scambler, G., & Hopkins, A. (1990). Generating a model of epileptic stigma: The role of qualitative analysis. *Social Science & Medicine, 30,* 1187-1194.

Schneider, J. W., & Conrad, P. (1980). In the closet with illness: Epilepsy, stigma potential and information control. *Social Problems, 28,* 32-44.

Schwandt, T. A. (1997). *Qualitative inquiry: A dictionary of terms.* Thousand Oaks, CA: Sage.

Silverman, D. (1998). The quality of qualitative health research: The open-ended interview and its alternatives. *Social Sciences in Health, 4*(2), 104-118.

Strauss, A. (1995). Notes on the nature and development of general theories. *Qualitative Inquiry, 1,* 7-18.

Thorne, S. E. (1991). Methodological orthodoxy in qualitative nursing research: Analysis of the issues. *Qualitative Health Research, 1*(2), 178-199.

Thorne, S. E. (1997). The art (and science) of critiquing qualitative research. In J. M. Morse (Ed.), *Completing a qualitative project: Details and dialogue* (pp. 117-132). Thousand Oaks, CA: Sage.

Thorne, S. E., Reimer Kirkham, S., & MacDonald-Emes, J. (1997). Interpretive description: A noncategorical qualitative alternative for developing nursing knowledge. *Research in Nursing & Health, 2,* 169-177.

Winton, M. A. (1992). Letter to the Editor. *IMAGE: Journal of Nursing Scholarship, 24*(2), 162.

Waxler-Morrison, N., Hislop, T. G., Mears, B., & Kan, L. (1991) Effects of social relationships on survival for women with breast cancer: A prospective study. *Social Science & Medicine, 32,* 117-183.

Comment:

Looking Inward

Forgive the researchers, O Wise Ancestors, for they do not always know what they do, because they sit in their universities and do not look into the eyes or see the faces of those they research.

We must educate the researchers to see that we are a people who must be involved from the beginning of any research. We must be in an equal partnership with involvement and a decision-making process. In our project, a very successful component is the moral and ethical guidelines (Code of Research Ethics) that empower all the community members and researchers to work together in a successful relationship. Through that empowerment comes the ownership and the commitment to work together for a healthier community.

As Onkwehonwe (the Real People), we ask our Ancestors to help us to "look inward" to ourselves, our culture, and our spirituality for a healthy lifelong journey.

Amelia Tekwatonti McGregor
Kahnawake, Canada

Editor's Note: Adapted by permission of Amelia Tekwatonti McGregor.

7

Community-Based Research

Negotiating Research Agendas and Evaluating Outcomes

NANCY GIBSON
GINGER GIBSON
ANN C. MACAULAY

Community-based research approaches, known variously as participatory research (PR), participatory action research, action research, and so forth, are strategies for creating knowledge that is relevant to a community's needs and interests. Community-based research is strengthened by a process in which research goals and community partners are made explicit at the outset. This goal identification process increases both the level of success of the research process and its relevance to the community. By acknowledging personal, professional, and organizational goals, a common agenda can be negotiated that focuses on the outcomes of the project (Israel, Schurman, & Hugentobler, 1992) and provides a framework for evaluation.

Community-Based Research: An Ethical Approach

Community-based research is a strategy for democratizing the research process (Meyer, 2000). It is a strategy that satisfies various communities' demands to have a voice in the research done in their communities and to participate as equal partners (Boston et al., 1997; Smith, 1999). Participatory research models negotiate a balance between the development of valid generalizable knowledge and knowledge that is meaningful to the community (Argyris & Schon, 1991; Macaulay et al., 1999). Participatory research can be conducted with people who have a strong sense of being a community, who share a history, and who have mutual geographical, cultural, social, political, or economic interests

(Macaulay, Commanda et al., 1998; Macaulay, Delormier et al., 1998; Macaulay et al., 1999). Characteristics of participatory research include

- extensive collaboration between defined researchers and the community at each research stage, from identifying the problem to applying and disseminating results;
- a reciprocal educational process for community members and researchers;
- shared power and control of the agenda and of research products; and
- an emphasis on taking action on the issue under study.

This approach also can serve to enhance scientific understanding by incorporating the knowledge and expertise of community members (Meyer, 2000; Susman & Evered, 1978) and by blending scientific inquiry with education and political action (Dickson, 2000). Sharing control of science can be a major stumbling block for some academic researchers, who argue that without proper training (within an academic discipline), science cannot be adequately served (Cancian, 1993). In other words, the use of unqualified community participants may impede the research. Short-term training, they argue, cannot prepare people to collect valid data. Critics also maintain that responding to research questions coming from communities dilutes the mandate of science to develop new theories, and that community involvement threatens academic freedom to publish. Furthermore, many conventional research models do not readily allow for community-level collaboration. However, the Inuit Tapirisat of Canada notes that the legacy of conventional research in northern communities includes many different sorts of failures: exclusion of the study community from the research process, inaccessibility of results, inappropriate interpretation and dissemination of results, and lack of benefit to the communities (Inuit Tapirisat of Canada, 1993). These failures have resulted in feelings of being used and betrayed in the research process and an unwillingness to participate in future research endeavors.

Collaboration between academic colleagues, nonprofit organizations, and corporations is not uncommon. Collaboration that includes a mix of these groups and the community is a relatively new approach (Barr & Huxham, 1996). In the words of Susan McDaniel, however, "Growth occurs at the boundaries of academic disciplines, much like in Alexander Fleming's petri dishes" (McDaniel, 2000, p. 2). To ignore the edges is to risk missing important opportunities for the expansion and development of science. The objective of participatory research is to create knowledge that is both relevant to community needs and reflects the interests of the community. For many types of research, we argue that this objective can best be met by including the community and the other stakeholders in the research and collaborating with them as equal partners throughout the process. Functioning at the academic boundaries and integrating community perspectives creates difficulties for conventional models of evaluation. Thus, it is incumbent upon us to explain to our colleagues, peers, and critics how our participatory action work can be assessed (Mays & Pope, 2000). The approach suggested here is a tool that can be applied throughout a research project as an integrative mechanism that guides research agendas; however, it also can be used retroactively to produce a comprehensive evaluation based on explicit goals. Both applications will be discussed. Hagey (1997) observes that "research utilization is both process and product in participatory action research" (p. 2); hence, evaluating the process can be as important as assessing the outcomes. Using this agenda-based evaluation model, it is possible to measure the process of negotiating the goals of a community-based research project as well as evaluate the stakeholders' perspectives of the project's effectiveness. Multimember research teams can include community members, community leaders, health care providers, government funders, and industry representatives. Our case studies provide examples of applying this approach in situations ranging from health-risk communication research to program and service delivery research, illustrating the broad range of potential agendas.

The Agenda-Based Evaluation Model

Rationale

Whether stated or not, every research project includes both formal and informal goals. Most projects begin with formally stated goals that are often weighted toward the most powerful organizational partner on the research team. Although they may remain hidden, the personal and professional goals of each participant, whether academic scholar, government funder, community member, or industry employee, influence the level and direction of participation as well as the establishment of the formal shared research agenda (Whyte, 1991). Found (1997) observes that participatory research participants are assumed to be operating with the best of intentions; however, this assumption will not necessarily result in empowerment unless participant motivation is examined more closely and structured to ensure cooperation. He found that suspicion, jealousy, cynicism, and other factors seemed to contribute to a lack of motivation in some of the participatory research projects he reviewed. Unrecognized or unacknowledged goals can lead to tension within the research team and, in extreme cases, to the collapse of the research process. We all operate first as individuals and second as professionals and organizational representatives. Our choices are governed not only by our personal goals but also by our ethical principles. In cross-cultural and/or interdisciplinary situations, communication regarding these issues can be complex and lead to misunderstanding. The agenda-based evaluation model permits the expression of ethical principles and the integration of these principles into the research design. This proactive strategy can signal potential conflicts and help the research team avoid situations where varying goals are not addressed until they become problems and threaten the integrity of the research (Ervin & Dawkins, 1996). A process for identifying agendas and establishing a working environment while conducting continuous evaluation is described below (see Table 7.1), with case examples to illustrate variations in application. The case studies illustrate many, if not all, of the steps for community-based evaluation. In each case, we attempt to articulate the application of at least one of the steps.

Step 1. Establishing Evaluation as a Goal

Many approaches and techniques for evaluating research outcomes, both during and after completion of the research project, are revealed in the literature (Greene, 1994). Methods range from formative to summative, with many variations (Chess, 1999). Most evaluation techniques are designed to measure the effectiveness of either the research process itself or the outcomes of a project, and some projects have adopted multimethod evaluation approaches (Flynn, 1995). An important part of establishing evaluation as a goal is to identify the whole agenda. This is the starting point of collaboration with the community. A multimethod evaluation is currently being conducted at the Northeast

TABLE 7.1 Nine Steps to Community-Based Evaluation

Step 1	Establishing evaluation as a goal
Step 2	Identifying the partners
Step 3	Understanding contextual factors: drawing the outer circle
Step 4	Establishing trust and mutual respect
Step 5	Clarifying constituency and representation
Step 6	Identifying individual agendas
Step 7	Identifying competing agendas: research and power
Step 8	Negotiating the shared research agenda
Step 9	Comparing agendas and outcomes

Community Health Centre in Edmonton, Canada. A team of professional consultants is evaluating the actual programs; scholars are collecting and analyzing stories from the client community and using scales to measure perceived levels of service and ownership; other researchers are assessing the documented trail of goals, jointly identified by the research partners, that influence the outcomes of the research; and still others are measuring staff responsiveness to innovative changes and preparing a historical account of the Centre from its roots in a community lobby in the 1970s to the present. PR evaluation models, however, rarely address the varied agendas of the partners throughout the research process (Found, 1997), particularly when it involves community members.

Step 2. Identifying the Partners

Community-based research often involves multiparty teams with diverse backgrounds and educational experience that represent different and potentially conflicting groups with disparate organizational mandates. Stoeker (1999) points to the potential conflict between the academic perspective (the project as research) and the community perspective (the project as community development). Often, community participants are self-selected, representing a narrow band of the community. Efforts to be as inclusive as possible are strengthened by making agendas explicit. The approach suggested here recognizes and accommodates the various agendas in community-based research, and it helps

participants develop research agendas (Found, 1997) that contribute
to the entire process. Identifying all appropriate partners at the outset,
in consultation with the various stakeholders, is an important step.
Overlooking a source of relevant expertise can jeopardize the project.
Furthermore, each time a new person joins the group, there can be a
ripple effect, with time lost as everyone adjusts to new relationships.
Unwieldy as it may seem, it is important to ensure that all relevant partners are as involved as they want to be and in roles that are appropriate
to their positions in the project.

**Step 3. Understanding Contextual Factors:
Drawing the Outer Circle**

In evaluating community-based research, it is often difficult to assess
the influence of invisible contextual factors on the project. For each
community, there is an outer circle of unique factors that affect overall
community status: for example, geography, history, culture, politics,
environment, and economics. The agenda-based evaluation model can
accommodate these factors (see Figure 7.1). The outer circle of experience is unique to each community and must be considered within a
time continuum. The history of the community, particularly the political history, is a good example. Much community-based research is
related to issues resulting from power and economic differentials, with
implications for policy, access to program funding, and therapeutic
outcomes. For example, in the community-based tuberculosis (TB)
study (Case Study 3), the historical experience of each of the identified
high-risk populations, aboriginal and foreign born, is vastly different,
and yet, this experience was found to bear directly on adherence to
preventive therapy. Geography is another factor that contributes to the
outer contextual circle. If a rural community has had uneven delivery
of health services over time, confidence in service providers can be
eroded, causing distrust among the research team members. Quality,
source, and importance of formal education within the community
may also be peripheral factors influencing the research issue, as may access to employment or future funding. The process of identifying these
contextual factors with the full participation of all stakeholders, including the community, contributes to the depth and validity of the research and indeed helps to confirm the decision to use the PR approach
and methods in a particular setting (Vakil, 1994).

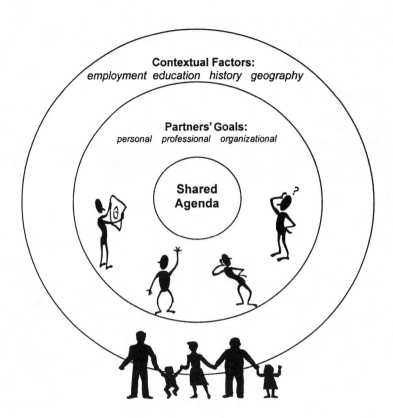

Figure 7.1 Agenda-Based Evaluation Model

Step 4. Establishing Trust and Mutual Respect

Community-researcher relationships should be established early in the planning process. These relationships are facilitated and strengthened by written agreements that outline the formal obligations of each partner throughout the research process (Gibson & Gibson, 1999; Macaulay et al., 1999; Macaulay, Delormier et al., 1998). This includes negotiating the research question, the ethical principles, the requirements and methods of evaluation, ways of accommodating differences of opinion, and plans for dissemination of the results. The process of jointly developing a mission statement and written agreement can promote detailed discussions and negotiations. Also, it can help stakeholders reflect on the goals of the research and recognize and share their own personal goals. The process promotes respect for communities, a relatively new concept in research ethics (Weijer, Goldsand, & Emanuel, 1999), and collaborative empowerment. Application of these concepts can transform traditional power relationships through a democratization process and ensure recognition of the roles and goals of all collaborators (Himmelman, 1996). The empowerment process is multilateral in that the creation of an open and equitable forum can promote the interests of all partners (Fetterman, Kaftarian, & Wanderson, 1996).

Step 5. Clarifying Constituency and Representation

People become involved in research for a variety of reasons, and participatory models tend to base participation on the assumption of constituency. This is a shifting concept, however, and there are levels of representation that are not always easily identified. There are gatekeepers in communities who act as individuals but claim to represent a particular community. As Weijer et al. (1999) observe, "Any vibrant community will have multiple and even conflicting interpretations of its own traditions and values. Selected representatives may not be able to speak adequately for the diversity of viewpoints of community members" (p. 277). The authors suggest that a mechanism for broad-based community consultation adds validity to the process. Among professional collaborators, there is a potential for split loyalties to a profession (e.g., medicine, nursing, or law) and to the community. Degrees of representation vary, depending on many community- and employment-embedded factors. An appreciation of the degree of representation of each partner and the nature of the constituency will increase the probability that recommendations will be adopted. This also helps to identify gaps in expertise and representation.

Step 6. Identifying Individual Agendas

To date, few evaluation methods identify the full range of goals and objectives of the partners in a community-based project (Chess, 1999). As Sink (1996) notes, "A major challenge in facilitating collaboration is dealing with individual representatives' idiosyncrasies, egos, personal agendas and interpersonal quirkiness" (p. 106). Many motivations underlie community-based research, ranging from conventional academic investigations to advocacy research. Recently in Canada, court-ordered studies are being designed as a result of settlements favoring community claims of environmental encroachment (Provincial Court of Alberta, 1999). Acknowledging the underlying agendas of the partners increases both the likelihood of success of a research project and the level of commitment of the collaborators. Each partner's agendas (personal, professional, and organizational) will influence their roles in a research project. Stoeker (1999) identifies three roles that can be played by an academic in PR: the initiator, the consultant, and the collaborator. These roles can be influenced by professional goals, such as gaining new knowledge about an issue of interest or experience in using participatory methods to benefit a community or even increasing income or experience in a new research environment. Other professional reasons may include completion of a degree or fulfilling training requirements. A community leader's agenda might include the personal goal of improving the health of the community and the organizational objective of increasing the visibility of the community with health care providers and/or funders. Personal reasons may also include achieving higher status in the community. Organizational agendas may include extending the consulting network of the university/company. Even though shared goals are often altruistic, personal and professional goals may be more specifically focused, although they need not be contradictory to the overall research objectives. Reticence in expressing personal goals is to be expected and respected. Not all personal goals may be shared, and some may be articulated later in the process. In a carefully structured and reflexive research setting, however, where issues and principles are revisited throughout the research process, an atmosphere of trust can be established that permits the honest sharing of personal and organizational goals by all stakeholders, an essential step in successful evaluation.

Step 7. Identifying Competing Agendas: Research and Power

Health problems can usually be linked to political or economic inequities, or both. Power and income inequities are clearly linked to health status (Wilkinson, 1996). Thus, research agendas often include the commitment to effect change, for example, to improve the health status of the community. Participatory action research is an approach in which the commitment to effect changes through research is explicit and part of the research design. If the political allegiance of various partners is in conflict, the outcome of the research may be less than satisfactory. When academics and/or funders are initiators of the research project, power tends to rest there unless specific steps are taken. This is where the process of acknowledging the various goals of each partner can make a difference, not only to the research process itself but also to the outcomes. Consider an industrial representative with split loyalties: for example, a personal loyalty to improve the health of the community and its organizational responsibility to protect the interests of a corporation's investment. Positive tensions between partners' agendas can lead to productive relationships. Openly acknowledging these goals and aligning them with those of other participants can lead to innovative strategies for addressing the apparent contradiction. Meeting both the agendas for this industrial representative could mean, for example, that the company would play a more sensitive role in the community as a result of the research.

The example of the Boston Healthy Start Initiative (Plough & Olafson, 1994), with the overriding goal of decreasing infant mortality, highlights the tensions and challenges of building partnerships between a large city health department, a coalition of community-based, government and social service agencies, community leaders, and residents. The federal funding agency imposed tight timelines, creating additional complexity:

> Sharing power was the major challenge and working out governance took significant time and energy. . . . Many community participants were keenly aware of this and thus appropriately skeptical about the ability of a large city health department to be an equal partner. A key component of the effective mobilization was to mobilize against the dominance of this governmental partner. (p. 229)

The end result of this successful 2-year project was decreasing levels of infant mortality and the creation of over 100 jobs and community-based programs based on the linkages developed inside this research.

Step 8. Negotiating the Shared Research

Most research projects begin with an issue, question, or set of related questions intended to collect information and/or to solve a problem. A research team is assembled, with representation from all stakeholders, and it is assumed that all partners on the team are committed to the original issue. However, effective research with sustainable results will include a process of negotiation and continual evaluation that acknowledges as many agendas as possible and weaves them into a research design acceptable to all. The process involves identification of agendas, negotiation of the shared goal(s), and an element of compromise. Community-based research must meet the research needs of the community, but it should also strive to achieve the goals of the partners. Research that is not balanced in its design might be influenced negatively by interpartner tension and invisible agendas. This can affect the outcomes and the sustainability of the project, limiting the commitment and willingness of the partners to the project (Bracht et al., 1994). Developing a mission statement and revisiting it throughout the process provides a framework for evaluation. The process becomes an ongoing part of the research and a strategy for marking progress toward the shared research goals. If conflicting goals emerge, scenarios can be discussed to anticipate various outcomes: for example, a plan for disseminating sensitive findings to the communities, organizations, and professions in an acceptable and appropriate fashion. Not all the goals of each partner or participating organization will be achieved completely, but through the process of negotiation, the achievement and sustainment of consensus and commitment are possible.

Step 9. Comparing Agendas and Outcomes

Whether or not a community-based research project has followed the above steps in negotiating a common agenda, the agenda-based evaluation model can still be used as an approach for outcome evaluation. Retrospective evaluation of the goals of community-based research includes a study of the degree of consistency and level of consensus in setting and achieving common goals throughout the research process. It also includes an assessment of the influence and level of achievement of the individual goals of the participants. This process can be multimethod, using tools such as scaled surveys and meeting evaluations. Qualitative methods can include participant interviews and focus group or feedback sessions with the research team. The process may be led by an external facilitator or by one of the partners, but in either case, inclusion of the research team is paramount. An evaluation could examine the perceived effectiveness of each step of the research process from the perspective of the group as a whole, each individual participant, and the community at large. Implicit in such an evaluation are the completion of the goals, the identification of the challenges/barriers encountered during the project, and the strategies that led to success.

Found (1997), in a meta-analysis of 145 participatory research projects funded by the International Development Research Centre, felt that the evaluation component of most projects was weak, and he strongly suggested that a participatory-evaluative mechanism should be developed in association with all participants. Developing a worksheet of goals with all partners is one way of negotiating the common research agenda and evaluating effectiveness of the process (see Table 7.2).

Case Study No. 1. The Kahnawake Schools Diabetes Prevention Project, Steps 6, 7, 8, & 9

The Kahnawake case illustrates the identification of individual agendas, the discussion of competing agendas, and a final negotiation of a shared agenda. The research team compared agendas and outcomes in a perceived-ownership survey and found that most of the research team felt a strong degree of ownership over the process, suggesting that agendas and outcomes were well matched.

The Kahnawake Schools Diabetes Prevention Project (KSDPP) (1997) is a community health promotion project, using participatory research, for the primary prevention of Type 2 diabetes. Kahnawake is a Mohawk community (population 7,500) 15 kilometers from Montreal, Canada, with a high prevalence of diabetes. KSDPP began in 1994 using a participatory research model in which the researchers formed a partnership with the community of Kahnawake. The original grant proposal was written by a small group of Kahnawake community leaders and researchers from health and education together with invited academic

TABLE 7.2 Making Goals Explicit

Partner	Personal Goals	Professional Goals	Organizational Goals	Included in Common Goal?	How Well Achieved?
Community leader	Maintain water quality for community	Recognize community issues Enhance skills of community	Raise funds for community	Maintain water quality	
Industry representative	Learn about research process Maintain water quality	Achieve project goals successfully	Protect interests of corporation Keep apprised of changes in water quality standards	Maintain water quality	
University researcher	Complete degree Learn about PR Maintain water quality	New knowledge of PR Expand research network Explore publishing opportunities	Expand organizational expertise in evaluation Establish linkages with community partners New sources of outside funding for research Develop evaluation techniques for field Systematically document evaluation so that process may serve as a model for others	Maintain water quality	
Government funder or representative	Gain research experience	Establish trust with organizations Successful advancement of project	Assure responsible expenditure		

researchers from neighboring universities. The proposal included recommendations from the community elders that this project focus on elementary school children. Once funding was secured, Kahnawake formed a Community Advisory Board (CAB) to represent the voice of the community. This volunteer board was and continues to be open to all interested people, and it includes representatives from other community organizations and individuals from the private sector, whose ages range between 24 and 74 years. The intent of this participatory research project is to develop and maintain an equal partnership between researchers and CAB, with shared power and control for decision making from research design to dissemination of results.

In the language of the researchers, the long-term goal of KSDPP is the primary prevention of Type 2 diabetes. Short-term goals are to target two of the known risk factors associated with Type 2 diabetes onset, physical inactivity and unhealthy diet, and to achieve ecological changes in the community in order to facilitate these behaviors. The CAB transformed these concepts into a vision statement, saying that in the future,

> All Kahnawakeronon are in excellent health. Diabetes no longer exists. All the children and adults eat healthily at all meals and are physically active daily. The children are actively supported by their parents and family who provide nutritious foods obtainable from family gardens, local food distributors and the natural environment. The schools as well as community organisations maintain programs and policy that reflect and reinforce healthy eating habits and daily physical activity. There are a variety of physical activities for all people offered at a wide range of recreational facilities in the community. All people accept the responsibility to cooperatively maintain a well community for the future Seven generations. (Community Advisory Board of the Kahnawake Schools Diabetes Prevention Project, 1994)

This vision statement represents the negotiated agenda between researchers and the community. Thus, the agenda is shared between the partners, written in ways that are appropriate for both scientific and lay communities, and incorporates the Mohawk values of community, family, and tradition.

For further clarification of the roles and to formalize the guidelines of the research process, the researchers and community jointly negotiated a written Code of Research Ethics to guide the process from the design, implementation, analysis, and interpretation of data to the dissemination of results. This code was written by three partners: members of CAB, academic researchers from neighboring universities, and community researchers. Community researchers are the project staff and investigators who, because of other concurrent positions in health and education, hold dual roles in Kahnawake. The Code of Research Ethics (Kahnawake Schools Diabetes Prevention Project, 1997) includes a description of the overall research principles and research partnership and establishes research goals and objectives. It acknowledges the following points: the different obligations of the academic and community researchers and the community partner; the degree of confidentiality; the strategy for the evaluation process; the interpretation and control of data, knowledge of where data are filed, and current and future use of the data; responsibility for resolving issues arising from the research; and joint dissemination of the results in lay and scientific terms to both the communities and the scientists. This code includes some unique features: (a) it recognizes the difference between academic and community researchers; (b) new researchers can only be incorporated into the team after meeting and being accepted by all partners and only if they agree to abide by these research ethics (for instance, data cannot be given to a student for analysis without prior knowledge and acceptance); and (c), to act as a safeguard at the time of dissemination, all results must first be shared with the community of Kahnawake before being disseminated outside the community. Also, in the case of any dissent in the data interpretation, there is no veto, but a written agreement is developed in which both researchers and community members will document their own interpretation, with both interpretations being disseminated and published concurrently.

In our experience, this written Code of Research Ethics has been invaluable and served the project well for the last 6 years (Macaulay, Delormier et al., 1998). It is also our belief that the 8-month experience of developing this written agreement and the frank discussions that were necessary to achieve consensus forced all the team members to carefully decide on the essential elements of the research process and their own personal goals, beliefs, and commitments. We recommend that every research/community partnership should take the time to discuss and develop their own written agreements because the journey itself is "even more important than the arrival" (McGregor, 2000). This is part of the trust-building process that is essential in establishing and maintaining a partnership.

To evaluate the partnership process and transfer of ownership of this project to the community, at 2 and 5 years, KSDPP administered a perceived ownership survey adapted from Flynn (1995) to the CAB, project staff, researchers, and the Mohawk Supervisory Board. At two years, ownership of this project was perceived to lay first with the Mohawk project staff. At five years, however, ownership was perceived to be shared between the project staff and CAB, indicating early transfer of ownership to the community. It is interesting to note that all these partners perceived themselves to have a "moderate amount" or "a lot" of influence in project-related decision making, a hallmark in shared decision making. At both times, researchers were perceived to have the least ownership, yet they were satisfied with this position. These unpublished data are currently being interpreted, disseminated, and written up by a joint researcher/community team.

Negotiating agendas, which are subject to evaluation and revision as part of the research process, helps to ensure that the community and researchers are equal partners (Mittlemark, 1990). A key element of KSDPP involved developing flexibility and realistic expectations about what each partner could and could not contribute. Just as participatory research enhances validity by including context, so too is the validity of the research relationship enhanced if the context of each partner is understood. The exercise of defining the strengths, limitations, and resources that can be brought together contributes to the establishment of trust, enhances mutual respect between researchers and community, and facilitates community understanding of research, ownership of KSDPP, and involvement for future health care decisions.[1]

Case Study No. 2. Alberta Tuberculosis Study: Establishing the Foundational Principles, Steps 3 & 5

When the manager of a TB clinic noticed disproportionate levels of the disease in some communities, a research team, which included representatives of many of the affected constituencies, was drawn together. Through the inclusion of people from the cultural groups disproportionately affected, the contextual factors affecting community involvement in TB prevention and control were identified.

The manager initiated this multifaceted research project because of her interest in the diversity of her patient population and the impact that culture had on the type of cases being seen. In 1996, approximately 80% of her clients were foreign born, and 16% were aboriginal. The manager approached a potential research team, including an anthropologist (with an academic institution) and a practicing family physician/researcher. These individuals invited a Community Advisory Committee (CAC) to guide the investigation. Included on the CAC were people who shared the cultural backgrounds of the six major immigrant groups and various aboriginal groups represented in the TB patient population. All were leaders in the province and well respected in multicultural and/or aboriginal organizations.

The project began with a workshop that included the research team and the CAC to address the joint development of the research question. Concepts of culture were examined, and a generic accommodation of culture as a factor, rather than as culture as specific framework, was adopted. The CAC clearly advised against using ethnicity as an isolated factor. To seek out common cultural factors that could influence program and policy development, the research question thus became "What are the cultural factors that influence the prevention and treatment of TB in immigrant and aboriginal populations in Alberta?" The group initially recognized the need to agree on the underlying ethical principles to guide the research. The process whereby these foundation principles were forged was also the process whereby trust was established within the team.

These principles, reflecting an ethical stance that is consistent with the personal, professional, and cultural goals of each of the various partners, are often revisited. The research project is now well into the second year of a three-year process. With this focus, the team selected appropriate research methods. Participant Action Research most closely fit the group's ethical principles, and it quickly became the selected methodology. Community research associates were selected and recruited to conduct qualitative interviews in their own cultural communities (2 from each of 10 communities), which is consistent with the principles of empowerment and capacity building. During their training sessions, the community research associates also reviewed and revised the foundation principles, thus becoming part of the team and developing a strong sense of ownership and commitment to the research process.

Case Study No. 3. The Raritan Basin Watershed Study: A Process Evaluation, Steps 1 and 2

This case study serves to illustrate the up-front commitment of a group to formative and ongoing evaluation. Through this evaluation, the group also managed to clearly identify partners who needed to be involved in this study.

In 1999, a group of stakeholders came together to form the Raritan Watershed Management Project Team. Their goal was to characterize and assess the sources of pollution in a 1,100-square-mile watershed in New Jersey. Stakeholders included the basin's water supply authority, the state environmental protection agency, three nonprofit watershed community organizations, the U.S. Geological Survey, builders and developers, the Farm Bureau, and a university nonprofit center, among others. The Center for Environmental Communication at Rutgers University was invited to routinely evaluate the group's progress toward goals, which are sometimes conflicting. Formative research to identify group goals included

- gauging participant satisfaction with the process and products of meet- ings using evaluations (see Table 7.3);
- periodic checking in with a range of participants to get an in-depth sense of their level of satisfaction or to check on why they were not participat- ing months after they signed up; and
- evaluating needs and resources with respect to the watershed management data and process through a 3-stage participatory needs and resources assessment.

The academic team made sure evaluation was experimental and adap- tive and became involved, because a literature review of stakeholder involvement in watershed management had revealed little outcome or process evaluation (Chess, Hance, & Gibson, in press). As a result, guid- ance for watershed managers was largely based on individual narratives and rarely on systematic evaluations of multiple perspectives. As the academics also worked and lived in the watershed, their commitment was common with many other groups, that is, maintaining water quality. Through interviews with the most active members of the group (roughly 45) during the needs and resources assessment, the personal, professional, and organizational goals for each interviewee were identified. Results of these interviews were circulated, and the stake- holder group identified common goals and agendas. The most active stakeholders were found to have different goals than the less involved characterization committee. These findings served as a warning flag to the group, allowing individuals to reach out to the less involved group regarding needs and goals.[2]

Conclusions

The primary purpose for conducting community-based research is often to meet the community's needs in an empowering and equitable

TABLE 7.3 Example of Meeting Evaluation

Watershed Management Project

Thank you for taking the time to provide feedback on this meeting. Your comments will help improve future meetings. **All responses will be kept anonymous**—only summarized results will be reported.

1. **I felt this meeting was well organized** [circle one]

   Strongly agree　　Agree　　Neutral　　Disagree　Strongly disagree

2. **The pace of the meeting was:** [circle one]

   Too fast　　　Just right　　Too Slow

3. **I felt this meeting was productive** [circle one]

   Strongly agree　　Agree　　Neutral　　Disagree　Strongly disagree

4. **The information presented at this meeting was useful to me** [circle one]

   Strongly agree　　Agree　　Neutral　　Disagree　Strongly disagree

4a. If you answered "disagree" or "strongly disagree" to Question 4, please explain why the information presented was not useful to you.

5. **Did this meeting increase your understanding of the Raritan Watershed Management Project?**　　yes/no [circle one]

6. **Have you visited the Raritan Project's new website (www.Raritanbasin.org)?**　　yes/no [circle one]

   If you answered "yes" to question 6:
6b. **What did you like most about the site?**

6c. **What do you think could be improved?**

7. **Additional comments?** *[use back of form if necessary]*

Please write down your name and phone number if you would like a CEC researcher to call you and discuss in confidence your thoughts on the Raritan Workgroup process or if you have any suggestions for questions you would like to see on the evaluation forms in the future.

fashion. Plough and Olafson (1994) observe that "the proposed 'cure' [or outcome] must be demonstrated to be more helpful than the application of the same funds directly as income to the client or community organizations" (p. 221). This criterion for research is stringent in that the evaluation process must be perceived by all partners to add value, in this case by guiding collective decision making throughout the research process.

The dynamic model presented in this chapter is designed to guide the research process while it facilitates ongoing (process) evaluation. Articulating and negotiating the agendas of all the partners is an essential component of successful researcher-community partnerships, and the overall agenda includes the complex intertwined professional, organizational, and personal agendas of each player in the partnership. We have presented a 9-step model that evaluates outcomes by focusing on process, trust, and potential conflicting interests throughout the research period. As Found (1997) has observed, emerging PR approaches hold considerable promise for sustainable research projects, which will in turn require new forms of planning and evaluation. The agenda-based evaluation model is a contribution to that end.

Notes

1. With acknowledgments to Mary McComber and Amelia McGregor (Community Advisory Board), and Margaret Cargo, Ojistoh Horn, and Lucie Levesque (researchers).
2. For more information on the Raritan Basin Watershed Management Project, please see www.raritanbasin.org.

References

Argyris, C., & Schon, D. (1991). Participatory research and action science compared. In W. F. Whyte (Ed.), *Participatory action research* (pp. 85-98). Newbury Park, CA: Sage.
Barr, C., & Huxham, C. (1996). Involving the community: Collaboration for community development. In C. Huxham (Ed.), *Creating the collaborative advantage* (pp. 110-125). London: Sage.
Boston, P., Jordan, S., MacNamara, E., Kozolanka, K., Bobbish-Rondeau, E., Isherhoff, H., Mianscum, S., Mianscum-Trapper, R., Mistacheesick, I., Petawabano, B., Sheshamush-Masty, M., Wapachee, R., & Weapenicappo, J. (1997). Using participatory action research to understand the meanings Aboriginal Canadians attribute to the rising incidence of diabetes. *Chronic Diseases in Canada, 18*(1), 5-12.

Bracht, N., Finnegan, J. Jr., Rissel, C., Weisbrod, R., Gleason, J., Corbett, J., & Veblen-Mortenson, S. (1994). Community ownership and program continuation following a health demonstration project. *Health Education Research, 9*(2), 243-255.

Cancian, F. (1993). Conflicts between activist research and academic success: Participatory research and alternative strategies. *American Sociologist, 24*(1), 92-117.

Chess, C. (Ed.). (1999). *Evaluating environmental public participation: Methodological questions.* New Brunswick, NJ: Center for Environmental Communication.

Chess, C., Hance, B., & Gibson, G. (in press). Adaptive participation in watershed management. *Journal of Soil and Water Conservation.*

Community Advisory Board of the Kahnawake Schools Diabetes Prevention Project. (1994). *Vision statement.* To obtain a copy, write to KSDPP, Box 1000, Kahnawake, Quebec, Canada J0L 1B0.

Dickson, G. (2000). Participatory action research: Theory and practice. In M. Stewart (Ed.), *Community nursing: Promoting Canadians' health* (2nd ed., pp. 542-563). Toronto, ON: W. B. Saunders.

Ervin, N., & Dawkins, C. (1996). Agency and research team co-operation: An exploration of human territoriality. *Journal of Advanced Nursing, 23,* 728-732.

Fetterman, D., Kaftarian, S., & Wanderson, A. (1996). *Empowerment evaluation: Knowledge and tools for self-assessment and accountability.* Thousand Oaks, CA: Sage.

Flynn, B. (1995). Measuring community leaders' perceived ownership of health education programs: Initial tests of reliability and validity. *Health Education Research, 10*(1), 27-36.

Found, W. (1997). Evaluating participatory research supported by the International Development Research Centre. *Knowledge and Policy, 10*(1/2), 109-133.

Gibson, N., & Gibson, G. (1999). Articulating the agendas: Negotiating a collaborative model for public health research. In D. Wall (Ed.), *Securing northern futures: Developing research partnerships* (pp. 109-114). Edmonton, AB: Canadian Circumpolar Institute Press.

Greene, J. (1994). Qualitative program evaluation: Practice and promise. In N. Denzin & Y. Lincoln (Eds.), *Handbook of qualitative research* (pp. 530-544). Thousand Oaks, CA: Sage.

Hagey, R. (1997). The use and abuse of participatory action research [Guest Editorial]. *Chronic Diseases in Canada, 18*(1), 2.

Himmelman, A. (1996). On the theory and practice of transformational collaboration: From social service to social justice. In C. Huxham (Ed.), *Creating the collaborative advantage* (pp. 19-43). London: Sage.

Inuit Tapirisat of Canada. (1993). *Negotiating research relationships in the North.* Background paper for workshop on guidelines for responsible research. Yellowknife, NWT, September 22-23, 1993.

Israel, B., Schurman, S., & Hugentobler, M. (1992). Conducting action research: Relationships between organization members and researchers. *Journal of Applied Behavioural Science, 28*(1), 74-101.

Kahnawake Schools Diabetes Prevention Project. *Code of research ethics.* (Copyright 459302). (1997). To obtain a copy, write to KSDPP, Box 1000, Kahnawake, Quebec, Canada J0L 1B0.

Macaulay, A., Commanda, L., Freeman, W., Gibson, N., McCabe, M., Robbins, C., & Twohig, P. (1998). *Responsible collaboration with communities: Participatory research in primary care. A policy statement for the North American primary care research group.* Retrieved May 12, 1999, from the World Wide Web: views,vcu.edu/views/fap/napcrg98/exec.html.

Macaulay, A., Commanda, L., Freeman, W., Gibson, N., McCabe, M., Robbins, C., & Twohig, P. (1999). Participatory research maximizes community and lay involvement. *British Medical Journal, 319,* 774-778.

Macaulay, A., Delormier, T., McComber, A., Cross, E., Potvin, L., Paradis, G., Kirby, R., Saad-Haddad, C., & Desrosiers, S. (1998). Participatory research with Native community of Kahnawake creates innovative code of research ethics. *Canadian Journal of Public Health, 89*(2), 105-108.

Mays, N., & Pope, C. (2000). Qualitative research in healthcare: Assessing quality in qualitative research. *British Medical Journal, 320,* 50-52.

McDaniel, S. (2000). Leaky boundaries: Bodies, borders and well-being. *Henry Marshall Tory Chair Public Forum,* University of Alberta, February 7, 2000.

McGregor, A. (2000). *Kahnawake School District Prevention Project.* Personal communication.

Meyer, J. (2000). Qualitative research in healthcare: Using qualitative methods in health related action research. *British Medical Journal, 320,* 178-181.

Mittlemark, M. (1990). Balancing the requirements of research and the needs of communities. In N. Bracht (Ed.), *Health promotion at the community level* (pp. 125-139). Newbury Park, CA: Sage.

Plough, A., & Olafson, F. (1994). Implementing the Boston healthy start initiative: A case study of community empowerment and public health. *Health Education Quarterly, 21*(2), 221-234.

Provincial Court of Alberta. (1999). *Order pursuant to section 220 of the environmental protection and enhancement act.* Edmonton, AB: Provincial Court of Alberta, Criminal Division.

Sink, D. (1996). Five obstacles to community-based collaboration and some thoughts on overcoming them. In C. Huxham (Ed.), *Creating the collaborative advantage* (pp. 101-109). London: Sage.

Smith, L. (1999). *Decolonizing methodologies: Research and indigenous peoples.* London: Zed Books.

Stoeker, R. (1999). Are academics irrelevant? Roles for scholars in participatory research. *American Behavioural Scientist, 42*(5), 840-855.

Susman, G., & Evered, R. (1978). An assessment of the scientific merits of action research. *Administrative Science Quarterly, 23,* 582-603.

Vakil, A. (1994). Of designs and disappointments: Some limits to participatory research in a third world context. *American Sociologist, 25*(3), 4-20.

Weijer, C., Goldsand, G., & Emanuel, E. (1999). Protecting communities in research: Current guidelines and limits of extrapolation. *Nature Genetics, 23*(3), 275-280.

Whyte, W. (1991). Comparing PR and action science. In W. Whyte (Ed.), *Participatory action research* (pp. 97-98). Newbury Park, CA: Sage.

Wilkinson, R. (1996). *Unhealthy societies: The afflictions of inequality.* London: Routledge.

IV

The Nature of Analysis
and Interpretation

Dialogue:

Confirming Evidence

MEADOWS: I am definitely interested in the area of replication, and I'd like to take on some writing in this area. I initially hoped I would have an abundance of literature that suggested various things about replication that I could argue and put forward from my perspective or your perspective. However, when you look in literature, you'll find that there's very little about replication in a qualitative area. After an extensive search, I think we found about 10 papers that mentioned replication of sorts and about 6 of which actually talk about replication. But quite often, they will say things such as "We're replicating a study in Boston of HIV patients," and that's it. There's nothing about the original study. There is no definition of what they are talking about when they use the word *replication;* there's no evidence, in fact, to show that they're replicating anything—it's just that they use the word. There are a couple of texts or collections talking about replication, but they quite often are from a quantitative perspective. And in fact, my richest source about replication is Jan Morse's chapter in this book. So it's sort of a sorry state of affairs and I've been looking for some help.

I was reading a recent proposal in which I sort of restated or resituated what I'm doing as part of my women's health study, the WHEALTH project. I wanted to describe it to people who will be reading my proposals in a way that would be understandable. I had to move from the way I talked about it previously—as a series of stages and phases that people just were unable to work their way through—to talking about a series of studies on various subpopulations of women's health. So I began to think that what I'm doing is actually replicating my study over and over again into subpopulations, but then again, reflecting back on what Jan wrote—a part of what would be said, I think, is "Naughty, naughty, you shouldn't be doing that."

MORSE: I would say it's not replication because you're doing it in this group, and you're doing it in this group for different cultures, and you're extending the study.

SWANSON: With Strauss, he had NIH-funded grants and a research team. So he collected data from a variety of sites, including hospitals, home care agencies, etc., using both formal and informal interviews and also participant observation. The analysis by the team was extensive and very comprehensive. Now, someone like Roberta Durham is very typical of our doctoral students who come out. She did a very small study. Anselm said, "Your first grounded theory study should be nothing more than interviews with about 20 participants, and it would be better if you also did participant observation; not everyone does that." So she interviewed 25 women, nearly all Caucasian and middle-upper-class women, and looked at how they managed preterm labor at home. She wasn't funded extensively, as this was her dissertation work. Once it was completed, she decided that she needed to do another study and decided to interview low-income African Americans, a high-risk population for preterm labor. So she went after that and found that the theory held; however, the conditions were vastly different because people had no support, and so forth. Now she's on sabbatical this year in Glasgow, Scotland, and she's doing a cross-cultural piece, looking at where it is with the health care system, how it's different. But can she afford to go out and do that huge monstrous thing? No. She's got to do it a piece at a time. Some people call that replication, some people don't.

MORSE: It's not replication. It's not, it's just not. It's extending your study. I definitely think it doesn't make any sense to replicate. If someone else has done the study properly, because it's good, it should hold. On the other hand, if you have some reason to suspect there's something wrong with the findings of the study, then that's justification for you to do another study.

MEADOWS: But what about different cultures, different health care systems?

MORSE: You can't just have a conglomerate of patients in your sample. Quality of studies is quite important: they have a few blacks and a few

Hispanics, and qualitative research does not work there. If you believe in culture, you have to saturate your sample to capture cultural differences. Some studies in journals have nine whites and one Hispanic—I don't even know how they pick their sample. So we have problems with major funding organizations. NIH, for instance, requires through their minorities' regulations that you include minorities. So if you are putting in for a major grant, you have to have separate studies for different cultural groups.

SWANSON: Anselm [Strauss] never reported demographics.

MORSE: I know, I know.

SWANSON: He said that it wasn't important.

KUZEL: You've clarified some of this, but I wanted to ask when this work is thought of as replication and when is it not replication. What is your kind of way of thinking about it, and how do you define the term?

MORSE: Well, if Lynn [Meadows] is in Calgary and does a study of breast cancer, and I see it and I think that it's a good study and I'm up here in Edmonton, there's no sense replicating because the population is more or less the same—the population, the disease, etc. If I did do the study, would it not be a replication? Why would I want to do it?

8

Constructing Evidence Within the Qualitative Project

LYNN M. MEADOWS
JANICE M. MORSE

The arguments centering on the semantics to ensure rigor and all it entails are becoming stale and unproductive. If a contribution to knowledge, evaluation of research, and education of the scientific world can be made by qualitative researchers by using traditional terms, we must now embrace that opportunity. In this chapter, we consider the critical issue in qualitative research: the rigor within and the resulting credentials of individual projects. We argue that each study should be an addition to existing knowledge through its contribution to theory, explanation of a phenomenon, or addition to methods used in qualitative inquiry. Ideally, one project should accomplish all these goals, but more often studies attain only one of these goals. But to truly qualify as a good and valuable piece of qualitative research, *it must do at least one* of these. Studies that are isolated from relevant literature, are questionable methodologically, and/or are based on faulty design and analysis *do not add to qualitative evidence.*

Indeed, at a workshop leading to this volume, the term *immature study* was used to describe studies that reflect work that has been done (and even published) but does not currently meet the criteria necessary to add to qualitative evidence. This chapter is targeted toward a discussion of techniques of internal validation that will add to the understanding of what constitutes rigor and thus is a contribution to qualitative evidence.

This chapter is written with full awareness of current and past debates regarding the uses of traditional techniques and nomenclature for establishing rigor in research, including reliability, validity, and validation. Leininger (1994) writes, "The importance of preserving and maintaining the purposes, goals, and philosophic assumptions of the qualitative research paradigm and of using qualitative research methods and criteria appropriate to the paradigm . . . [leads to the conclusion that] the use of quantitative criteria such as validity and reliability remains inappropriate for qualitative studies" (pp. 112-113). The rejection of orthodox nomenclature has been largely a North American habit. Researchers in the United Kingdom (e.g., Hammersley, 1995) and Europe (e.g., Kvale, 1989) have continued to use traditional terminology, including "reliability" and "validity." In 1999, however, Morse argued convincingly that by not using the traditional, quantitative evaluative criteria and terminology, we are losing ground in the world of evidence.

Maxwell (1992) discussed five types of understanding (i. e., validity) that may emerge from a qualitative study: (1) descriptive (what happened in specific situations), (2) interpretive (what it meant to the people involved), (3) theoretical (concepts and their relationships, used to explain actions and meanings), (4) generalizable (extension of findings to other persons or settings), and (5) evaluative (judgments of the worth or value of actions and meanings). Although our discussion is not grouped into those categories, they are useful reminders of the many facets addressed through qualitative research questions. Another useful discussion in the debate is the distinction between "validity" and "validation" in a qualitative research context. Validity is a static term and suggests the extent to which the research findings represent reality (Morse & Field, 1995, p. 244). Validation emphasizes "the way in which a judgement of the trustworthiness or goodness of a piece of research is a continuous process occurring within a community of researchers" (Angen, 2000, p. 387, following the example of Mishler, 1990). Kvale (1989) further clarifies the concept: "Validation becomes the issue of choosing among competing and falsifiable explanations" (p. 77). This then demands an examination of the use of standards used in quantitative research and their application to a project. The stance taken here is that for qualitative evidence to take its rightful place in the world of science, the criteria used for the evaluation of its merits must be made transparent. In using the terms *validity, validation,* and *verification,* we consider that we are building on past arguments and moving the discussion forward.

This chapter is organized according to three components of rigor inherent in the research process. First, we discuss strategies of verification or ways to ensure validity that are used in the process of conducting research. Next, we address the ways researchers may evaluate validity during the process of inquiry that are external to the strategies required for actually doing a project. Finally, we briefly examine the means to

TABLE 8.1 Components of Rigor

Terms	*Verification*	→	*Validation*	→	*Validity*
Process	Strategies internal to inquiry		Within project evaluation		Outcome
Means	Design Bracketing Saturation Methodological cohesion		Inter-rater reliability Member →checks Audit trail Computer-assisted analysis		Trustworthiness
Source	Investigators		Investigators		External judges and standards

ensure that standards of validity of the completed project have been achieved (which, of course, is the goal of the researcher for the project itself) and standards used by external evaluators. This topic is addressed further in Chapter 9. Strategies for verification, evaluation of validity, and determining if the project as a whole is valid are listed in Table 8.1.

Strategies for Verification

Strategies of verification are those techniques that contribute to the validity of a project and are implemented in the actual research process. Even though these techniques are discussed separately and sequentially here, it is vital to acknowledge that qualitative research is iterative, not linear. Therefore, good studies use design and implementation processes that move back and forth between recruitment, sampling, data collection, analysis, and back again, and constantly validate the nature and progress of the process and results. In that way, data are checked in a systematic way, focus is not lost, the "fit" and "work" of the analysis and interpretation are monitored, and the internal validity of a project is consistently and stringently monitored. The result is a study that adds to our substantive knowledge, honors those whose experiences and time were contributed, and is worthy of publication. Verification strategies complement each other, so that evidence incrementally creates a valid project. *Incremental evidence* refers to the compounding of evidence achieved by verification. Many of the within-project techniques to ensure verification of findings are standard methods used to control the threats to validity and to ensure reliability. We discuss several of these techniques: using literature reviews, developing study design, bracketing, adequate and appropriate sampling, and ensuring methodological coherence.

Situating the Project: The Literature Review

It has been endlessly repeated that qualitative research is conducted when "little is known about the topic." This merely means that a study being targeted in the planned project has not been conducted, that few related studies were identified in the literature search, or that they are somewhat scarce. Formal knowledge is incrementally built. A research project does not exist in isolation. Even when conducting a one-shot project, the researchers are standing on the shoulders of giants and fitting their projects into a battery of published studies conducted by others. With luck, these single projects add a little new knowledge to the topic as a whole and to the general field of inquiry.

Study designs start with a literature review to explore what is currently known or not known about the topic or question under consideration.[1] Looking "educated" (Giorgi, 1986) is necessary. When lacunae are identified, the existing knowledge is temporarily put on hold in the researcher's mind while the data needed for the current study are collected, analyzed, and interpreted. Knowledge acquired from libraries or one's own experience is used to compare and contrast developing categories. Rather than to guide inquiry, it is used to inform the research so the researcher recognizes, compares, and contrasts one's own developing knowledge with what is already known.

Project Design

In qualitative research, as in other approaches, careful study design is a vital part of ensuring a good and rigorous outcome. The base is set on knowledge of the literature and refinement of the topic or phenomenon under inquiry in order to be able to focus the design on methods that will result in good and adequate data to answer the researcher's question or build his or her theory. Even when acknowledging the existing debate on purists' approaches to methods (e.g., grounded theory, phenomenology, ethnography, hermeneutics) or those that blend underlying philosophies and accompanying techniques for data collection, analysis, and interpretation, it is necessary to make decisions that do not violate the methods and that follow guidelines in a systematic way.

Regardless of the approach taken, consistency and clear explanation are the key to a good study design that provides a precise template for the study team to follow and later document for other researchers and reviewers. For example, grounded theory would be designed so that the process of seeking preventive screening can be captured, and the appropriate iterative procedures are undertaken through sampling, data collection, coding, and additional interviews. A second example: A semi-structured interview guide is used, recognizing that data are analyzed at the end of data collection. The researcher would not suggest that data analysis be further guided by theoretical sampling. The important point here is to maintain the integrity of the approach being used: If observation, document analysis, and interviews are being used, the purpose should be clear in the study design. Snapshot observations will not likely reveal a process; cultural beliefs and views will not likely be "discovered" from three interviews; a period of fieldwork will be essential.

Study design constitutes the plan for a project from beginning to end. However, it is not written in stone: The essence of naturalistic inquiry implies that we are working with real people in the everyday world, and all the nuances that occur in the research setting cannot be anticipated. If something does not work, and the necessary data are not being obtained, then strategies should be changed. Even the best design can face challenges at the implementation stages. These realities need not compromise the project, but they must be acknowledged and resolved. Sometimes they stall the project; sometimes a wonderful serendipity ensues. But this must be monitored and documented. Nevertheless, in order to maintain integrity of the project and demonstrate why design changes were made, there must be an initial study design, one based on clear knowledge of the point of the project and the path to be followed to its completion.

Bracketing

We have been taught not to contaminate our minds with the information obtained from others' research when we use qualitative methods. However, this does not mean that the investigator can approach the topic innocently, ignoring what is known about the topic and the results of others' research. Neither does it mean that the investigator is somehow expected to expunge this information from her or his consciousness. Bracketing means that the information learned about prior work is simply put on hold and is not used as a framework or conceptual scheme for the proposed study or observations. But it does provide an impetus for the ongoing inquiry—wheels need not be reinvented. It provides a comparative template to show the researcher what is the same and what is new in the process of inquiry, and it does provide a context in which to compare and to place results.

This is an important point, because some investigators have recommended that researchers need not bother going to the library before beginning a project (for example, see Glaser, 1998). Rather, they suggest that the library should be consulted later in the data collection, once the researcher "knows what is going on." The lesson here is that on every topic, a researcher will find information that is relevant to this topic and to the population. It means that when the study is completed and published, these findings will eventually find their place in the greater scheme of knowledge in the library, as it is discussed in a later chapter. This is only possible, however, when a study is done by researchers familiar with relevant literature and design—situated securely in knowledge that currently exists.

We cannot emphasize enough that a good researcher learns all there is to know before beginning inquiry. He or she systematically places that knowledge aside where it can be retrieved as necessary and uses it as a comparative template, something to test the emerging data and categories.

Sampling

Within each study, the process of qualitative inquiry proceeds in two ways: through replication and confirmation. Depending on the project design, the replication of data is described as "theoretical saturation," when theory generation is the goal, or "sampling to redundancy," when it is not. Data collection and analysis proceed until the researcher has collected adequate data—data from different participants, various contexts, and various circumstances and situations—that are similar and fit within the same category.[2] The type of purposive sampling (Patton, 1987) used in the project is part of the decision making for the study design. Techniques such as maximum variation (to get at as many aspects of a phenomenon as possible), homogenous sampling (that allows the researcher to "control" a condition, experience, or characteristic), or snowballing (participants identify others to be sampled) all have their own rationale and purpose (Kuzel, 1999; Kuzel & Like, 1991; Patton, 1987; Sandelowski, 1993). Again, making this process transparent and making it a component of design are part of the process of within-project validation.

Margaret Mead noted that the cardinal sign of saturation is that the investigator is bored. Once saturated, data collection for that category ceases unless the category itself is reanalyzed into subcategories. In this case, each subcategory should contain enough data to make it rich and descriptive. Although investigators cannot predict how many participants are required in a study to obtain saturation, the number depends on the scope of the study (hence the breadth of the interviews), the quality of the interviews and the appropriateness of participant selection, and the analytically driven style of data collection and analysis. In brief, the narrower the scope of the study, the fewer interviews required to reach saturation. High-quality interviews are obtained from "good" participants (i.e., those who have experience relevant to the topic, are articulate, and willing to report that experience and reflect on it) and analytically driven inquiry. Analytically driven inquiry is well paced and drives data collection. There is a synchrony between data collection and analysis; the investigator asks analytic questions of the data and actively (rather than passively) sorts data. In this way, step-by-step, saturation is deliberately sought, with data confirming pieces previously collected or pointing the investigator to new areas of data collection. Categories that are "thin" or inadequate become the focus of deliberate data collection until they are also saturated. The identification of negative cases allows for comparison and the expansion of the domain to include all variations, and in turn each of these negative cases is verified and saturated. Thus, qualitative inquiry *is verified during the process of theory construction,* both vertically by replication and laterally for completeness of topic.

Methodological Coherence

Methodological coherence is the adherence to the assumptions and consequently to the strategies within each particular method. Thus, at the most basic level, sampling strategies and indices for saturation must fit the particular method used. So must coding techniques and other components of the research process. One would not expect to find data collection analysis synchronic with semistructured interviews, where data are analyzed all at once; one would expect to find a basic social process (an analytic goal of grounded theory) in ethnography, and so forth.

Validation

Techniques that help in evaluating validity provide assurance to investigators that the study in progress is sound. Although there is utility in this assessment process, there is also a need for wise use: These techniques do not substitute for good enquiry and may, in fact, be unnecessary if enquiry is done properly. If used in a mechanical fashion, they may inhibit the development of a strong and creative study, thereby paradoxically weakening the very study they are expected to strengthen and creating a false sense of confidence in the project on the part of the researcher. The key to productive use of these techniques is a good understanding of their appropriate use as well as their limitations. We discuss here using multiple methods within the project, inter-rater reliability, computer-assisted data analysis, member checks, audit trails, and incremental evidence.

Using Multiple Methods

The intricacies of using multiple methods within one project provide both challenges and opportunities to researchers. The next chapter talks about triangulation of projects (not to be confused with using multiple methods to inform a single project). Within a project, the use of multiple methods can entail collecting data in a variety of ways (e.g., observations and interviews), combining types of data (e.g., unstructured interview and closed-ended survey data), combining analytic approaches (e.g., constant comparison, immersion/crystallization, matrices, manual analysis, and computer-assisted analysis), and/or analyzing the same data with two different methodological approaches (e.g., grounded theory and ethnography). The purpose of using multiple methods is to enrich the study, to provide as much data as possible to inform the question, and to do as thorough and complete an analysis as possible. Not every study design needs or dictates the use of multiple methods. Those that do have an added challenge of integrating the complementary components into a cogent and valid whole. Key questions to consider when combining methods are what each component contributes toward answering the central question of the project, if the multiple methods being used are appropriate, and how they fit together. The right blend can certainly enhance a study, but the wrong blend can discredit the project and undermine other efforts to ensure rigor and valid outcomes.

Inter-Rater Reliability

The term "inter-rater reliability" is often used to describe the advantage and replicability of coding and interpretation when more than one person is doing it. In qualitative inquiry, the use of multiple coders must be approached with caution, for multiple coders may not have the same theoretical background, knowledge of the literature, or intimate knowledge of the interviews and time to reflect on them as has the principal investigator. With unstructured interviews, decisions about the interpretive coding process may be based on the knowledge of the whole—knowledge that a second coder may not have had the opportunity to acquire. Therefore, in the process of coding unstructured interviews, it is unlikely that two coders will proceed in the same way. On the other hand, when coding semistructured interviews where questions have been asked in the same way consistently, coding may be constructed by several coders, provided that coders have been trained and features have been well defined. Miles and Huberman (1994) use the term *check-coding* (p. 64) to describe two researchers coding the same data set and discussing their initial difficulties, as well as confirming the meanings seen in the data.

Using Computer-Assisted Data Analysis

Software programs that assist in the process of data summary, analysis, and interpretation are relatively new to qualitative research. These tools can be invaluable to the process and can expedite the completion of a rigorous project. However, beware of the assertion that "the data were analyzed using..." followed by the name of a program as if that in itself ensured rigor and the software program itself carried a pedigree for qualitative research excellence (Meadows & Dohendorf, 1999). The data are analyzed only and always by the researcher. It is the expertise and experience of the researcher/research team that ensures validation—not the use of a program that can produce models, colors, summaries, sorts, and the like. A computer program does only what it is told to by a researcher. Poor design, sloppy implementation, and inadequate sampling cannot be saved by complex tools available through computer programs or theoretical models generated graphically by these programs. Validation is enhanced by the use of these programs, but not ensured by it.

Member Checks

Member checks are traditionally seen as an opportunity to gain insight and share opinions, reactions, and clarifications (Borkan, 1999). Participants can also provide occasional additions to insight/interpretation and confirm interpretation by the research team (Crabtree & Miller, 1999). Member checks are a useful tool for reflection by participants or key informants on the work done by the researcher as one source of information on the topic. However, blind adherence to and faith in member checks to validate the work that is the responsibility of the research team does not truly enhance the validation process. Indeed, one may find it difficult to imagine that the opinion of a single participant outweighs the expertise of the researcher/analyst (Morse, 1998). Member checks provide an opportunity for the researcher to examine summaries of interpretations, open them to lay scrutiny, and reexamine their analytic process as one of the many steps in the research process. However, dependence on lay validity in the guise of member checks can keep data shallow and detract from the project.

Audit Trails

An audit trail is a "documentation of the researcher's decisions, choices and insights," including subjective interpretations; it "assists the researcher in demonstrating theoretical rigor" (Morse & Field, 1995, p. 147). Basic types of documentation for the audit trail are contextual documentation, methodological documentation, analytic documentation, and personal response documentation (Rodgers &

Cowles, 1993). Although there is a history of using audit trails as a criterion of rigor in qualitative research (Halpern, 1983; Lincoln & Guba, 1985; Rodgers & Cowles, 1993), the development of the field of qualitative research has now reached a stage where this record of the research process is likely most useful in the context for which it is named: an audit of the project.

As a standard practice of good research and, in particular, of qualitative research, a record of meetings, changes to protocols, sampling and recruitment strategies, method of transcription (e.g., verbatim or not), and the evolution of coding and interpretation are routinely kept. Therefore, while an audit trail is usually a de facto part of the study, it is not explicitly put forward for examination as the project is disseminated. The likely exceptions to that occur during the defense of graduate theses or in the teaching process with people new to qualitative research. An audit trail is primarily used in the literature not as a criterion but as a technique (along with other techniques such as member checks, peer debriefing, triangulation, etc.) that should be employed to safeguard against investigator bias and help to ensure that the criteria have been met.

Validity

The process of within-project validation begins as a project is conceptualized and developed and continues throughout the research process. It was argued earlier that achieving validity in a project is also a process, one that begins with strategies internal to the project (e.g., verification), then continues with those that are part of the process of evaluation within the project. Validity is one of the outcome goals of a project. It is achieved through the process of demonstrating trustworthiness, which in turn addresses both reliability and validity. Reliability traditionally implies that some research finding can be replicated or repeated, that is, that an outcome or findings are not unique. Validity implies that the findings are real and that there is little or no reason to doubt their truth. Taken together, characteristics of validity, reliability, and evidence of a study or project completed under conditions of rigor establish the trustworthiness of a project. Trustworthiness in turn is open to scrutiny external to the project researcher, and in some forms of dissemination should serve as a guide for others seeking to do quality qualitative research. The key to this sanctioned external evaluation is the presentation of evidence that supports the project's conclusions.

Incremental evidence is the systematic layering of evidence. It implies that as the analysis progresses and data pieces and categories begin to fit together either laterally or vertically within the project, the researcher becomes increasingly more certain of the rigor of the conclusions. Incremental evidence is compiled through the process of asking analytic questions about data (thus ensuring the acceptance of the most reasonable explanation), bracketing of what is known from the previous literature (but then reflecting on it), saturation of data (or the constant verification of data), and seeking negative cases (to ensure maximum variation and a complete description of the domain of inquiry). This process may have to address the challenge of negative cases or examples that do not fit the findings but help clarify the limits and meaning of the primary pattern (Patton, 1987, p. 160). In some cases, the research will have to verify findings by going back to data and exploring parameters and circumstances under which the finding holds true. New leads or original findings need to be verified, situations where the researcher decides to follow her or his nose must be examined for methodological cohesion, and techniques for validation must be routinely implemented and evaluated. Finally, as results and interpretations are confirmed and their parameters assessed and/or theories tested, the literature must be revisited. This ensures that the researchers take the final step in the within-project validation to test assertions that a contribution is being made to qualitative evidence through a mature project that meets established standards of rigor in research. The most significant feature that makes qualitative research a systematic and rigorous process is the iterative data collection and data analysis. Inherent in this process is the cognitive work of inquiry, which is the essence of analysis and the part that is least discussed. It is not passive but hard work, and not haphazard but systematic.

Conclusions

Good qualitative research is good science: It is rigorous and attends to traditional indicators and measures of excellence such as reliability and validity—even in spite of ongoing debates about the place of "quantitative benchmarks" in qualitative research. People involved in good qualitative research recognize that adhering to these standards is not a retreat to quantitative traditions but a necessary step in becoming part of the cumulative body of scientific knowledge from wherever the research project lies along the continuum of scientific methods. Step-by-step, qualitative research is verified in the process of development against the phenomenon itself and tested by implementation and by processes of comparison with the results of others. These systems of built-in checks and balances prevent qualitative inquiry from producing fictitious and erroneous results and provide us with a confidence that far exceeds mere opinion.

Our products provide structures, causal explanations, and explanatory or predictive theory that make sense of diverse and chaotic observations. Such explanations are not developed numerically—this numerical certainty, usually considered hard evidence, is not usually useful to the qualitative researcher. Not having the certainty of numerical indices of reliability and validity, qualitative researchers must rely on other mechanisms to ensure that the end result of their research is correct, reliable, relevant, succinct, intelligible, and useful. The standards of verification, validation, and validity are key components of the process of enhancing validity in qualitative research and adding to the established body of scientific knowledge.

Notes

1. We disagree with the recommendation by Glaser (1998) that this is neither reductionist nor a threat to the use of induction if the investigator brackets the information; moreover, according to him, it expedites inquiry.

2. One common error is to consider data saturated when only a few participants have been interviewed, sometimes when each has been interviewed multiple times. Saturation of data obtained from few informants is not saturation. Rather, using techniques of following negative cases proximate saturation: It is saturation of data that is important.

References

Angen, M. J. (2000). Evaluating interpretive inquiry: Reviewing the validity debate and opening the dialogue. *Qualitative Health Research, 10*(3), 378-395.

Borkan, J. (1999). Immersion/Crystallization. In B. F. Crabtree & W. L. Miller (Eds.), *Doing qualitative research* (2nd ed., pp. 179-194). Thousand Oaks, CA: Sage.

Crabtree, B. F., & Miller, W. L. (1999). Researching practice settings: A case study approach. In B. F. Crabtree & W. L. Miller (Eds.), *Doing qualitative research* (2nd ed., pp. 293-312). Thousand Oaks, CA: Sage.

Giorgi, A. (1986). Theoretical justification for the use of descriptions. In P. Ashworth, A. Giorgi, & A. de Konig (Eds.), *Qualitative research in psychology* (pp. 3-22). Pittsburgh, PA: Duquesne University Press.

Glaser, B. G. (1998). *Doing grounded theory: Ideas and discussions.* Mill Valley, CA: Sociology Press.

Halpern, E. S. (1983). *Auditing naturalistic inquiries: The development and application of a model.* Unpublished doctoral dissertation, Indiana University.

Hammersley, M. (1995). Theory and evidence in qualitative research. *Quality and Quantity, 29,* 55-66.

Kuzel, A. (1999). Sampling in qualitative enquiry. In B. F. Crabtree & W. L. Miller (Eds.), *Doing qualitative research* (2nd ed., pp. 33-46). Thousand Oaks, CA: Sage.

Kuzel, A. J., & Like, R. C. (1991). Standards of trustworthiness for qualitative studies in primary care. In P. G. Norton, M. Stewart, F. Tudiver, M. J. Bass, & E. V. Dunn (Eds.), *Primary care research: Traditional and innovative approaches* (pp. 138-158). Newbury Park, CA: Sage.

Kvale, S. (1989). To validate is to question. In S. Kvale (Ed.), *Issues of validity in qualitative research* (pp. 73-92). Lund, Sweden: Student-litteratur.

Leininger, M. (1994). Evaluation criteria and critique of qualitative research studies. In J. M. Morse (Ed.), *Critical issues in qualitative research methods* (pp. 95-115). Thousand Oaks, CA: Sage.

Lincoln, Y. S., & Guba, E. G. (1985). *Naturalistic Inquiry.* Beverly Hills, CA: Sage.

Maxwell, J. A. (1992). Understanding and validity in qualitative research. *Harvard Educational Review, 62*(3), 279-300.

Meadows, L. M., & Dohendorf, D. (1999). Data management and interpretation using computers to assist. In B. F. Crabtree & W. L. Miller (Eds.), *Doing qualitative research* (2nd ed., pp. 195-220). Thousand Oaks, CA: Sage.

Miles, M. B., & Huberman, A. M. (1994). *Qualitative data analysis* (2nd ed.). Thousand Oaks, CA: Sage.

Mishler, E. G. (1990). Validation in inquiry-guided research: The role of exemplars in narrative studies. *Harvard Educational Review, 60,* 415-440.

Morse, J. M. (1998). Validity by committee. *Qualitative Health Research, 8*(4), 443-445.

Morse, J. M. (1999). Myth #93: Reliability and validity are not relevant to qualitative inquiry. *Qualitative Health Research, 9*(6), 717-718.

Morse, J. M., & Field, P. A. (1995). *Qualitative research methods for health professionals* (2nd ed.). Thousand Oaks, CA: Sage.

Patton, M. Q. (1987). *How to use qualitative methods in evaluation.* Newbury Park, CA: Sage.

Rodgers, B. L., & Cowles, K. V. (1993). The qualitative research audit trails: A complex collection of documentation. *Research in Nursing and Health, 16*(3), 219-226.

Sandelowski, M. (1993). Rigor or rigor mortis: The problem of rigor in qualitative research revisited. *Advances in Nursing Science, 16,* 1-8.

Dialogue:

Extending Findings to Practice

MORSE: The problem is that qualitative researchers are generating *theory*, and then they expect it to be implemented somewhere else. But all they have developed is a theory. And people say, "Well, qualitative research gives us insight." But that is not enough. They are not pushing their research far enough to get at implementation, because the strategies or interventions were incomplete [in the first study]. They have not enough to implement.

KUZEL: But people would not even label it as insightful unless it had a practical impact.

MORSE: That might be so. But the practical impact remains theoretical.

KUZEL: I am saying that I, as a practitioner, might appear to exhibit the same behaviors, but now I attach a different meaning or significance, or there is a different affect or experience in doing my work than there was before. This is important to me. Then it has had a practical impact. It does not have to be visible to the patients.

ESTABROOKS: I think Cochrane has a perspective that is quite limited in that regard. But if we look historically, that is how the ideology got built. They want to know the exactness of the intervention and how big it is. Not that that is not important, but that happens to be where they started and where the ideology got built from.

MADJAR: There is a message that needs to come through here, and that is that the process is still important. And that seems to be what is completely lost. The Cochrane approach misses out when it stresses that the only thing that is measurable is the outcome.

RAY: Process and context.

MADJAR: And the intervention and the outcome. And what happens in the middle is a black box that doesn't seem to matter. And I think that qualitative research has a tremendous strength in contributing to the understanding of the process. To patients the process matters.

A clinician who has a heart, who listens, and who understands may not get a different outcome from the patient's response to the antibiotic, but the patient is going to have a qualitatively different experience. Whether it is measurable or not, it still matters.

9

Qualitative Verification

Building Evidence by Extending Basic Findings

JANICE M. MORSE

In qualitative inquiry, how do we really *know* what we know? How can we be sure enough to make recommendations based on qualitative inquiry when *measurement* is disregarded? How *solid* is qualitative inquiry? How can we be *certain* when qualitative researchers dispute the very existence of an objective reality and base their research on perceptions, beliefs, and self-reports? These questions are the conundrum of granting agencies seeking to fund qualitative research; they are the enigma of qualitative researchers everywhere when their methods are challenged, and they are the bane of clinicians wanting to establish evidenced-based practice. In Chapter 8, Meadows and I explored strategies to ensure optimal rigor is developed during the conduct of the project. Although verification of qualitative inquiry takes place primarily when the project is being conducted, processes of verification also occur after the project has been completed.

In this chapter, I will explore strategies that continue to build evidence within a research program once the initial project is completed. My goal is to describe strategies that continue to contribute to the solidity of the research within a research program during processes of application and implementation and as the findings from the first project are incorporated into the literature or are used in meta-synthesis and meta-analysis. Exploring results that contradict or fail to confirm previous findings provide justification to continue inquiry and to determine under what contexts and conditions the previous results are supported or not supported.[1] Extending the findings to the level of implementation makes the results readily available for the practice arena and answers the "so what" questions. These are systems of built-in checks and balances that prevent qualitative inquiry from producing fictitious and fickle results and provide us with a confidence that far exceeds Cochrane's category of "mere opinion."

Thus, this chapter complements Chapter 5 on *standards* (goals for achieving rigor) and Chapter 8 on the means for achieving rigor within a research project. I maintain that qualitative research is not complete at the end of the initial project; basic findings may be extended to enhance the certainty of results as the project continues to be established as knowledge during the process in which the findings are implemented and transformed for clinical utilization. I will discuss how investigation continues as the findings are used and explain three major methods by which the results may be modified or expanded from the original study. First, investigation may continue *within the research program* by fitting projects together and by using different methods to examine different aspects of the original topic and techniques of methodological triangulation to fit the findings of these divergent studies together, thus enabling the development of a more comprehensive theory. Theory may also be built by linking concepts to develop a more comprehensive qualitatively derived theory. Second, as the results are incorporated into the literature, they become incorporated into a class of studies pertaining to a certain topic. Techniques of *meta-synthesis* or *meta-analysis* may be used to further expand the scope of the theory or to move it to a higher level of abstraction. And finally, we will explore why an initial project may not provide results developed adequately for implementation, thus requiring that the investigation continues, for instance, by implementing an intermediate step, such as *developing assessment guides* from a qualitatively derived theory before results can be used clinically. We will discuss *qualitative outcome analysis* (QOA)—how implementing the results of a study produces a new area for investigation and how, if the results support the original study, this provides new data that supplement and support the original model. These three methods, their definitions and outcomes, are summarized in Table 9.1.

Incremental evidence refers here to the compounding of evidence that occurs over multiple studies within a research program by means of the implementation of a study into the clinical area or the analysis of multiple studies. As the analysis progresses, data pieces and categories begin to fit together either laterally within the project or vertically as studies are completed and complement each other. It is through the systematic layering of evidence that the researcher becomes increasingly more certain and the study more powerful. Each of these pieces

TABLE 9.1 Incremental Evidence: Approaches, Methods, Definitions, and Examples of Outcomes for Extending Basic Findings

Approaches	Methods	Definitions	Examples of Outcomes
Developing a research program	Project fit	Examining two or more projects to determine a comprehensive perspective of a phenomenon	Increased understanding—when projects overlap, data should be consistent and verified
	Methodological triangulation	Conducting two or more complementary projects on the same topic, often using different methods	Results provide information from differing perspective or on different aspects, thus providing a more complete description or enabling a more comprehensive theory to be developed
	Theory construction	Exploring related concepts that parallel, transect, or link and, using qualitative inquiry, incorporating these concepts into the same theory	Development of a more comprehensive theory
Analyzing multiple projects	Meta-synthesis	Combining several similar qualitative theories into one; techniques such as "label soothing" are used	Coherent theory at the same level of analysis
	Meta-analysis	Utilizing and reanalyzing several qualitative studies with a similar focus to develop a new, higher-level theory	Theory at a higher level of abstraction and with greater scope, level of generalization, and explanatory power
Verifying by implementation	Developing assessment guides	Transforming research for clinical utilization, such as developing assessment guides	Provides the means for direct clinical application of qualitative theory
	Qualitative outcome analysis	Exploring and documenting the strategies used in the application of qualitative research, and exploring efficacy	Enables the inquiry to extend directly into the clinical arena and to develop and test intervention strategies

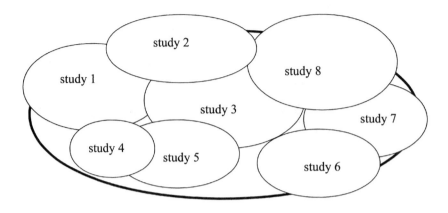

Figure 9.1.1 Descriptive Studies Conducted in Various Contexts, Addressing the Same Concept or Phenomenon

incrementally supports or builds onto the researcher's understanding of the phenomenon and provides a new or expanded perspective on the topic.

Developing a Research Program

Project Fit

What do I mean by projects "fitting together"? Different projects addressing the same topic may produce similar findings, with the concepts overlapping. Despite the fact that concepts may overlap, they may not be *exactly* the same, as they may have been conducted in different settings, with different participants, or under different conditions. Different investigators may have selected different concept names for similar concepts, and the studies may vary in scope. Figure 9.1.1 shows a number of descriptive studies using the same method addressing the same phenomenon (shown with the dark circle), and Figure 9.1.2 illustrates triangulation, when different methods have been used to elicit different perspectives of the same phenomenon.

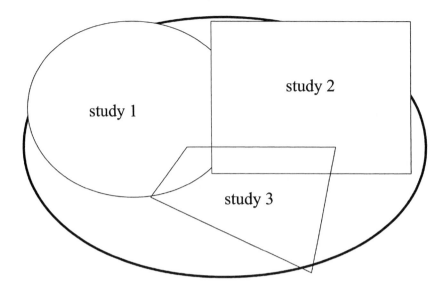

Figure 9.1.2 Triangulated Studies

However, when reading these similar studies, it may sometimes be clear that two studies overlap somewhat, thereby verifying each other in some respects. On the other hand, if these two projects butt, that is, fit with very little overlap, they may address adjacent characteristics of the phenomenon. As the number of studies addressing a certain topic increases, a concept or phenomenon becomes better understood, is perceived to be more pervasive or universal, and its complexity is revealed. The domain of the concept or phenomenon is covered as these studies "fit" together, ideally with little overlap or duplication. For instance, at present there are many studies on the experience of caregiving (see Figure 9.2): studies examining caregiving by spouses for persons with different diseases (e.g., Alzheimer's disease, AIDS, stroke, and so forth) that fit together on the *disease dimension*; studies examining caregiving in families with Alzheimer's or a stroke in different ethnic groups that fit together on a *provider dimension*; studies on caregiving for an infant or a disabled child (compared with caregiving for a spouse) fit together, informing us about *dimensions of different relationships* in caregiving. These studies provide us with information about *the landscape of*

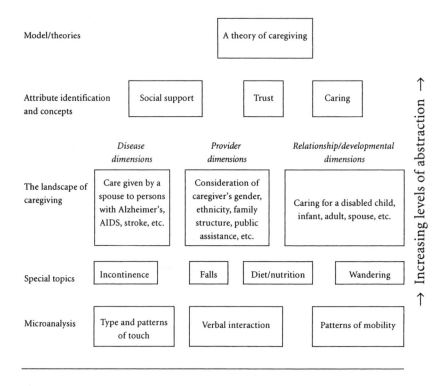

Figure 9.2 Levels and Dimensions of Research About Caregiving

caregiving. But we may also explore caregiving on a more microanalytic scale, examining the types of touch or types of support used by the caregiver during caregiving. Alternatively, we may explore caregiving laterally, examining the type of support needed by the caregiver; we may focus on a special topic in caregiving, such as incontinence management or the effects of wandering in a spouse with Alzheimer's disease; we may explore the concept of caregiving more abstractly, identifying the attributes of caregiving; or we may construct a model or a theory of caregiving that will apply to caregiving relationships in general. How these studies fit together is the prerogative of the researcher, guided by the research question or goal. The important point is that each study contributes in some way to the overall scheme or development of the knowledge base.

For the researcher, this broad perspective of completed research means that one's research program is a deliberately constructed agenda targeted toward a goal of understanding an area. For the Cochrane reviewer, because qualitative studies do not intentionally replicate, it means that all projects on a general topic must be retrieved to explore the phenomenon in its entirety. For the clinician, who wants to implement the research, it means that a cluster of studies should be pulled and explored and those selected for utilization implemented cautiously, perhaps in conjunction with qualitative evaluation, such as QOA. It means that it is inadequate to implement studies based solely using "evidence-based reviews": These summaries simply do not contain enough information for the researcher, the critic, or the clinician to analyze. They may simply be used to point the clinicians to studies that may possibly be clinically pertinent and useful.

Complementary Projects: Methodological Triangulation

Frequently, when the research topic is broad in scope or complex, more than one study must be conducted to explore the concept or phenomenon. These projects use different methods, sometimes different qualitative methods, or, quite often, a mixture of qualitative and quantitative methods. These *triangulated* projects require that the researcher *compare the results,* fitting them together like pieces of a puzzle, to obtain a comprehensive understanding of the phenomenon. These pieces, even if obtained from different research perspectives, verify each other, since they are complementary, perhaps by virtue of their overlap, and provide a more complete, broader understanding of the phenomenon.

Principles of Triangulation The triangulation of completed studies that address the same topic provide complementary perspectives of a phenomenon so that a more complete understanding is obtained (see Morse, 1991). These complementary perspectives verify each other, provide information about what is *not* known, and sometimes provide tension, or conflicting results, that must be resolved in future studies. The projects are studies complete in themselves, but the results enable several perspectives or levels of analysis to be obtained, thus confirming as well as broadening the overall scope of the expanded theory.

When proposing a triangulated study, the researcher must first be very aware of the dominant thrust of the inquiry: That is, he or she must consider if it is for discovery (i.e., induction) or for testing (i.e., deduction). If the thrust of the project is inductive, in which case the primary mode of inquiry is qualitative, the notation of QUAL indicates an inductive theoretical drive. If the project uses a theoretical framework and the primary mode of analysis is quantitative, then the theoretical drive is deductive and the notation of QUAN is used. Next, the researcher must indicate if the two projects will be conducted simultaneously or sequentially, with a plus sign (+) indicating simultaneity and an arrow (—>) indicating sequentiality. The possible forms of triangulated studies are the following:

- QUAL + qual (for two qualitative studies conducted simultaneously, with the qualitative study being dominant);
- QUAL + quan (for a simultaneously conducted qualitative and quantitative study providing supplemental findings in a qualitatively driven project);
- QUAL > quan (for conducting a qualitative study followed by a supplemental quantitative study in a qualitatively driven project);
- QUAN + qual (for simultaneously conducting a quantitative and a supplemental qualitative study in a quantitatively driven project); and
- QUAN —> qual (for conducting a quantitative study followed by a supplemental qualitative study in a quantitatively driven project).

Most important, note that it is the *results* of the projects that inform each other using the project as a whole. Because of this, each project is considered a separate entity until its completion. Unless the researcher is combining two *qualitative* projects, data are not shared. (However, as described later, provided the same assumptions for sampling are followed in each study, participants may participate in both studies.)

Let us consider the circumstances in which triangulation might be used. Sequential triangulation is used by and large when questions emerge or remain unanswered during the first study. QUAN→ qual triangulation is used when the quantitative study reveals surprising results or when it is clear that the instrument used has not been entirely satisfactory (e.g., when respondents have written comments in the margins, making it clear that the instrument did not capture the experience adequately). In this case, a separate qualitative sample should be drawn with participants who may or may not have participated in the first study, and this sample should be selected purposefully, which is congruent with qualitative sampling techniques. QUAL —>quan studies are conducted most commonly to test the qualitatively derived framework and to obtain normative data. Obviously, in this case, the qualitative sample is too small and does not meet the quantitative criteria of randomization; therefore, a new sample should be drawn from the population for the quantitative study.

For simultaneous triangulation, QUAL + quan is performed when it is necessary, for descriptive purposes, to quantify some aspect of the phenomena of interest. For example, it may be advantageous to administer an anxiety scale for documenting the exact level of anxiety of the participants, rather than just state that the participants were anxious. Therefore, the quantitative instrument may be administered to the qualitative sample *if* normative data are available for the interpretations of scores. If not, then it is necessary to obtain a separate, randomly selected sample, which, by chance, might include some of the qualitative participants.

QUAN + qual studies are conducted when some component of the study does not lend itself to one form of measurement. Again, participants included in the qualitative portion may or may not be participants in the quantitative component; nevertheless, the sample must be selected purposefully, according to the principles of qualitative inquiry.

Methodological triangulation, therefore, assists with the verification of inquiry by ensuring completeness of the research and confirmation of the parts that overlap in the deliberate ongoing inquiry. Since inquiry is deliberate, the key to success is an awareness of the thrust of the research (induction or deduction) and of the assumptions that underlie qualitative or quantitative research (which must not be violated), as well as careful attention to research design issues.

Theory Construction

Between Projects Researchers must always be aware of the completed work of other investigators, in particular those reported in the literature. Regular updating of bibliographies is essential for determining how one's study fits with the literature. Researchers must be able to assess how their project contributes to knowledge in general. But it is more than that. Researchers should be able to use their completed study as a template to assess similarities/differences between their study and those documented in the literature, which will help them determine the contribution of their study to knowledge in general. Similarities between their own findings and the work of others is indicative of validity. Differences between their study and the work of others may be due to error on their part or on the part of other investigators, differences in context or population, or other factors. The important task is to identify the differences and to try to account for them. Finally, comparison with the literature will provide information about which findings from the study *are new* and enable the investigator to address the significance of their study.

Concept Analysis Using the literature to analyze and develop a concept is an important type of verification that "pushes" knowledge forward (see Morse, 2000b). Initially, all the literature (both qualitative and quantitative) describing a certain concept and its definitions, both explicit and implicit, the characteristics or attributes of the concept, its boundaries, and the preconditions for outcomes is retrieved and summarized. Then the literature is sorted, if possible, into different schools or theoretical perspectives. Next, analytic questions derived from the literature as a whole are asked, using the literature as data.

Examples of such procedures are Hupcey's (1998a, 1998b) analysis of social support, which revealed logical inconsistencies between the definitions and the utilization of the concept in research. An analysis of caring (Morse, Bottorff, Neander, & Solberg, 1991; Morse, Solberg, Neander, Bottorff, & Johnson, 1990) revealed that although caring appears as a concept with a consistent meaning, it was used in five different ways, each with its own assumptions, antecedents, and outcomes. Caring was perceived to be a human trait, a moral trait, an affect, an interpersonal interaction, and a therapeutic intervention. Furthermore, caring could be manifest in multiple ways (Morse, Bottorff, Anderson, O'Brien, & Solberg, 1992): as first-level responses, such as sympathy, pity, consolation, compassion, commiseration, or as second-level (learned) responses, such as empathy or compathy.

Second-Order Integration Second-order integration is the linking of two related but different concepts (Morse & Penrod, 1999). Reality is complex, and one threat to validity is the simplistic depiction of complex processes. Rather than describe a complex process concept by concept, we need to be able to develop models and theories that will use linkages, transections, and interactions of related concepts.

In addition to increasing the validity of models by linking concepts, the process permits verification of the original concepts. The process of linking itself validates the original concepts and increases their utilization. For example, linking the concept of suffering with hope strengthens our understanding of both "coming out of suffering" and the role of hope. Furthermore, linking the two concepts forced the concept of uncertainty to the fore, further enriching the clinical usefulness of the findings from research.

Linking concepts is achieved by "opening" different concepts and examining the processes by which they evolved. Identifying the common processes in the two concepts provides the linkage points. Comparison of the processes, conceptual attributes, or categories in both concepts will reflect the interaction of the two concepts. Data should be referred to whenever possible, and if, by using this new lens, data appear thin, new data should be collected. Thus, using processes of fit, data from the two studies confirm the points of interception and attain understanding of the interaction and response of the two concepts. New or revised theoretical models may then be redeveloped and redrawn.

Analyzing Multiple Projects

Although *replication* per se is neither a useful nor sensible approach to qualitative inquiry, qualitative work is now becoming so commonplace that there are enough qualitative studies on one area to reanalyze these works as a whole. Using these completed works *as data* expands the context and focus of the original studies, thus producing a stronger and broader theory, which verifies and incrementally builds qualitative work.

Meta-Synthesis

Meta-synthesis is the examination of a collection of qualitative studies that have been published on a common area. For example, Jensen and Allen (1996) conducted a meta-synthesis of studies of the illness experience. Adequate studies of caregiving for the patient with Alzheimer's or the person with AIDS now exist, and one may wish to collect these studies and conduct a meta-synthesis. Referring again to Figure 9.2, a meta-synthesis could be conducted with each of the studies in "the landscape of caregiving" category, on a special topic, or on the specific concepts.

There can be problems with the meta-synthesis of studies: For instance, studies might have been developed using different methods and, as a result, may not easily "fit" together. For example, how does one fit grounded theory into a phenomenological study? As grounded theory depicts a process, use this as the framework and use the phenomenological study to illustrate a particular stage in the process. Of course, the best (and easiest) way to approach meta-synthesis is to select studies that share a common methodology.

Another problem with meta-synthesis is the practice of qualitative researchers to select labels for their categories from the data in their own study (and indeed this is the recommended practice). However, if the study produces a category that is the *same as* or similar to another investigator's category, qualitative researchers tend not to use the one already published by the first study but rather select their own emic label. This results in the emergence of multiple labels for the same categories or processes, confusion in the literature, and theoretical congestion (Morse, 2000a). Therefore, one of the important functions of meta-synthesis is that of "label smoothing" or standardizing a particular process or behavior. This, of course, must be done with care, so that variation and important detail are not lost and the emerging study is not just a simplification of the topic. If this occurs, then it is possible that meta-synthesis could be a source of invalidity. However, if done properly, the meta-synthesis will become a seminal article, widely referenced and widely used.

Meta-Analysis

Meta-analysis is similar to meta-synthesis except that the results in meta-analysis present a new theory, developed to a higher level of abstraction. For this reason, the literature selected may be broader than that selected for meta-synthesis. For instance, the literature on caregiving for AIDS patients may be combined with the literature on Alzheimer's patients and then with other caregiving literature (for example, on the topic of mothers caring for infants, chronically ill children, and so forth) to produce a general theory of caregiving. The process of developing the theory will "shake off" contextual features associated with the illness or the relationship, so that the essential nature and process of caregiving remains.

Referring to Figure 9.2 again, meta-analysis may include studies conducted with a *landscape of caregiving* topic, developing a category (such as social support or trust) to the conceptual level. Then these concepts may be used to develop a theory of caregiving. In this way, meta-analysis moves the study to a higher level of abstraction and to a theory that becomes broader in scope and more generalizable.

Again, the problems remain with selecting the methodological form of the emergent theory and determining the most appropriate labels for categories. These are researcher decisions that should be done wisely and with care. The final results will be an important contribution to the field—one that goes beyond the significance of the original studies. As qualitative research becomes more mainstream, it is probable that meta-analyses will become increasingly used, and this will be the means by which reviews are conducted in qualitative inquiry, equivalent to techniques of statistical meta-analysis in quantitative inquiry. However, there is one problem with conducting a meta-analysis of qualitative studies: At this time, there are very few research areas that have enough studies for an adequate meta-analysis.

Verification by Implementation

In qualitative inquiry, researchers frequently do not develop their studies to the level required for clinical application. Most studies produce findings that only "inform" or enlighten the clinician, enabling him or her to understand what is "going on," but not what to do about the problem. Therefore, these studies remain theoretical, providing at best a framework for interpreting practice or patient behavior rather than pragmatic interventions with outcomes that may be observed or measured. Furthermore, findings that remain at the basic level of inquiry are not usually suited for Cochrane reviews because they do not contain interventions per se.

Why do we have this reticence to develop research pragmatically? One part of the problem is that qualitative researchers have yet to develop a means for implementation of their research findings. This is probably the most unexplored part of the qualitative methodology and the part most urgently in need of development. Another (and related) part of the problem is that our system for funding research does not provide adequate budgets for the development of the study to the level of clinical application. When qualitative investigators submit proposals, they cannot promise or predict what the outcomes will be, let alone whether or not the findings will be suitable for implementation. Reapplication for continuation funding is a slow and clumsy process, and it is an inefficient way to obtain the relatively small amount of funding needed to complete the project—albeit the most significant part. We are at the point in our development where funding agencies need to take risks when funding qualitative researchers, as they do for our colleagues in the hard sciences, and provide qualitative researchers with enough funding to learn by trial and error, to develop new methods, and to continue the research as far as needed.

Verifying and Extending Findings Through Application

If the qualitative study has identified an intervention, then qualitative methods (perhaps in conjunction with quantitative measures) may be used to evaluate the outcomes, identify unanticipated outcomes, and assess the clinical feasibility of implementation. Control of bias, for instance, in the case of the researcher "seeing" expected results, may be addressed in part by using a researcher with less investment in a positive outcome. However, often qualitative findings are so pragmatic that even the outcomes are obvious. For instance, my own research into patient falls contains a qualitative component, using nonparticipant observation and observing how patients moved about in their hospital rooms (Morse, 1997). It was evident that hospital rooms were organized and constructed for the convenience of the staff (i.e., for the ease of moving gurneys [patient trolleys] rather than the ease of patient movement). There were no handrails or stable furniture for the patient to use as support between the bed and the bathroom. The patient lockers were on wheels, there were handrails only in the bathroom, and the distance between the bed and the bathroom was often more than 10 feet. The obvious intervention was to construct a path using handrails between the bed and the bathroom to assist with ambulation. Evaluation on the increased safety for patients could be assessed qualitatively by observing that patients no longer needed to "dive" for the doorway and quantitatively by measuring the reduction in falls. This was a qualitative finding that could be implemented, and the effectiveness of its implementation could be evaluated quantitatively.

Development of Assessment Guides

Transforming Results: Developing Useful Products I mentioned previously that qualitative researchers tend to cease investigation at the stage of theory development. As these studies explain but do not directly inform practice by identifying interventions, they are not considered optimally useful. One way to further develop the results is to transform the theory (for instance, grounded theory) into an assessment guide. Using such a guide, the clinician can determine or more easily locate the patient in the trajectory. This process thus transforms the theory into an assessment instrument.

When researchers have developed a grounded theory, they have usually developed an understanding of the process. At very best, this process "informs" practitioners; that is, it enlightens them as to what is going on, but it does not provide information about strategies on how to assist patients to move through the process itself. For example, I and Doberneck developed an understanding of the process of attaining hope from despair (Morse & Doberneck, 1995). By using each of the identified stages, this process became a question(s) for assessment, with indices used to determine whether or not each stage has been reached.

Despite the usefulness of such an assessment guide, the level of implementation is not complete without one further study. For any data collected where study is of the phenomenon itself and data about the *intervention(s)* have been identified serendipitously, one further step is required—that of QOA—to verify the implementation of the theory as an assessment guide, to identify strategies that might be used to facilitate or alter the trajectory as measured by the assessment guide, and to verify the use of the interventions themselves.

Verification via Ongoing Evaluation: QOA

Qualitative Outcome Analysis (QOA) (Morse & Penrod, 2000) verifies the results of a study by implementing and evaluating the model

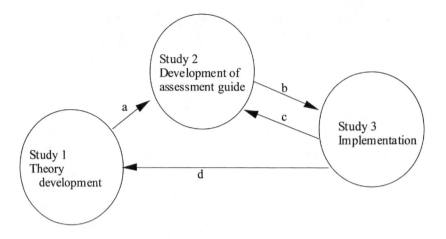

Figure 9.3 Interaction Relationship Between the Research and Implementation of Clinical Research

and interventions identified from prior studies as well as identifying and evaluating additional interventions. QOA uses elements of participatory action research and qualitative evaluation techniques. Briefly, when using QOA, the clinicians learn about the theoretical model and then learn how to use the assessment guide. They are prepared as data collectors in the techniques of observation, interviewing, and recording field notes. While using the assessment guide, they learn to record their own intervention strategies and their patients' responses, thus serving the dual role as an intervention and a researcher. Additional confirmation regarding the intervention is obtained from the patient and another nonparticipant observer. In this way, the intervention strategies are further identified and tested, and the original theory is verified.

Let us summarize this important process of verification by implementation. Developing the assessment guide is only one outcome of theory development; it is listed as *a* on Figure 9.3. Using QOA (Figure 9.3, pathway *b*) and the assessment guide may in turn result in the modification of the assessment guide (pathway *c*) or the theory itself (pathway *d*). This iterative process illustrates the important contribution that the informed utilization of results in the clinical area can make to research and to knowledge development in general.

Conclusions

In this chapter, I have illustrated how qualitative research is verified after the first project is completed by comparing the results of other studies using techniques of meta-synthesis and meta-analysis, by examining for overlap and fit, and by using processes of transformation, implementation, and utilization. All of these processes are techniques of validation, modification, and utilization. Although they are techniques that are primarily in the control of the researcher (or clinician-researcher teams), they are important in this volume because they are alternatives to the Cochrane review process of validation. As alternatives, they are equally important and reveal that clinicians may be confident of research findings without the necessity of meta-analysis or triple replication of studies.

Note

1. It is important to recall that qualitatively derived theories are not normally "tested" quantitatively following their completion, but rather are tested as they are constructed during the initial project itself. Neither are qualitative studies verified by replicating the initial research project, for such a replication is a threat to validity, as it violates the tenets of induction.

References

Hupcey, J. (1998a). Clarifying the social support theory-research linkage. *Journal of Advanced Nursing, 27,* 1231-1241.

Hupcey, J. E. (1998b). Social support: Assessing conceptual coherence. *Qualitative Health Research, 8*(3), 304-318.

Jensen, L. A., & Allen, M. N. (1996). Meta-synthesis of qualitative findings. *Qualitative Health Research, 6*(4), 553-541.

Morse, J. M. (1991). Approaches to qualitative-quantitative methodological triangulation. *Nursing Research, 40*(1), 120-123.

Morse, J. M. (1997). *Preventing patient falls.* Thousand Oaks, CA: Sage.

Morse, J. M. (2000a). Theoretical congestion. *Qualitative Health Research, 10*(6), 715-716.

Morse, J. M. (2000b). Exploring pragmatic utility: Concept analysis by critically appraising the literature. In B. Rodgers & K. Knafl (Eds.), *Concept development in nursing* (pp. 333-352). Philadelphia: W. B. Saunders.

Morse, J. M., Bottorff, J., Anderson, G., O'Brien, B., & Solberg, S. (1992). Beyond empathy: Expanding expressions of caring. *Journal of Advanced Nursing, 17,* 809-821.

Morse, J. M., Bottorff, J., Neander, W., & Solberg, S. (1991). Comparative analysis of the conceptualizations and theories of caring. *IMAGE: Journal of Nursing Scholarship, 23*(2), 119-126.

Morse, J. M., & Doberneck, B. M. (1995). Delineating the concept of hope. *IMAGE: Journal of Nursing Scholarship, 27*(4), 277-285.

Morse, J. M., & Penrod, J. (1999). Linking concepts of enduring, suffering, and hope. *IMAGE: Journal of Nursing Scholarship, 31*(2), 145-150.

Morse, J. M., & Penrod, J. (2000). Qualitative outcome analysis: Evaluating nursing interventions for complex clinical phenomena. *Journal of Nursing Scholarship, 32*(2), 125-130.

Morse, J. M., Solberg, S. M., Neander, W. L., Bottorff, J. L., & Johnson, J. L. (1990). Concepts of caring and caring as a concept. *Advances in Nursing Science, 13,* 1-14.

V

The Nature of Utilization

Dialogue:

Does It Make a Difference?

ESTABROOKS: One of the reasons we can't find examples of use is that people don't know about use, which is a separate problem from "Should it be used" or "How can it be used." Qualitative researchers should be held to the same standard as other researchers in terms of disseminating their work to appropriate target populations.

MADJAR: The key question in my mind is "Does qualitative research make a difference?" When one of my postgraduate students went back to report the findings of her study, she found that they had changed an important aspect of their practice.

OLSON: But did she actually write about that?

MADJAR: Well, you see, this is the problem. And I think that if other people read the work, they may change their practice, but nobody will know, and that is part of the problem as well. Part of what she described was the impact on the intensive care unit patients of having the ward round conducted just far enough from the bed that they could not be part of the conversation. And then people would walk away as a group, and the patient would still not know what was going on. So they stopped doing that, and now they discuss patients in the office, and when they come to the bedside, they talk with the patient.

OLSON: Where would you publish the impact of your research? The problem with it of course is . . . how would you even know? It might surface in audits. It wouldn't be a research study. If you tried to submit it to a research journal, somebody would say, "Did you have ethical clearance to collect these data?"

MORSE: Where does the researcher's responsibility stop? And often it's not the nurses' decision anyway. . . . It takes an administrative decree to make it happen.

10

The Nature of Outcomes

JANICE M. SWANSON

In this chapter, I discuss issues about the nature of outcomes. Despite the existence of a growing body of literature on outcomes, which is drawn largely from quantitative research and which is used to support the trend toward Evidence-Based Practice, I take an alternative position. That position accepts that

- quantitative outcomes, in and of themselves, are not the sole indicators of evidence to support practice;
- outcomes drawn from qualitative research may be used to support a trend toward the use of theory, generated from qualitative research, as legitimate evidence to support practice; and
- the use of evidence from quantitative studies and the use of theory from qualitative studies can be linked and mutually shaping.

This alternative position is supported through examination of issues such as the role and origins of theory. Using the example of experimental epidemiological studies, I further contend that there is a need for sociocultural solutions that call for use of outcomes as evidence for practice from quantitative studies and the use of theory from qualitative studies.

Outcomes

Webster (1979) defines outcome as "that which comes out of or results from something else; the issue; the result; the consequence" (p. 1270). Outcomes most often addressed in the literature are results from quantitative research that have been measured and have been verified through rigorous randomized control clinical trials (Gray, 1997).

However, the notion of outcomes or results from qualitative research and how outcomes may play a role in achieving health in a population is not discussed as often in the literature.

Quantitative Outcomes and Evidence-Based Practice

The trend toward Evidence-Based Practice stresses selecting outcomes of interventions based on the best evidence derived from research and other sources and documenting those outcomes. Much has been written about Evidence-Based Practice and measuring outcomes (Welch, 1997) in, for example, medicine (Huber, 1991) and nursing (Flynn, 1999; Hilton, 1997). Nursing developed the Omaha Classification System, which is a research-based system that includes a method for evaluating client outcomes. The Problem Rating Scale for Outcomes uses a Likert Scale to rate outcomes, such as knowledge, behavior, and status, following interventions in relation to identified problems (Martin, Leak, & Aden, 1992). In the present cost-conscious era in the delivery of health care, outcomes have been found to be increasingly useful for addressing issues that involve practice (Johnson, Hayslip, Sims, Smith, Keen, & Burrows-Hudson, 1995) and administration, such as client outcomes achieved through differentiated practice models (Anderko, Uscian, & Robertson, 1999) and cost-effectiveness (Cutler, 1996). Despite the increased attention to outcomes, the adoption of the best approaches to clinical practice is, however, often inadequate (Carruthers, 1999). The complexity of the challenge is enormous and can be seen, for example, in Ray and Mayan's reviews (see Chapter 3) of the many stakeholders on and off the scene and their competing agendas. The bottom line is that the evidence-based care given by practitioners must make a difference in the health of the individuals and the population for which care is provided. The dilemma rests in the best use of the evidence in a context-laden clinical scene where many highly varying circumstances and ideologies compete (for an overview, see Chapter 2).

Qualitative Outcomes and Evidence-Based Practice

The results or outcomes of qualitative research have been referred to in the health and medical literature in less overt ways.[1] Quantitative research is more likely to be used in medicine as a means for obtaining quantifiable answers to specific questions, whereas qualitative research is more likely to be used by some social scientists to understand human behavior (Peat, Toelle, & Nagy, 1998). Nevertheless, qualitative methods have been and are being used by a small but growing group of researchers in medicine, and many social scientists also employ quantitative methods. Traditionally, qualitative research outcomes have been seen as less concrete in application and use than have quantitative research outcomes. Qualitative research findings have typically been considered of value to practitioners insofar as they stimulate holistic thinking about common problems. These findings provide a contextual sea, rich in detail, that often present a social process encountered by people who are struggling to live with a common condition or disease (see Chapter 11, this volume; Swanson, Durham, & Albright, 1997). Initially, a qualitative study may have preceded a quantitative study, suggesting hypotheses that could then be tested quantitatively. Or a qualitative study may have followed puzzling or contradictory findings revealed by a quantitative study (see Chapter 9). Currently, the use of both methods simultaneously may lead to information necessary to address contemporary health problems. Rather than just measuring the characteristics of participants pre- and postintervention, a qualitative study may also be used to carry out program evaluation by describing the process(es) that occur as participants enter, go through, and exit from the black box of the intervention (Swanson & Chapman, 1994).

The following summary reports research that used both quantitative and qualitative research methodologies in the approach to managing an infectious disease, schistosomiasis, in two Nile Delta villages in Egypt.

Combining Methods to Manage an Infectious Disease: Schistosomiasis in Egypt

An example of an interdisciplinary study that combined the fields of epidemiology and anthropology is a study carried out by el Katsha and Watts (1997). In this 5-year study, the authors carried out an intervention in the study of schistosomiasis in two Nile Delta villages in Egypt. The development and use of theory in this study was critical to the outcome desired, that is, the control of schistosomiasis. This study points out the importance of combining these two approaches to research to create theoretically driven practice *and* Evidence-Based Practice.

In this study, the authors developed an interactive theoretical model using concentric circles extending outward from household as core, surrounded by village, surrounded by community, then district, then regional, and then national circles to show the discourses, viewpoints, and interests across all levels regarding the persistence of schistosomiasis in Nile Delta villages. This theoretical approach stands in stark contrast to the preexisting unified, top-down view of what ought to happen, as depicted by Van Ufford (1993).

The authors call into question the traditional approaches to disease control, which are often based on assumptions that the people conducting the research are in possession of the necessary knowledge whereas the people being studied are ignorant of the necessary knowledge. Instead, the authors state that "the situated practice of local people, and of health and other local staff involved in schistosomiasis control, should be recognized as knowledge which researchers need to take into account alongside their own culturally based scientific knowledge and their ignorance of local practice" (p. 847). Blaming people for risk behaviors without understanding how those behaviors are interpreted by the people might lead Western researchers to blame people for the wrong behaviors. Likewise, failure to seek treatment locally might not be perceived as wrong by the local people when the local health service is considered to be irrelevant to what they feel they need.

Schistosomiasis is a persistent major rural health problem, which has been linked to selected human behavior in close proximity to water resources such as in the areas of Egypt under irrigation; growing rural population and environmental problems, such as lack of provision for drainage and a high water table, have contributed to problems of schistosomiasis control in the Nile Delta (Watts & el Katsha, 1995). Schistosomiasis can be transmitted to humans in different ways, including exposure to the disease agent via water contact, water that has been contaminated by infected humans who have shed the disease agent, infective miracidia, and by the broad diffusion of the disease agent from one site to another through a mobile population (Watts, 1991).

In this study, the authors combined a social science approach to the study of human behavior, primarily anthropology, and a biomedical approach, primarily epidemiology. El Katsha and Watts (1997) describe a set of qualitative and quantitative research methods that were used in this interdisciplinary study. Qualitative research strategies used included observation and participant observation, structured discussion in households, in-depth interviews, and focus groups. Quantitative data collection methods were also used and included a baseline household census, laboratory confirmation of schistosomiasis using stool specimens, water and snail studies, and biological and chemical tests of water quality.

The two villages in the study are situated north of Cairo, are experiencing marked growth and rapid urbanization, and have canals that flow through the settlements. The study progression is presented below.

Quantitative research methods included traditional biostatistical, biomedical, and epidemiological approaches. A baseline census was conducted of the two villages to provide data necessary for the epidemiological investigations. A pilot study indicated that the strain of disease, *S. haemotobium,* had a prevalence rate of <1%; thus, further studies of incidence, prevalence, and reinfection were carried out for *S. mansouri* only. Stool specimens from the residents living in all the study houses were collected and analyzed, and cases that were positive were treated. Further testing during years 2 and 3 yielded reinfection and incidence rates. For 3 years, water and snail studies were carried out at known water contact sites in both villages. Water samples were collected, and biological and chemical tests were conducted.

Qualitative data collection methods were those commonly used in ethnographic fieldwork. Participant observation and structured discussion were carried out in households. Observation of water contact activity such as grain washing and in-depth interviews provided data of actual behavior rather than relying solely on self-reported behavior. Focus groups addressing water contact practices were held with schoolchildren, young farmers who worked in the fields, adult men and women, and local schoolteachers. In-depth interviews were conducted with key informants, both male and female teachers, village leaders, and health workers at local village levels as well as at the district and regional levels. In addition, the research team monitored selected activities, including diagnosis, treatment, and record keeping at a rural health center. The study incorporated female villagers and health and education staff from the local areas into all phases of the study to provide a gender-sensitive protocol in order to assess the needs and abilities of people in the traditional male-dominated village setting and to also contribute to a view that would differ from primarily male-oriented biomedical models.

The findings of the quantitative phase of the study were reported first. Following the baseline household census, a pilot study was conducted that showed that more than 99% of cases were *S. mansoni*. Stool specimens were collected from all residents in the sample houses, and positive cases were treated. In years 2 and 3, an epidemiological survey was conducted that documented the extent of the disease in the villages, both incidence and reinfection rates, and found that the prevalence of *S. mansouri* was 8% in one village and 25% in the other. Prevalence rates for the disease a year following treatment indicated that the disease transmission in both villages was ongoing. Water and snail studies were then carried out.

The findings of the qualitative portion of the study were then reported and revealed that despite knowing the risk of exposure to schistosomiasis, most villages that used the canals for domestic, agricultural, or recreational purposes did so because they thought they had few alternatives. For example, although major sources of contamination in both villages were found to be pipes that carried sewage from latrines into canals and sewage effluent that was dumped into canals, villagers felt they had good reasons to continue to use the canal. For example, grain was washed in the canal by women, standing waist-deep in the canal water, because it only took 2 hours, whereas washing grain at home took 2 days. Many washed clothes in the canal, especially large items such as bedding and mats, because they required large amounts of water, a practice that occurred even in households with piped-in water and drainage. Clothes were washed in the canals, including infants' clothes, which were soiled with fecal material, and utensils and dishes were also washed in the canals. Even when older women refrained from washing clothes or utensils in the canals, their younger daughters were likely to do so. As stated by one educated woman with both sewage links and water in her home, "We are like fish, if we leave the canal we will die" (el Katsha & Watts, 1997, p. 851). Teenage girls took pride in purposely washing utensils in the canal so that they could demonstrate their potential to become clever housewives (p. 851). Young children played and older children swam in the canals.

Economics also played a distinctive role. For example, some women again used the canals following the installation of sewer systems in their homes to lower the cost of water bills. The high cost of other amenities such as emptying a septic tank prevented women from washing at home, thus filling the tank needlessly. Increases in charges for water in rural areas had recently doubled at the time of the study, noticed by villagers because rates were no longer highly subsidized. In addition, an extra charge of 50% of the water bill was assessed households with a sewerage connection. Agriculture, which played an important part in the economy, also was an important factor in the spread of the disease, not only to farmers but to women and girls who frequently used the canals to wash vegetables.

The Ministry of Health in Egypt has offered free diagnostic services and treatment using a one-dose drug, praziquantel. These services were available not only for adults but also were offered to children in schools. The study identified problems in the delivery of health services using one of the rural health centers. First, health providers' knowledge of the disease was outdated, comparable to that of 20 years earlier. Furthermore, the staff members were screening for the wrong strain of schistosomiasis, that is, for *S. haemotobium,* rather than for the more prevalent strain, *S. mansouri.* Urine and stool specimens, necessary for diagnosis, were not routinely collected from all villagers visiting the health center, as required, unless the physician determined that the patient had certain signs and symptoms. Furthermore, the recording system was inadequate to provide follow-up to positive cases, and outreach and education activities for the community were not encouraged.

In keeping with the theoretical approach to the study, the study team investigated and found that integration of the various actions needed to control the disease was problematic due to the various authorities involved. Overall, the team reported that little horizontal integration occurred at the regional and district levels by the ministries of health, education, and irrigation. In turn, at the village level, little contact was made between the health units and the villagers and the village council, which impaired delivery of necessary local services such as water and sewerage systems, sewage evacuation, and collection of rubbish.

Yet, almost all villagers had heard of schistosomiasis. They lacked knowledge, however, of the symptoms of the most frequently found strain, *S. mansouri,* and thus did not seek treatment. Some villagers sought out alternative sources of treatment, for example, from private doctors or clinics, especially if they felt that their needs were not being responded to by the public clinics. The research team carried out an intervention as a result of the investigation. They trained the health center staff by updating their knowledge of the disease to improve their performance and to facilitate a more satisfactory protocol for diagnosing and providing treatment to schoolchildren.

Conclusions of the study indicate the gulf between the disease control strategies at the higher, official levels in the government and the reality of continuing disease transmission at the village level, exacerbated by the absence of a role for community groups or individuals at the local level. The authors recommend the development of effective control strategies via community participation as in a separate action research project carried out by selected members of the research team in other villages. In these other villages, the researchers acted as facilitators, encouraging the local people to take action by using their own knowledge and resources to set goals to improve village water supplies and removal of solid waste (el Katsha & Watts, 1993).

This theory-driven study reinforces the need for what the investigators state is "integrated research and implementation strategies" (el Katsha & Watts, 1997, p. 846).

Application at the Individual Level—Schistosomiasis Application of the findings of the study at the individual level do not address the problem of the spread of schistosomiasis in villages located along canals. Application of the findings of the study at the individual level were based on Evidence-Based Practice, that is, using epidemiological studies. The organism suspected of causing the outbreaks was identified, and a clinic model of practice with individuals was instituted to control the spread of the disease and to eliminate it. In fact, relatively accessible forms of screening and affordable, one-dose treatment were offered through the rural health centers. Prior to the initiation of the study, this model was applied and was not successful in containing the spread of the disease. During the initial phase of the study, this model was intensely studied and applied; indeed, people with the disease were identified and treated. Surveillance then established that despite the Evidence-Based Practice, the disease was continuing to spread. Flaws in this practice model based on epidemiological studies were identified during the study. For example, the authors report in their findings that the knowledge that the clinicians had about the disease was 20 years out-of-date. The clinicians were testing villagers for the wrong strain of schistosomiasis, thus failing to identify many cases in the village. In addition, the villagers were not seeking care at the rural health centers but were going elsewhere, seeking care from private sources. Even when villagers were screened for the proper strain of schistosomiasis and treated during the initial phase of the study, over time, the disease recurred among the population of villagers. Thus, the Evidence-Based Practice of individual clinical care was insufficient to treat the population for the disease.

Application at the Population Level—Schistosomiasis During the second fieldwork phase of the study, in which an ethnography was carried out, the investigators identified many sociocultural practices and beliefs among the population that involved water contact with infected sources that would lead to cases of the disease. Through study of the gulf between continuing disease transmission at the village level and disease control strategies at ever higher, official levels of government, the investigators were able to identify many gaps in policy and practice that had an impact on the local village people and resources to improve village water supplies and remove solid waste. The investigators developed an interactive theoretical model to show the discourses and viewpoints across all levels—from household to nation—regarding the continued presence of schistosomiasis in the delta villages. The investigators' findings show the importance of the situated practice of the villagers as knowledge that is needed to address the problem. This knowledge must be recognized as valid and necessary knowledge to control a local health problem, knowledge that must fully stand alongside scientific knowledge, which, if used alone to address a problem, may be culturally biased. Thus, the second phase of the study added the critical theoretical base, which led to the recommendation of theoretically driven practice in which community individuals and groups would have a role, using their own knowledge and resources, to set goals and carry out interventions to control the disease. This recommendation was applied at the population level through action research in other villages by the investigators (el Katsha & Watts, 1993).

Types of Qualitative Outcomes in Research

The outcomes of qualitative research are not variables that can be measured in clinical or other settings. Rather, the outcomes of qualitative research are varied and include theories, process(es), and categories or concepts. As stated by Glaser (1978), they are conceptual and thus are ideas that may have many indicators. These indicators are analyzed from the data, which include accounts of people's lives, observations, and so forth. Narratives are important because humans are largely bound by language and speech, which are used to convey our experience. In keeping with the diverse accounts of people's lives, these conceptual ideas are heavily contextualized and can handle much diversity. They are not finite but are transferable to other areas. Thus, these concepts can be integrated into a theory. The results or outcomes of qualitative research are myriad; one attempt to categorize them may be to view them as (a) instrumental, (b) pragmatic, and (c) theoretical.

Instrumental: A contrivance or means to elicit better quantitative research outcomes.

Qualitative research approaches have been used instrumentally, that is, as a means to elicit better quantitative research outcomes. Their instrumental use is valid because it brings a needed perspective to the development of better quantitative studies. For example, qualitative research may assist in identifying variables that can be investigated in a quantitative study, as in Black and Thompson's (1993) study of physicians' attitudes toward medical audit. Although British physicians' responses to surveys indicated they desired audit by peer review, audits were not forthcoming via observational reports. Interviews of the physicians and observation of clinical meetings resulted in 19 reasons why the physicians were unsupportive of audit, the majority of which had not been addressed in the previous quantitative study. This paved the way for subsequent quantitative work that could more realistically address the range of responses of the physicians to audits. In another example, qualitative approaches have led to better instrument development, for example, in a study developed to improve questionnaire modules for assessment of peripubertal breast cancer risk factors in adult Hispanic and Caucasian women (Hatch et al., 1999). Authentic phrases, items, and contexts from each ethnic group were integrated into questionnaires designed to elicit retrospective recall of a critical time period.

Pragmatic: Practical, matter-of-fact feedback, for example, about programs and interventions (pre, during, post), as well as other practical uses.

The pragmatic or practical outcomes of qualitative research approaches are evidenced in the area of formal program planning, program development, and program evaluation (Carey, 1997; Greene, 1994). For example, the complex or hidden nature of the problem that the program is supposed to address may be an important outcome of qualitative research, necessary for judicious program planning. Campbell and Williams (1999) use a case study approach in a study of HIV prevention efforts in the Southern African mining industry. The authors highlight, through analysis of the responses to HIV/AIDS by the various players in the mining sector, how the many and varied contextual factors must be addressed. These contextual factors underline the need for a broad social and developmental approach to HIV/AIDS rather than an approach that addresses the individual biomedical and behavioral level or HIV/AIDS as a human rights issue. An example of a new, more integrated approach to HIV management is suggested that uses a community approach and networking strategies at higher provincial and national levels.

Thus, as Rist (1994) has pointed out, the social construction of problems is particularly valuable as an outcome of qualitative research. Other areas of value include community and organizational receptivity to programs and program monitoring. As Rist (1994) states, "Social conditions do not remain static" (p. 552). Therefore, the very problems that the intervention was designed to address may change in nature over the course of the program; problems and conditions need to be studied using qualitative methods to answer such questions as "Is the program still appropriate? Are services being delivered? Changed? Why is there attrition? Low morale? What is the institution's capacity to deliver the program?" Both anticipated and unanticipated outcomes can be studied, such as backstage issues, staff conflicts, and turnover.

Health services research is another area in which examples of practical outcomes of qualitative research approaches exist. For example, Gulitz, Hernandez, and Kent (1998) used qualitative methods to identify both patient and provider barriers to breast and cervical cancer screening among older women. In another example, Cohen, Mason, Arsenie, Sargese, and Needham (1998) analyzed focus group data and report nurse practitioners' mixed reactions to managed care organizations, including their invisibility as legitimate providers in these MCOs. Caine and Kendrick (1997) report findings from a study in which clinical directorate managers were interviewed about their role in facilitating Evidence-Based Practice. In addition to the identification of factors such as budget, policies, and goals of the Trust, the authors found the managers failed to use their position and authority to further the use of Evidence-Based Practice in the clinical setting.

Theoretical: A vision or representation of reality.

The theoretical outcomes from qualitative research are the outcomes with perhaps the greatest potential. These types of studies, which generate theory, are few in the health care arena and are undervalued by the Evidence-Based Practice movement. Qualitative studies may generate theories or may generate concepts or categories, which are the building blocks of theories (Swanson, 1986). Common qualitative approaches to generating theory include grounded theory, a method developed by Glaser and Strauss (1967; Strauss & Corbin, 1990), which describes a social psychological process used to alleviate a social psychological problem. Thus, process or multiple processes may be the outcomes of this type of qualitative study. An example of a grounded theory study is Durham's (1999) study of the process of how women negotiate the restriction of activity placed on them by their physicians in the management of preterm labor. Although knowledgeable about the importance of bed rest to ensure a healthy full-term infant, the women were unable to carry out the demands of this regimen due to many situational imperatives occurring in their lives. They set and reset priorities on a daily basis to economize motion; they used three major strategies to manage the restriction of activity: *testing* (their limits), *cheating* (engaging in forbidden activity), and *piggy-backing* (doubling up a permissible activity, such as going to the bathroom, with a forbidden activity, such as sweeping the bathroom floor) (Durham, 1998). The substantive grounded theory, "negotiating activity restriction," is a description of the basic social process that women find they must go through to process the basic social problem placed on them by their physicians, that of restricting them during later pregnancy largely to bed rest. The theory suggests that women cannot take to their beds during a high-risk pregnancy. Rather, they enter a process of negotiating activity restriction as they set priorities to economize motion. The theory has implications for practitioners. As well, it calls into question traditional approaches to patient education and compliance in the management of preterm labor.

The Role of Theory

What role does theory play and why is it important? These questions are important to, among others, clinicians and policy makers as well as investigators. To answer these questions and to show their importance, it is necessary to discuss the role of theory.

Theory is derived from the Greek *theoria*, meaning "a looking at, contemplation, speculation, theory" (Webster, 1979, p. 1893); it is defined by Webster as "a mental viewing; contemplation . . . an idea or mental plan of the way to do something." Thus, it is an idea or vision of some reality. Much has been written about theory both by quantitative as well as by qualitative investigators (Morse, 1997). Kaplan (1964) notes that theories are symbolic constructions of reality. Morse (1997), using different words, states that "theory is not reality, but our *perception* or organization of reality, perhaps closely resembling reality, but *not* reality per se. It remains a representation of reality, malleable and modifiable" (p. 171).

How Do We Get Theory?

Morse clearly delineates the differences between quantitatively derived theory and qualitatively derived theory (Morse, 1997). According to Morse, quantitatively derived theory is derived from a process of reasoning and making deductions using available knowledge and one's experience prior to designing the research study. Data are then collected, which are used to test the theory, either supporting the theory or failing to support it. Although the theory is derived without the use of empirical data, previous research results may be used in the development of the theory. Qualitatively derived theory, on the other hand, is derived from empirical data through analytic procedures. One important distinction between the two is that quantitatively derived theory is formulated prior to the collection of data and is hypothetical, using conjecture, whereas qualitatively derived theory is formulated during the joint collection and analysis of data and is a representation of the empirical world. Prior assumptions held by the investigator and disciplinary differences, whether using quantitative or qualitative research methodology, nevertheless have great impact. For example, procedures for verification of hypotheses that are generated vary greatly between a quantitative and a qualitative study.

Uses of both quantitatively derived theory and qualitatively derived theory are different; they do different things. For example, quantitatively derived theory tends to adopt models that are mechanistic, to move more to systems, and to simplify for measurement. Quantitatively derived theory works very well, for example, with physiological data, whereas qualitatively derived theory works better, for example, with sociological data, for getting at the messiness of reality. Again, as stated by Madjar and Walton (Chapter 2, this volume), evidence used by the practitioner in a clinical or community setting most often requires more than physiological indices.

How Does One Get From Data to Theory?

Simply stated, there is a gap between data and theory that both quantitative and qualitative investigators must bridge. To bridge this gap, both types of investigators build a bridge, commonly called concepts (Burns & Grove, 1999). A concept describes and names a phenomenon. As Chenitz and Swanson (1986) state, in discussing Kaplan's work (1964), "Concepts are theoretical terms used to denote abstract material or phenomena and are related to the facts at the empirical level and to the abstract constructs about those facts at the theoretical level" (p. 4).

Quantitative investigators use a preselected concept that best fits the components of their quantitatively derived theory. Thus, these concepts must be highly structured and uniformly measure the phenomenon. Examples include valid and reliable measurement instruments such as questionnaires or physiological tests. These instruments measure elements that are called variables, that is, elements that are measurable and vary from one instance to another, that is, data. Burns and Grove (1999) give the example of palmar sweating as a variable. In their example, palmar sweating is a variable that may be used as an indicator of anxiety, a more abstract term that they label a concept. The concept, anxiety, is more abstract than the variable, palmar sweating. The variable, palmar sweating, is but one indicator of many of the variables that may be used to indicate the concept, anxiety.

Both quantitative and qualitative investigators develop their own concepts. Quantitative investigators, for example, may label a concept based on a group of similar variables that cluster together statistically in the analysis of numerical data. On the other hand, qualitative investigators may label a concept as it develops from the narrative data. This is done by coding the data and clustering similar codes and giving them a super-code name, or as in grounded theory, the super-code is called a category (Chenitz & Swanson, 1986; Glaser & Strauss, 1967; Strauss & Corbin, 1990). In using grounded theory, for example, data such as narrative data from interviews and field notes from observation or participant observation are analyzed through processes of analysis that use coding and categorizing to generate concepts (larger categories) that are the explanatory building blocks of the qualitatively derived theory. Types of coding may vary, and the reader is directed to texts on analysis pertaining to the particular type of qualitative research methodology in use. For example, in grounded theory, open coding usually commences by reading the narrative line by line and comparing incident with incident; codes are jotted over the incident or in the margin (Glaser & Strauss, 1967). Memos are written on the nature of the codes as they occur. Coding is a very involved process and includes asking questions of the data, making constant comparisons between incidents in the same interview or in different interviews, and naming as a category those codes that are alike. On the other hand, depending on the analyst's ability and the type and density of the data collected, open coding may begin with examining sentences or paragraphs or even examining entire documents rather than with examining data line by line.

Evidence-Based Medicine is an effort to ensure best practices and thereby improve the chances for best outcomes. Although measurable outcomes are derived from quantitative research, the many and varied incidents that occur in the life of an individual patient in the clinical setting or to a population in a community may preclude a fit with the selected measurable outcomes. The use of qualitative evidence in practice is an effort toward ensuring that practitioners provide health care that is conceptual. Thus, a practitioner can be flexible and apply ideas from qualitative research findings at a higher conceptual level to

TABLE 10.1　Components and Outcomes of Quantitatively and Qualitatively
　　　　　　　Derived Theory

	Data	Bridge	Theory
Quantitatively Derived Theory	Data	Measurable Concept(s)	Support or Fail to Support Preselected Theory
Qualitatively Derived Theory	Data	Codes [Categories]	Generated Theory

other conditions encountered in practice, such as varied contexts or changing conditions in clients' lives.

Evidence-Based Practice

Epidemiology

A major source of research to support Evidence-Based Practice is from epidemiological research. It is important to examine the nature of epidemiological research and its relationship to Evidence-Based Practice, to theory, and to the clinician, as well as current issues in epidemiology, in order to better understand epidemiology's relationship to qualitative research methodology.

As originally defined, *epidemiology* is "the study of the distribution and determinants of diseases and injuries in human populations" (Mausner & Kramer, 1985, p. 1). The discipline of epidemiology is the science of the distribution in the population of various states of health and how this distribution is affected by environmental conditions, lifestyles, and other factors. Once a causal agent of a particular disease or illness is identified, then public health officials can plan to prevent or control it. Most epidemiological research is disease oriented and focuses on abnormalities in structure and/or function of body systems or pathological states (Inhorn, 1995).

Uses of Epidemiology

Epidemiology has many uses. It can be used to determine the natural history of a disease, the etiology of a disease, the identification of risks and syndromes, the classification of disease, differential diagnoses, planning clinical treatment of individuals, surveillance of the health status of groups or populations, community diagnosis of health problems in a neighborhood or a community, planning and evaluation of health services for a community, and public health interventions at a population level. An example of a public health intervention at the population level is the removal from the market of Rely© brand superabsorbent tampons, which were linked to the occurrence of toxic shock syndrome, the subsequent monitoring of rates of the illness, and its drop in frequency in menstruating women (Morbidity and Mortality Weekly Reports, 1990).

Epidemiology and Evidence-Based Practice. Epidemiology is the discipline that has traditionally provided the scientific evidence for the practice of public health: "a science concerned with health events in human populations" (Valanis, 1992, p. 3). The definition of epidemiology is changing, however, and tends to reflect states of health as well as illness and stresses the role of epidemiology in providing data to ensure appropriate and timely interventions in clinical practice. For example, Valanis (1992) gives the following definition:

> Epidemiology is the study of the distribution of states of health and of the determinants of deviations from health in human populations. The purposes of modern epidemiology are to (1) identify the etiology of deviations from health, (2) provide the data necessary to prevent or control disease through public health intervention, and (3) provide data necessary to maximize the timing and effectiveness of clinical interventions. (p. 7)

Most notably, research that is used to guide interventions in practice is randomized clinical trials (RCTs), which are the products of epidemiological investigations.

Epidemiology and Theory The theoretical basis for the discipline of epidemiology includes the following axiom: "Disease does not distribute randomly in human populations" (Stallones, 1980, p. 80). Many epidemiological studies, however, appear to be atheoretical. Indeed, epidemiology has long been criticized for being atheoretical and empirically based with an emphasis on methods (Krieger, 1999; Smith, 1978). Smith, in 1978, called for an integration of frameworks in epidemiology to include the social, political, and biological. Krieger (1999) has noted that epidemiology has diverted its attention from concepts to methods and technique. Bhopal (1999) points out a key focus in an ongoing controversy about the role of epidemiology as "the increasing inability of epidemiology to solve socially based public health problems" (p. 1162). Susser and Susser (1996), responding to the concerns about lack of attention to concepts, called for a paradigm shift, for a new paradigm in which they vision a multilevel eco-epidemiology, which would be inclusive of a molecule to the macroenvironment. Yet Kuhn (1996), in a treatise on the philosophy of science, commented on the limits of a paradigm. He suggests that some of the more predominant problems identified by a scientific community might reside outside the realm of that scientific community based on solutions that would stem from use of other current methods. In effect, Kuhn suggests that a paradigm can insulate a scientific community from problems that are socially important but not reducible to conceptual terms and instruments supplied by the paradigm.

Theories, when named and used in epidemiological studies, such as the theory of reasoned action (Ajzen & Fishbein, 1980), are applied to individual behavior and are time and unit bound, examining the impact of social and demographic variables at a point in time. Exceptions, such as core group theory, a major concept in sexually transmitted disease (STD) epidemiology, has been applied to control selected SDTs in populations in selected countries with variable outcomes (Brunham, 1997). Both the theory of reasoned action and core group theory consist of preselected concepts; research is conducted that tests each theory and either supports the theory or fails to support it.

Epidemiology and the Clinician The focus of epidemiology differs from the focus of clinical practice. Although epidemiological research may evolve out of initial observations made in practice, clinical practice focuses on the individual and the health of the individual. The epidemiologist, however, focuses on the health of the group of which the individual is a member; this group may be small, as in a family, or this group may be large, as in a nation. Thus, the clinician describes the disease or condition in the individual, whereas the epidemiologist describes how a group of individuals or a population is affected by the disease or condition. Thus, epidemiology provides data for decision making to clinicians as well as to public health professionals. Traditionally, however, epidemiology is considered a basic science of public health, whereas basic sciences for medicine and other health professions such as nursing have traditionally included sciences such as anatomy, physiology, biochemistry, and genetics (Valanis, 1992).

Clinicians contribute heavily to the generation of epidemiological knowledge through careful clinical workups of their patients, by making astute observations, and by carrying out careful examinations and laboratory tests. In fact, clinicians are often critical to the first step in the epidemiological progression (see below), that is, case definition, as their routine contact with patients allows them to observe patterns of any abnormalities in patients and to raise questions. The identification of initial unusual cases have been the cornerstone of many epidemiological investigations, as in the case of Tourette's Syndrome and AIDS (Swanson, 1994), which have, among other outcomes, led to knowledge of the natural history of the disease and have directed efforts to control the disease. In turn, clinicians often use epidemiological knowledge in their practice not only to make a differential diagnosis but also in terms of choosing the best treatment, the duration of treatment, and in specifics such as the amount of medication to be prescribed. Furthermore, the identification of risk factors for specific diseases, such as breast cancer, a result of epidemiological investigations, can lead to preventive action initiated by the clinician on the part of patients, to screening, and to early diagnosis.

Issues in Epidemiology There are many issues in epidemiology. Among them is the focus of epidemiology: on the one hand, a narrow focus on the individual, whereas on the other hand, a very broad focus on the population, including the multiple contexts of major health problems, be they social or even political in nature. How knowledge from epidemiological studies is used by the clinician, then, is an important issue.

A common criticism of epidemiology by qualitative researchers is that it is reductionistic and positivistic (Inhorn, 1995). However, as Inhorn points out, epidemiology is population-based and is interested in a level of analysis far beyond that of the individual:

As the history of epidemiology shows, since its inception more than a century ago, epidemiology has considered the political-economic nature of numerous health problems, including the historical development of diseases rooted in ecologically disruptive development schemes. Thus, for at least some broad-minded epidemiologists, political-economic analyses of health problems are nothing new—despite their "reinvention" within the so-called "critical" social sciences. (p. 287)

Epidemiology: Public Health Specialty Versus Relationship to Biomedical Clinical Practice Epidemiology and its sister science, biostatistics, have long been considered the "statistical subdiscipline of biomedicine" (Inhorn, 1995, p. 286). Epidemiology, however, has long been associated with public health, traditionally is considered a public health specialty, and is taught in schools of public health at the graduate level. It is not routinely offered in schools of medicine, and physicians interested in public health, and especially international health, must receive additional training in epidemiology in a school of public health or elsewhere, such as the Centers for Disease Control and Prevention in Atlanta, Georgia. Furthermore, epidemiology involves very different models of disease and uses very distinct and different units of analysis and models of causality (Inhorn, 1995). In fact, problems arise when clinical medicine tries to translate epidemiological knowledge into clinical practice, because epidemiology is public health-based and population-focused research that does not involve intervention at the clinical level. Yet, the model of epidemiology, particularly in its progression to the gold standard, the RCT, is espoused by Sackett, Rosenberg, Gray, Haynes, and Richardson (1996) as the ultimate indicator of evidence for practice. On the other hand, epidemiology, because it has been given less emphasis by clinical medicine and may not be a core topic taught in medical schools, might not be easily understood by the clinical practitioner.

Perhaps one critical issue is to distinguish between epidemiology and public health. Savitz, Poole, and Miller (1999) point out the clear distinction between epidemiology and public health: "Epidemiology is a science; public health is a mission that is implemented through societal action" (p. 1158). The Institute of Medicine, Committee for the Study of the Future of Public Health (1988) has defined *public health* as "the fulfillment of society's interest in assuring the conditions in which people can be healthy" (p. 40). Thus, public health is the "organized community efforts aimed at the prevention of disease and promotion of health" (p. 41), and people engaged in public health are local, state, and federal health department personnel, policy makers, politicians, and other workers whose activity affects the health of the public (Savitz et al., 1999). Those in the field of public health draw on epidemiologic findings to carry out their mission. This becomes problematic when epidemiology fails to solve ongoing public health problems, as in the case of tobacco use. Savitz et al. (1999) point out that many public health efforts may be successful without research evidence, whereas, on the other hand, carefully designed public health efforts that are built on research evidence may fail. Public health is viewed as being "far more complex than merely applying epidemiology" (p. 1158). Although epidemiologists have a responsibility to study public health problems and to communicate their findings to public health workers, public health workers cannot base their actions solely on epidemiologic evidence. Despite strong epidemiologic evidence in an area, the lack of an immediate response by public health workers or no response at all may well be the rational response, due to the existence of a host of other considerations that have to be addressed, such as economic considerations, cultural differences, ethical concerns, and the political situation. The public health professional cannot address the problem alone. Complex problems demand complex answers; thus, many disciplines need to be involved to address the complexities of, for example, the problem of smoking. The public health worker accumulates knowledge from a vast array of sources, only one of which is epidemiology, and uses that knowledge to plan, implement, and evaluate public health programs and to be involved in setting and carrying out public health policies. The public health worker also needs information from a host of what Savitz et al. (1999) term the public health sciences. These include varied sciences such as anthropology, sociology, political science, economics, clinical medicine, toxicology, nutrition, sanitary engineering, industrial hygiene, policy analysis, risk assessment, and molecular biology. Although Savitz et al. believe it is wrong to mix the roles of scientist and activist, promoting a specific public health agenda, major public health problems have been addressed by scientists in the role of activists in the United States and in other countries. To feel that scientists only do science and that policy makers only make policies drawing on evidence from both scientific as well as nonscientific considerations limits the fact that the research act is a political statement;

it is a challenge of the nature of the status quo in a field of study. Thus, scientists are particularly sensitized to the nature of the problem and the complexities of the issues and, with activists and others, are in a position to advocate for necessary change.

Epidemiology and Qualitative Methods: Compatible or Incompatible?

Traditionally, epidemiology has been associated with number-crunching computer-based research methods, without human interaction, whereas qualitative research methods are highly interactive with people in natural settings. Most epidemiological studies, however, are observational rather than experimental. For example, historically, John Snow, an anesthesiologist and epidemiologist in the 19th century, was concerned about cholera, a major problem in England at the time (Rosen, 1958). Although nothing was known about the biology of the disease, using observations and recording of those observations, he demonstrated that removing the pump handle to a well that served as a resource for water from a polluted area of the Thames in London decreased the number of new cases of cholera. Thus, he demonstrated that cholera was a transmissible disease, caused by contaminated water, which was contrary to prevailing theory that it was caused by a miasm or cloud that hung low over the city.

The Progression of Epidemiological Studies

The progression of epidemiological studies is as follows:

1. Case study, in which an unusual condition is identified.
2. Descriptive epidemiology describes the distribution of selected health outcomes by person, place, and time (who, where, and when).
3. Analytical epidemiology searches for the determinants of identified patterns.
   A. Cross-sectional studies.
   B. Case-control studies using subject selection based on outcome status.

C. Cohort studies using subject selection based on variables of interest and followed over time to observe some health outcome.
  a) Retrospective studies using existing historical records such as medical record review.
  b) Prospective studies using subject selection and follow-up over time.
D. Experimental studies using interventions to test measures of prevention, treatment, policies, drugs, techniques, or materials.
  a) RCTs usually test the efficacy of a medical intervention (i.e., treatment) for disease in individual patients.
  b) RCTs usually test the efficacy of an educational policy, or programmatical intervention in a group, community, or region.

Commonalities Between Epidemiology and Qualitative Methods Talking with people is the most common method of data collection used by epidemiologists. Although there are many types of interviewing, talking with people is basically the same strategy used most commonly by qualitative researchers to collect data (Inhorn, 1995). Besides interviewing, epidemiologists have other data collection activities in common with qualitative researchers; for example, they do archival research and review medical and other records. They also use case studies. Inhorn points out that epidemiologists actually have fewer varieties of methods to choose from than do anthropologists and are more concerned about establishing "normative methodological standards" (p. 287). It is true, however, that epidemiologists tend to use more formal interviews, which may be standardized schedules, yet their interviews may nonetheless be very in-depth. Sample sizes may be larger in epidemiological studies; however, they may be quite small in epidemiological studies in the fields of, for example, genetics or isolated environmental disasters. Despite these similarities, differences between epidemiological and qualitative studies do exist in areas such as the use of theoretical bases (or lack thereof), purposes of studies, techniques used in data collection and analysis, and the role of subjects, which qualitative researchers tend to refer to as informants because they "inform" the investigator about their lives through interviews and at times by consenting to firsthand observation by the investigator and because they are not passive subjects, acted upon for purposes of the research.

Need for a Paradigm Shift: Theoretically
Driven Practice and Evidence-Based Practice

Contributions of Epidemiological Research
Versus Continuing Public Health Problems Worldwide

Epidemiology with all its shortcomings has nevertheless made marked contributions to the field of public health, specifically in disease prevention and health promotion. Marked gains have been made in the health of the American population, for example, in striving to reach the national goals set forth in the document *Healthy People 2000* (Department of Health and Human Services, 1995). Furthermore, epidemiology drives the health agenda of ministries of health worldwide.

It still remains that marked shortcomings exist in the health of the American population as well as in all other countries. For example, infectious disease, chronic malnutrition in some populations, occupational toxins, both natural and human-made disasters, environmental degradation, and political turmoil continue to be a problem in many developed countries as well as in developing countries. In the United States, deep-seated problems such as greater disparities in health outcomes in persons of color versus Caucasian persons, community violence, drug use, institutionalized racism, and poverty continue to plague the nation's health, despite concerted research and public policy efforts.

Outcomes: Individual Medical Interventions
Versus Sociocultural Solutions

It is important to note that not all problems have received adequate research attention. When RCTs have been conducted to yield evidence for practice, not everyone is eligible to participate in the trials, which leaves many people out of the trial (Stokols, Allen, & Bellingham, 1996). Most notably, according to Stokols, Allen, and Bellingham, those left out are low-income, marginalized groups such as immigrant groups and people of color, especially people who do not speak English. In addition, not all programs tested in a clinical trial are successful. Many people drop out, especially people with low incomes. Better-educated persons with higher incomes are more motivated to complete a program. Once a program is complete, others experience rates of high relapse. To address high attrition and high relapse, there is a need to look at contextual factors.

The Research Question and the Missing "Why?"

To address the many and varied determinants of health from the social and political arenas as well as the biological and psychological arenas, it is necessary to examine (a) conditions at both the micro and macro levels *and their interplay;* (b) multiple actors on the scene and their *interaction and movement over time;* (c) multiple contexts and changing contexts in which the interaction occurs over time; and (d) positive and negative consequences. This information should then be used to generate social processes that explain the "why" of both individual and population-based behaviors. Inhorn's (1995) insights regarding the potential contribution from anthropology can be extended to potential contributions from other qualitative research methodologies as well:

> If epidemiology is to be faulted in any way, it is for failing to go beyond mere identification of behaviors to attempt culturally meaningful explanations and contextualizations of those behaviors.... In other words, epidemiology asks "who," "when," "where" and "how" questions, without posing the crucial anthropological "why" question. (p. 288)

The "why" questions asked by anthropologists and other qualitative researchers are most often asked using an indirect approach in an attempt to elicit meaningful explanations and contextualizations of behaviors.

Sociocultural Solutions Inhorn (1995) further cautions, in her commentary regarding the contributions of anthropology to epidemiology, that

> while our contribution is greatly needed, we should be wary that social and cultural processes do not become reduced to factors which are translated *only* into individual health promotion. Rather, we must ensure that our understandings are more general in application and have relevance to health protection research and health policy issues. It is here that our strength as medical anthropologists lies in that the application of our knowledge needs

to be directed primarily towards socio-cultural solutions rather than medical interventions. (p. 288)

Theory: The Missing Link in a Paradigm Shift

Clearly, what is needed is what Stokols et al. (1996) call for: a paradigm shift. This paradigm shift would be away from a focus on individual behavior to a focus on process and ecological formulations of interdependencies between the socioeconomic, cultural, organizational, political, environmental, psychological, as well as biological determinants of health. This would include political systems and communities, as well as community coalitions.

A focus on process and interdependencies calls for a focus on multiparadigm research and theory as Evidence-Based Practice, as seen in the earlier summary of schistosomiasis in the Nile Delta in Egypt. The generation and use of theory from qualitative research is most important. Below is an example of a study in which the researcher claimed to use grounded theory to address the problem of anemia in immigrants in Great Britain, but in fact, the author did not successfully use this method, since her findings consisted of "facts" rather than concepts or theory.

An Example—Anemia

Chapple (1998) used grounded theory data collection and analysis methods to explore why women of South Asian descent (Pakistani, Indian) experience a high rate of iron deficiency anemia while living in Great Britain. The author used semistructured in-depth interviews with 30 women who stated they experienced menorrhagia and also interviewed Christian women of British descent who were affiliated with a mother and toddler group in a nearby village. The author stated that the qualitative data were analyzed using grounded theory methodology (Strauss & Corbin, 1990). Findings that were reported, however, were not a social-psychological process or even conceptual categories as is common to the grounded theory methodology. Instead, the findings were reduced to four statements of fact with headed sections, such as "Many Women of South Asian Descent Value Heavy Menstrual Periods" (p. 202) and "Dietary Modifications May Exacerbate Iron Deficiency" (p. 205). Each section was supported by anecdotes and commentary, which were full of facts. For example, women of South Asian descent thought blood was dirty and impure, and thus, they valued a heavy menstrual flow, which they believed would cleanse them of this impurity. Scanty periods were thought by the women to have consequences such as weight gain and pain. When they experienced heavy blood loss, they avoided "hot" foods, such as eggs, fish, and meat, which were valuable sources of iron. They also avoided seeking medical attention due to few female general practitioners and the embarrassment they experienced being examined by a male physician from their own culture. The author's conclusion was that "attitudes to menstruation and menstrual blood may help account for the relatively high levels of iron deficiency anemia" in these women (p. 199). Recommendations were to study other cultural groups.

Although the author presented a most interesting and useful study, the reporting of data that was not analyzed using grounded theory methodology, a common qualitative research methodology, which she purported to use, imposed a severe limitation on the study. Had concepts/categories and a grounded theory (i.e., process) been generated and reported, the contribution of the study to knowledge generation would have been enhanced. Furthermore, its ideas and conceptual thinking could have been used by practitioners in other settings facing problems of care with other immigrant groups. As Glaser (1978) notes, "Good ideas contribute the most. . . . Findings are soon forgotten, but not ideas" (p. 8). Chapple is not alone; other examples of missed opportunities to generate conceptual thinking can readily be found in the literature (e.g., Cohen et al., 1998; Power, 1996).

Conclusions

Need for Theory

Although outcomes from qualitative research approaches are many and varied, and necessary, as evidenced in the examples of instrumental outcomes and pragmatic outcomes, the generation of theory and theoretical concepts/categories is of primary importance. Glaser (1978), in a commentary on why one should generate grounded theory, asks,

Why bother, when in each area of life there are people in the know. These people are so knowledgeable that they think they can predict, explain and understand just about everything that happens in their terrain, field, area or world. . . . They run the world on their "know."

What the man in the know does not want is to be told what he already knows. . . . First, what the man in the know, knows is empirical, experiential and descriptive; his knowledge is non-theoretical. From the analyst's point of view what this "know" is are indicators that have yet to be conceptualized. The analyst gives the knowledgeable person categories, which grab many indicators under one idea and denotes the underlying pattern. One idea can then handle much diversity in incidents. Once ideas can be seen as conceptual elements that vary under diverse conditions, action options are provided the man in the know. Before this conceptualization, and integration, empirical incidents are seen as linked to finite situations. Now this finite social basis of knowledge can be flexibilized to apply [to] other general conditions. . . . With substantive theory the man in the know can start transcending his finite grasp of things. His knowledge which was heretofore not transferable, when used to generate theory, becomes transferable to other areas well known to him. His knowledge which was just known but not organized, is now ideationally organized. (pp. 12-13)

Finally, Glaser (1978), in his summary, states, "Concepts are easier to remember than incidents, especially fewer concepts which are integrated in a theory in the place of a multitude of unintegrated incidents. Thus his capacity to know is potentiated" (p. 13).

What Glaser says so well may raise the notion that theory is evidence and that the best use of evidence is when theory and evidence are linked and mutually shaping. Theory *is* evidence for practice. As stated by el Katsha and Watts (1997), "The situated practice of local people . . . should be recognized as knowledge which researchers need to take into account alongside their own culturally based scientific knowledge" (p. 847). Raising that "situated practice" to a conceptual level is the job of the researcher, the reflective practitioner of medicine, nursing, public health, and many others, so that there is a broader understanding than already exists, one with "grab" and utility.

Need for New Models

The need for new models is evident in the literature. Even the epidemiological literature is seeking new models that will generate "process." For example, Koopman and Lynch (1999) feel that epidemiology is limited because it usually treats populations not as systems of inter-acting individuals but as "collections of independent individuals" (p. 1120). These authors (1999) state that an "appropriate theoretical structure, which includes the determinants of connections among in-dividuals, is needed to develop a 'population system epidemiology' " (p. 1170). Disease transmission models could benefit by linking their model of interactions between individuals over a period of time to suf-ficient-component cause models that focus on "joint effects of multi-ple exposures in individuals" (p. 1170). Not only does this joint pros-pect include ways to measure degrees of connection between individuals, but it views individuals as being part of a system, and, as a result, it has the potential to yield "dynamic models of population pro-cesses" (p. 1174).

Need for Diversity and Tolerance

Questions must be asked about a structuralist orientation, particu-larly in response to postmodernism's call for diversity and tolerance for paradox. Perhaps the answer goes beyond replacing one paradigm with another, as in Kuhn's (1996) concept of "paradigm shift" and points out the need to examine "co-existence, juxtaposition, and inter-action of multiple paradigms" (Hlynka, 1991, p. 28).

Need for Investigators and Role Models

In addition, there is a need for generalist researchers who can do both qualitative and quantitative research: for example, researchers who can use both epidemiology and qualitative methods. Clearly, the idea that epidemiology is only one of several basic sciences of public health opens the doors to new interdisciplinary collaborations with fresh ap-proaches to examining population health (Krieger, 1999). For exam-ple, Krieger suggests that

> studying diversity of experiences among African Americans and other U.S. racial/ethnic groups in relation to varied forms of racial discrimination, rather than treating these groups as monolithic populations to be com-pared with White Americans, may well afford new insights into determi-nants of racial/ethnic inequalities in health. (p. 1152)

To accomplish this, Krieger (1999) believes it will take knowledge generated by a host of other disciplines, similar to those cited by Savitz et al. (1999), as "additional basic sciences of public health" (p. 1152).

Challenges exist in generating research that combines both quantitative and qualitative approaches to a research problem. First, research preparation typically occurs in a doctoral program, which is housed in a department within a discipline that may espouse only one approach or another. Pathways to learning either one approach or the other can increasingly be found in graduate schools in the United States. Using the dissertation level to learn the combined approaches to a health problem, however, may not be as readily available. For one thing, there are few mentors with expertise in both approaches, especially epidemiology and ethnography. To meet the needs for rigor in the process of learning to carry out each method, it may be necessary to take a more traditional approach; that is, a researcher may have to obtain skills in one approach at the doctoral level and then learn another approach during a postdoctoral fellowship.

Note

1. Although it is considered passé to do qualitative versus quantitative comparisons, in this context it is useful.

References

Ajzen, I., & Fishbein, M. (1980). *Understanding attitudes and predicting social behavior.* Englewood Cliffs, NJ: Prentice Hall.

Anderko, L., Uscian, M., & Robertson, J. (1999). Improving client outcomes through differentiated practice: A rural nursing center model. *Public Health Nursing, 16*(3), 168-175.

Bhopal, R. (1999). Paradigms in epidemiology textbooks: In the footsteps of Thomas Kuhn. *American Journal of Public Health, 89*(8), 1162-1165.

Black, N., & Thompson, E. (1993). Attitudes to medical audit: British doctors speak. *Social Science and Medicine, 36,* 849-856.

Brunham, R. C. (1997). Core group theory: A central concept in STD epidemiology. *Venereology, 10*(1), 34-39.

Burns, N., & Grove, S. (1999). *Understanding nursing research* (2nd ed.). Philadelphia: W. B. Saunders.

Caine, C., & Kendrick, M. (1997). The role of clinical directorate managers in facilitating evidence-based practice: A report of an exploratory study. *Journal of Nursing Management, 5*(3), 157-165.

Campbell, C., & Williams, B. (1999). Beyond the biomedical and behavioural: Towards an integrated approach to HIV prevention in the Southern African mining industry. *Social Science and Medicine, 48,* 1625-1639.

Carey, M. A. (1997). Qualitative approaches to evaluation. In M. G. Winiarski (Ed.), *HIV mental health for the 21st century* (pp. 291-304). New York: New York University Press.

Carruthers, S. (1999). Assimilating new therapeutic interventions into clinical practice: How does hypertension compare with other therapeutic areas? *American Heart Journal, 138*(3, Pt. 2), 256-260.

Chapple, A. (1998). Iron deficiency anemia in women of South Asian descent: A qualitative study. *Ethnicity and Health, 3*(3), 199-212.

Chenitz, W. C., & Swanson, J. M. (1986). *From practice to grounded theory: Qualitative research in nursing.* Menlo Park, CA: Addison-Wesley.

Cohen, S., Mason, D., Arsenie, L., Sargese, S., & Needham, D. (1998). Focus groups reveal perils and promises of managed care for nurse practitioners. *Nurse Practitioner, 23*(6), 48, 54, 57-60.

Cutler, C. (1996). Outcomes and cost-effectiveness: The payer's perspective. *Academy of Radiology, 3*(Suppl. 1), S33-34.

Department of Health and Human Services. (1995). *Healthy people 2000: Midcourse review and 1995 revisions.* Washington, DC: U.S. Government Printing Office.

Durham, R. (1998). Strategies women engage in when managing preterm labor at home. *Journal of Perinatology, 18,* 61-64.

Durham, R. (1999). Negotiating activity restriction: A grounded theory of home management of preterm labor. *Qualitative Health Research, 9*(4), 493-503.

el Katsha, S., & Watts, S. (1993). The empowerment of women: Water and sanitation initiatives in rural Egypt (Monograph No. 2). *Cairo Papers in Social Science, 16.*

el Katsha, S., & Watts, S. (1997). Schistosomiasis in two Nile Delta villages: An anthropological perspective. *Tropical Medicine and International Health, 2*(9), 846-854.

Flynn, L. (1999). The adolescent parenting program: Improving outcomes through mentorship. *Public Health Nursing, 16*(3), 182-189.

Glaser, B. (1978). *Theoretical sensitivity.* Mill Valley, CA: Sociology Press.

Glaser, B., & Strauss, A. (1967). *The discovery of grounded theory.* Chicago: Aldine.

Gray, J. (1997). *Evidence-based health care: How to make health policy and management decisions.* London: Churchill Livingston.

Greene, J. (1994). Qualitative program evaluation. In N. K. Denzin & Y. S. Lincoln (Eds.), *Handbook of qualitative research* (pp. 530-544). Thousand Oaks, CA: Sage.

Gulitz, E., Hernandez, M., & Kent, E. (1998). Missed cancer screening opportunities among older women: A review. *Cancer Practitioner, 6*(5), 289-295.

Hatch, M., von Ehrenstein, O., Wolff, M., Meier, K., Geduld, A., & Einhorn, F. (1999). Using qualitative methods to elicit recall of a critical time period. *Journal of Women's Health, 8*(2), 269-277.

Hilton, B. (1997). So—what's the fuss about outcomes and outcome evaluation? *Canadian Oncology Nursing Journal, 7*(1), 3-5.

Hlynka, D. (1991). Postmodern excursions into educational technology. *Educational Technology, 31*(6), 27-30.

Huber, M. (1991). Measuring medicine's effects: The outcomes management system. *Journal of Occupational Medicine, 33*(3), 272.

Inhorn, M. C. (1995). Medical anthropology and epidemiology: Divergences or convergences? *Social Science and Medicine, 40*(3), 285-290.

Institute of Medicine, Committee for the Study of the Future of Public Health. (1988). *The future of public health*. Washington, DC: National Academy Press.

Johnson, D., Hayslip, D., Sims, T., Smith, K., Keen, M., & Burrows-Hudson, S. (1995). Nurse's role in achieving patient outcomes. *ANNA Journal, 22*(2), 131-140.

Kaplan, A. (1964). *The conduct of inquiry: Methodology for behavioral science*. Scranton, PA: Chandler.

Koopman, J. S., & Lynch, J. W. (1999). Individual causal models and population system models in epidemiology. *American Journal of Public Health, 89*(8), 1170-1174.

Krieger, N. (1999). Questioning epidemiology: Objectivity, advocacy, and socially responsible science. *American Journal of Public Health, 89*(8), 1151-1153.

Kuhn, T. S. (1996). *The structure of scientific revolutions*. Chicago: University of Chicago Press.

Martin, K., Leak, G., & Aden, C. (1992). The Omaha system: A research-based model for decision making. *Journal of Nursing Administration, 22*(11), 47-51.

Mausner, J. S., & Kramer, S. (1985). *Epidemiology: Principles and methods*. Philadelphia: W. B. Saunders.

Morbidity and Mortality Weekly Reports. (1990). Reduced incidence of menstrual toxic-shock syndrome—United States, 1980-1990. *Morbidity and Mortality Weekly Reports (CDC), 29*(37), 441-445.

Morse, J. M. (1997). Considering theory derived from qualitative research. In J. M. Morse (Ed.), *Completing a qualitative project* (pp. 163-188). Thousand Oaks, CA: Sage.

Peat, J., Toelle, B., & Nagy, S. (1998). Qualitative research: A path to better healthcare. *Medical Journal of Australia, 21*(6), 327-329.

Power, R. (1996). Rapid assessment of the drug-injecting situation at Hanoi and Ho Chi Minh City, Viet Nam. *Bulletin on Narcotics, 48*, 35-52.

Rist, R. C. (1994). Influencing the policy process with qualitative research. In N. K. Denzin & Y. S. Lincoln (Eds.), *Handbook of qualitative research* (pp. 545-557). Thousand Oaks, CA: Sage.

Rosen, G. (1958). *A history of public health*. New York: MD Publications.

Sackett, D., Rosenberg, W., Gray, J., Haynes, R., & Richardson, W. (1996). Evidence based medicine: What it is and what it is not. *British Medical Journal, 312*, 71-72.

Savitz, D. A., Poole, C., & Miller, W. C. (1999). Reassessing the role of epidemiology in public health. *American Journal of Public Health, 89*(8), 1158-1161.

Smith, A. (1978). The epidemiological basis of community medicine. In A. E. Bennett (Ed.), *Recent advances in community medicine* (pp. 1-10). Edinburgh, Scotland: Longman.

Stallones, R. A. (1980). To advance epidemiology. *Annual Review of Public Health, 1*, 69-82.

Stokols, D., Allen, J., & Bellingham, R. (1996). The social ecology of health promotion: Implications for research and practice. *American Journal of Health Promotion, 10*(4), 247-251.

Strauss, A., & Corbin, J. (1990). *The basics of qualitative research*. Newbury Park, CA: Sage.

Susser, M., & Susser, E. (1996). Choosing a future of epidemiology, I: Eras and paradigms. *American Journal of Public Health, 86,* 668-673.

Swanson, J. M. (1986). Analyzing data for categories and description. In W. C. Chenitz & J. M. Swanson (Eds.), *From practice to grounded theory: Qualitative research in nursing* (pp. 121-132). Menlo Park, CA: Addison-Wesley.

Swanson, J. M. (1994). The value of short case-reports. *IMAGE: The Journal of Nursing Scholarship, 26,* 128.

Swanson, J. M., & Chapman, L. (1994). Inside the black box: Theoretical and methodological issues in conducting evaluation research using a qualitative approach. In J. M. Morse (Ed.), *Critical issues in qualitative research methods* (pp. 66-93). Thousand Oaks, CA: Sage.

Swanson, J. M., Durham, R., & Albright, J. (1997). Clinical utilization/application of qualitative research. In J. M. Morse (Ed.), *Completing a qualitative project: Details and dialogue* (pp. 253-281). Thousand Oaks, CA: Sage.

Valanis, B. (1992). *Epidemiology in nursing and health care* (2nd ed.). Norwalk, CT: Appleton & Lange.

Van Ufford, P. Q. (1993). Knowledge and ignorance in the practice of development policy. In M. Hobart (Ed.), *An anthropological critique of development* (pp. 135-160). London: Routledge.

Watts, S. J. (1991). Spatial aspects of human behaviour in relation to the transmission and control of parasitic diseases in tropical Africa. In A. Rais (Ed.), *Environment and health: Themes in medical geography* (pp. 119-120). New Delhi: Ashish Publishing House.

Watts, S. J., & el Katsha, S. (1995). Changing environmental conditions in the Nile Delta: Health and policy implications with special reference to schistosomiasis. *International Journal of Environmental Health Research, 5,* 197-212.

Webster, N. (1979). *Webster's deluxe unabridged dictionary* (2nd ed.). New York: Simon & Schuster.

Welch, J. (1997). Measures and meanings: Outcome measures in the management of sexually transmitted infections. *International Journal of STD/AIDS, 8*(12), 747-749.

Dialogue:

The Dilemmas of Replication

MORSE: Replication doesn't help if it's a terrible job, and if it's a good study, let it stand and build on it. The problem is that you see it over and over again—these articles written by masters' students and others—and in their findings they say that these findings confirm the findings of such-and-such and these findings confirm findings of so-and-so. But the trouble is, if they confirm the findings, then there is nothing new to report, and therefore they don't meet publication criteria.

MADJAR: I think because we've been adamant about saying that you don't do replication in qualitative research, people pretend that they're doing something new, even if what they say is "Well, I can't find in the literature a study done with this group of women." They ignore everything that anyone else has done and they say, "I'll call this new research." Then it doesn't really contribute to the literature or build on knowledge in another area. It simply sits there on its own.

MEADOWS: You know, I think we could do this as stakeholders and agenda analysis—why we have this myriad of little studies and what are the forces driving that.

ESTABROOKS: There is no paper written about what a good qualitative paper looks like, they don't know about transferability. . . . These things you spend weeks on when you are writing a grant, trying to turn these things into regular language. It's not acceptable language. What you need is something that says, "Most of the studies you read in the literature done by students take it to this level and it looks like this, and when you read a mature study that is done well, it looks like this." And give examples. "When you read a really fine watershed study, it looks like this," and give an example, although there are only a few examples. So that it's accessible to people. I find our language a real problem.

MORSE: I like the word *mature* study. I think we should use it in this book. I think it's very important. And it's a good word.

MEADOWS: I think the reason it's not out there is because it's extremely difficult to write it in a way that transcends methodology and philosophic presuppositions. Because when those pieces are there, then it's really impossible to tease out, because you're looking for different things. But you're talking about transcending the issues, and that's very difficult.

ESTABROOKS: But the quantitative folks think that we're hiding something, that it's fluff, and that we cover the fluff in language because of the language. It sounds like so much mumbo jumbo to others . . . and you really don't know.

SWANSON: But what about the Jeannie Kayser Jones study? A multisite study funded by NIH and looking at feeding patients in nursing homes. How people were dying in the nursing homes because they weren't getting fed. There wasn't enough staff, and unless friends and family were going in to feed them, they weren't eating and they were dying. This research team just went in and observed. And she would come in an hour later, and the patients would eat the cold spaghetti. If staff members fed it to them, they would eat it. They were ravenous, because no one was feeding them. The constraints of downsizing and bringing in nurses' aides and high turnover—and there's nobody for them. I think that there are some new issues. Some new things [beyond the work of Strauss] in the field of ethnography.

ESTABROOKS: That's a wonderful illustration of how even with an enduring special study the world changes, and there's going to be a time when there are differences.

SWANSON: Not only with patients but with staff members.

MADJAR: I think one of the important assumptions of qualitative research is that we are addressing human action in the context of the social world. Whatever that might be, we are not aiming to develop universal laws. This is not doing physics, this is not looking at the next law of thermodynamics. This is about understanding human behavior in a contextual way, a historical way.

Now if you accept that, you must accept that the studies always have to be done from time to time. I think we are stuck on the concept of replication because it suggests that if it's been done, it's been done forever. Whereas I think what you [Jan Swanson] are suggesting, and in fact illustrating very clearly, is that we really are saying we need to extend our understanding. We need to go back and reexamine some of these issues and these questions from time to time, and we have to keep developing what we know. Otherwise, I think we risk being accused of trying to generalize from a small single study in a different context, and I think that's really risky. That's really risky.

MORSE: Yes. But you have to have a good reason to [go back].

11

Using Qualitative Research in Clinical Practice

KÄRIN OLSON

Clinicians strive to make decisions based on the best and most complete information available. Until recently, most of this information came from research designed by individuals who held positivist worldviews.[1] What might happen if research methods facilitated the collection of data in the context in which it naturally occurred, the opportunity for study participants to speak in their own voice, the systematic acknowledgment of the influence of values on data analysis, the construction of theory based on observable data, and the careful description of unique and particular experiences? In this chapter, I explore benefits to be gained in clinical work by considering the previously inaccessible information now available through the use of methods that address the limitations of positivism. These methods fall broadly under the heading of naturalistic inquiry and are qualitative in nature. The clinicians whose studies will be discussed here used the findings of qualitative studies to explain processes underpinning the results of quantitative studies, to give a voice to the patient, to monitor treatment response, and to solve health care delivery problems with respect to organizational behavior, organizational processes, the implementation of change, and the elaboration of leaders' roles and functions. I argue that by using these methods in conjunction with traditional research approaches, as outlined by Miller and Crabtree (1994), the clinician may obtain a more complete understanding of problems faced in health care environments.

Filling Gaps in Clinical Knowledge

What kind of new information can be gained by changing one's worldview to incorporate the findings of qualitative research in clinical practice?

Explaining the Findings of Quantitative Studies

Qualitative studies can help clinicians explain the findings of quantitative studies. Clinicians are accustomed to reviewing quantitative studies in their area of specialization. Qualitative studies can be used to complement the findings of quantitative studies or provide additional insight in the processes that contributed to the outcome. For example, Marmoreo, Brown, Batty, Cummings, and Powell (1998) had read reports in the medical literature that only 11% to 15% of women age 50 years or older filled prescriptions for hormone replacement therapy (HRT). Were the remaining women simply noncompliant? The investigators used focus groups to find out how physicians could assist women with decision making regarding the use of HRT. The investigators learned that there were four spheres of influence that affected a woman's decision to use HRT: (1) her internal perceptions and feelings, (2) her interpersonal relationships (including her relationship with her physician), (3) external societal influences related to sexism and ageism, and (4) the consequences of the decision. The authors used this information to begin constructing a theory about how women made decisions about HRT use and noted that availability of this evidence could be used by physicians to structure a more directed conversation with female patients about whether they would like to use HRT or not.

On a similar note, Hunt, Arar, and Larme (1998) were interested in learning more about the reasons behind the failure of low-income individuals diagnosed with Type 2 diabetes to comply with treatment recommendations. Data were collected by interviewing individuals with Type 2 diabetes and their health care providers and by reviewing patient charts and relevant literature. The investigators found that even though physicians stressed the importance of motivation and glucose control, patient responses came from within a larger social context. The patients tried to follow the physician's recommendations, but when they did not get the desired benefit (a drop in blood glucose or an increased feeling of well-being), it was hard to remain committed to the original plan. These frustrations had to be endured in an environment lacking the social and economic resources that health care providers often assumed were present, and they had to be endured in conjunction with other competing social influences (not wanting to offend the cook!). Thus, rather than setting individuals up for successful management of their diabetes, health care providers inadvertently set them up for failure. By obtaining data from both the individuals with diabetes and their health care providers, the investigators were able to look at the similarities and differences between their perspectives and, from these data, to begin theorizing about ways clinicians could make their recommendations more useful. The investigators noted that clinical recommendations must be adapted to fit within the constraints of the social world of the individuals for whom they are intended. This is much more difficult (but also more realistic) than simply assuming that if only the low-income individual with Type 2 diabetes was motivated to engage in self-care, everything would be "fine."

Learning More About a Health Care Problem
From the Standpoint of the Patient

It would be unfair to say that researchers who use research methods shaped by a positivist worldview are uninterested in the point of view of the patient. Indeed, many such investigators could point to numerous interview schedules and questionnaires designed explicitly for this purpose. Still, one must stop and ask, "How (or from where) were the items generated? Whose voice is speaking?" Positivist research, with its emphasis on hypothesis testing, rests heavily on the need to "operationalize" concepts of interest. During this process, everyday experiences of participants become refocused through the lens of the investigator and defined in a way that can be measured with numbers. This "outsider" or etic view is a hallmark of the positivist worldview (Kerlinger, 1986). What happens to the parts of the experience left out of the operational definition? The results of projects in which data collection is constrained by operational definitions are understandably more narrow than qualitative projects in which the emphasis is on capturing the emic or "insider" voice and on as much experience as possible.

Consider the study undertaken by Chase, Melloni, and Savage (1997) about the experience of living with venous ulcer disease. Data indicating the huge economic impact of venous ulcer disease on health care systems around the world were readily available, but little information about the individual's experience of venous ulcers could be found. In order to obtain this information, the investigators conducted a phenomenological study of individuals who required weekly dressing changes at a surgical outpatient clinic. Four themes were identified: a forever healing process, limits and accommodations, powerlessness, and "who cares." The investigators noted that reliance on the "insider" view could help nurses anticipate the problems faced by individuals with venous ulcers and, recognizing the personal cost of the disease to the individual, provide more sensitive nursing care.

The addition of qualitative methods to the usual survey techniques traditionally used for needs assessments has led to the collection of rich, informative data that was previously inaccessible. For example, Killon (1995) used an ethnographic approach to study the special needs of homeless pregnant women. Study participants were identified through homeless shelter staff. The author outlined factors that contributed to becoming pregnant (e.g., need for intimacy, uncertain fertility) and showed that although these factors were not unique to homelessness, it was homelessness that was likely to intensify their significance. Once the pregnancy was established, the women had to manage all of the normal physiological changes (e.g., nausea, increased nutritional requirements), as well as occasional related health problems (e.g., urinary tract infections). Given the tremendous effort required to sustain survival on the street, health problems were not acknowledged until they were serious. The social context of the findings was carefully constructed. For example, the author noted that some of the participants were married. Since many shelters did not allow men and women to stay together, families were often separated. Thus, sexual encounters, when they did occur, were spur-of-the-moment and not conducive to the use of contraception.

As a public health nurse, I often puzzled over the apparent incongruence between individuals' health information and their behavior. To gain more insight into this phenomenon, I conducted a qualitative study of factors associated with doing and not doing a breast self-exam (BSE) and learned that the regular practice of BSE requires much more than knowledge of public health recommendations and technique. It also requires perceived social permission to touch your own body, a belief that early detection of breast cancer is associated with increased survival, a social role definition that includes "taking care" of oneself, and a careful reflection on the personal meaning of having breast cancer (Olson & Morse, 1996). When questions based on the study interviews were developed and administered to a large group of women, the factors identified in the qualitative portion of the study accounted for 49% of the variance (R^2) in BSE practice. On the basis of these factors, 84% of group members could be correctly classified with respect to their BSE practice status. The high degree of congruence between the findings of the qualitative and quantitative portions of the study is not surprising, since the sample for the qualitative portion was carefully chosen to ensure that participants were thoroughly enculturated. As a result, they knew the rules of their culture well and could speak for women in general as well as for themselves.

Monitoring Treatment Impact

Regardless of the discipline or specialty in which they work, clinicians generally agree that treatment response is as much about quality of life as it is about morbidity and mortality. A search of any literature database will show an exponential growth in the number of studies on quality of life since it was formally introduced into health care by the World Health Organization. Many investigators have recognized that the meaning of quality of life is different across diseases and have constructed disease-specific quality of life tools. Most quality-of-life tools recognize the multidimensional nature of quality of life by developing subscales related to some combination of functional status, physical symptoms, emotional well-being, and social well-being.

Quality-of-life scales are useful in a clinical setting when assessments must be done quickly. In a recent assessment of quality of life for new patients with gastrointestinal or lung cancer, the QLQ-C30 was used (Aaronson et al., 1993) to watch for changes in fatigue and other related symptoms that have an impact on quality of life in this population. After seeing a rapid decline in quality-of-life scores related to fatigue, we implemented a qualitative study to learn more about how fatigue was experienced by our patients and how it changed over the course of treatment (Olson et al., 1998).

On occasion, however, it becomes important to obtain a more detailed view of quality of life. Perhaps the scale results do not match the clinical picture. How can a person with a significant pathology have a score indicating "good" quality of life? In a study of quality of life in individuals with moderate to severe chronic asthma, Drummond (2000) invited participants to talk about the aspects of life that were important to them, about the things from which they derived "happiness" or "unhappiness," and factors affecting their quality of life. He learned that "emotionally-significant social relationships" were central to the definition of quality of life of study participants and that "having asthma," despite worries and fears associated with acute episodes, was relatively peripheral.

Using Qualitative Research to Solve
Problems in Health Care Delivery

In addition to the evidence generated by qualitative research regarding day-to-day clinical practice problems, qualitative research can also be used to solve practical problems that arise in the management of clinical environments. Because the findings of these studies "work" in the clinical environment, they are good examples of the relationship between qualitative research and pragmatic utility theories of truth. Hoffart and Bradley (1997) reviewed published qualitative research in the field of health care management and identified over 20 studies in four areas: organizational behavior, organizational processes, organizational phenomena, and leaders' roles and functions.

Understanding Organizational Behavior

Coeling and Wilcox (1988) used an ethnographic approach to study the work group culture on two nursing units. In this case, the unit of analysis was the nursing unit. Data were collected using participant observation and semistructured interviews with all staff members. The objective of the analysis was to identify the "rules" that should be followed if one wanted to "fit in." After the staff members had verified the rules for their unit, the investigators compared the rules between the two units. They discovered that the units differed with respect to how much they wished to work together, the use of a staff hierarchy, willingness to follow established standards, organization of time, and preferences regarding change. The authors outlined the implications of these

differences for hiring decisions, development of orientation procedures for new staff, and the implementation of organizational change.

Evaluating Organizational Processes

As health care resources become more scarce, managers are increasingly more often required to evaluate organization processes to ensure
quality and appropriate resources use. Traditionally, evaluation research relied on data generated by using survey methods. By adding
qualitative methods, evaluators are able to explore process issues in
sufficient detail to implement corrective action in a timely fashion.
Morse, Penrod, and Hupcey (2000) developed an approach called qualitative outcome analysis (QOA) for evaluating complex clinical phenomena. In this approach, clinicians use qualitative methods to evaluate the impact of interventions derived from qualitative research on
patient outcomes. In addition to helping staff assess the benefit of the
intervention in their setting, QOA also provides a systematic process
for monitoring the generalizability of qualitative findings.

Kerr (1996) was interested in evaluating programmatic changes implemented on a busy accident and emergency unit. On the basis of
work by McGuire (1990), which showed that clinicians were more
likely to adopt new practices if they had an opportunity to be involved
in all phases of the project, Kerr chose to use an approach based in action research. In informal settings, participants were encouraged to
discuss their work environment, identify areas requiring improvement, and generate solutions. The investigator shared the leadership
functions with the participants, occasionally taking on the moderator
role. The objective of the exercise, in addition to completing the program evaluation, was to enhance the self-critical skills of the participants to the point where they would be able to continue using action
research on their own, once the investigator left the setting. Although
the approach was time-consuming, it provided nurses with an opportunity to systematically observe their own practice, reflect on their observations, and implement desired changes.

In addition to providing information that organizations can use to
revise their programs, evaluation at an organizational level also provides evidence that can be used to support health care policy. Magilvy,
Congdon, and Martinez (1994) explored ways in which informal
support networks worked in conjunction with the formal health care

service in a rural environment in order to help frail elderly clients maintain their independence. The formal health care system, labeled the circle of continuity of care, included all hospital and community-based services used by the frail elderly. The informal caregivers of the study participants formed the circle of family and community support. The study focused on the ways in which these two circles were integrated. The investigators noted that nurses who lived and worked in rural communities were often part of both circles, since their clients were often also their neighbors. By studying the interrelationships between the two circles, the investigators were also able to identify individuals who had fallen through the cracks and determine the location of the gap. Most often, these gaps were in the formal circle.

Using principles of action research, Pearcey and Draper (1996) interviewed nursing staff to gain a better understanding of factors interfering with the adoption of research utilization in their hospital. Data were analyzed according to the stages of the Diffusion of Innovation model (Rogers, 1983). The authors were able to identify many barriers to research utilization that had been previously unnoticed. Of particular concern were the lack of time for research utilization manifested by the leader of the project and the perceived "top-down" fashion in which research utilization was implemented.

Qualitative research can be used to evaluate program planning initiatives, regardless of their size. Hoffart, Schultz, and Ingersoll (1995) used a case study approach with multiple data sources to evaluate the implementation of a professional practice model of nursing in a rural 53-bed hospital. Although many nurse executives implemented professional practice models in the 1980s in response to nurse shortages, only a few of these related to rural settings. This study, which ran in conjunction with a large quantitative study of the initiative, was designed to describe the processes that influenced the outcome of the initiative. The key elements of the model were control over practice, collaborative practice, continuity of care, continuing and inservice education, and compensation/recognition. The model was implemented by choosing two or three projects that emphasized these key elements. For example, nursing and medical staff collaborated in the development of clinical pathways for various diagnostic categories. These pathways included all daily treatment plans for both disciplines and were linked to the quality assurance program. Although many temporary roadblocks were encountered along the way, most of the projects started as part of the professional practice model implementation became a part of the ongoing operation of the hospital. The investigators commented on the link between organizational culture and the implementation of organizational change. The hospital in which this study was undertaken strongly valued a functional approach to both clinical and administrative work. This value influenced the way the clinical practice model was implemented.

Tracking the Impact of Organizational Change

In the course of managing health care environments, strategic initiatives are often established. However, the efficient operation of the programs stemming from these initiatives is sometimes compromised because of miscommunication. Given the extensive scientific and technical vocabulary that is part of the health care environment, this is not surprising. As the director of a strategic initiative in quality assurance, Jackson-Frankl (1990) wanted to ensure that all the individuals in her department, ranging from the chief nursing officer to the staff nurses, had a common understanding of quality, care, and quality of care. Interviews were conducted with a sample comprised of the nurse executive, assistant nurse executives, head nurses, and staff nurses. The author noted that the meaning of quality was not consistent among the participants, and outlined the implications of this finding for nurse managers. Qualitative studies frequently help investigators identify important side issues related to the main research question. In the case of the study conducted by Jackson-Frankl, the investigator found that study participants with less autonomy in the health care system became frustrated by the quality assurance initiative when the amount of time available or the educational level of the staff members was insufficient to address the quality assurance task at hand.

In the course of delivering health care, important philosophic issues frequently arise. Dill (1995) used qualitative research to highlight ethical issues related to discharge planning for older adults, with particular emphasis on the control of the patient over discharge decisions, the patient's ability to make decisions, and family involvement. This study is an example of the way qualitative research methods aid in discussions of ethical truth. Data were collected primarily using participant observation methods. The investigator noted that the patient's decision-making ability was most often questioned when the patient's wishes with respect to discharge were at odds with the views of the staff. Once the patient's ability to make decisions was questioned, the patient also began to lose control of the discharge decisions. The investigator also noted that although health care providers value the involvement of family in discharge planning, they do not always define family in a manner consistent with the definition of the patient. Hence, the willingness of a niece, who is *like* a daughter, to assist with discharge may be taken less seriously than that of a woman who *is* a daughter. Readers were reminded that the discharge process takes place in a larger social environment often lacking the resources to provide even the most basic accommodation for older individuals who are healthy, let alone those who are ill. This social environment weighs heavily on both the health care providers in geriatric settings and the older individuals for whom they are attempting to arrange a discharge to another setting.

Elaborating Leaders' Roles and Functions

Although most clinicians would readily agree that health care organizations are most efficient when they have good leaders, it is harder to describe what a good leader is like or what he or she actually does. Pederson (1993) used a qualitative study to learn more about the qualities of an excellent head nurse. Sixteen nurses were asked to describe an excellent head nurse with whom they had worked at some point in their career. Some of the participants were staff nurses, and others were head nurses. Interviews were analyzed using a content analysis approach. Conflict resolution skills were the most commonly mentioned characteristic. Staff members also noted that excellent managers were supportive of their staff, and that this support ranged from support during a family crisis to support for professional growth. Participants also identified a cluster of characteristics that were grouped under temperament. These included characteristics such as authenticity, honesty, reliability, sincerity, humor, and enthusiasm. Additional characteristics of an excellent head nurse included credibility, forward thinking ability, professionalism, and advocacy (for staff members and patients). The author noted that the participants downplayed the value of clinical expertise as long as the head nurse was able to provide this resource in other ways. Findings of this study could be used in the development of professional development programs designed to prepare individuals for middle manager positions or to design recruitment/hiring guidelines.

When Are the Findings of Qualitative Studies Ready for Implementation?

With the growth of the Evidence-Based Practice movement has come an awareness on the part of clinicians that the findings of some studies are ready for use in the clinical setting, whereas others are not. Clinicians want some degree of confidence that the findings are transferable. Before being able to fully appreciate the gains that can be made by incorporating the findings of qualitative research into practice, one must understand the differences between generalizability in quantitative and qualitative research methods. As Johnson (1997) noted, generalizability must be understood in the context of the chosen research method and the theory of truth to which one subscribes.

Quantitative research methods rest most heavily on correspondence theory, according to which, knowledge is objective and truth is singular in nature (Kirkham, 1995). The findings of a quantitative study apply to the study participants as a whole. For example, one could design a clinical trial to determine the most effective dose of a particular medication for a group of people with a common health problem. The decision regarding which dose was the best would have been mathematically determined and would have a proviso attached that informed the reader of the degree of confidence the investigators had in their conclusion. The usefulness of this kind of information is clear if one is responsible for laying out general treatment plans for large groups of people. Provided that the variables that could influence the outcome of the study were sufficiently "controlled," the findings would be considered generalizable to other groups like the one studied.[2] Stephens (1982) refers to this type of generalizability as horizontal generalizability.

Qualitative research methods, on the other hand, rest most heavily on coherence (internal consistency) and pragmatic utility (practical problem solving) theories of truth. Here, truth is subjective, and multiple truths exist simultaneously (Gould, 1999a; Gould, 1999b; Kirkham, 1995). Regardless of the method chosen, the structure of qualitative inquiry allows the investigator to gain information about the experience of each study participant as an individual. In grounded theory, the experiences of study participants are compared, looking for similarities and differences. Does A always follow B? What difference does context make? What is it like to live with condition X? What are the antecedents and consequences of A? Participants with opposing points of view are sought, and data collection continues until new information is no longer obtained. As data collection draws to a close, important themes emerge and hypotheses may be developed. In this sense, grounded theory applies to groups of individuals. By comparing and contrasting similar studies, investigators obtain sufficient data to begin building theories about the experience of the individuals studied. For example, Morse and Johnson used five studies of various illnesses, all developed using grounded theory, to construct the Illness Constellation Model (Morse & Johnson, 1991). The model traces the experience of illness from the initial suspicion that "something is wrong" to the end of the illness.

Qualitative methods such as case study and phenomenology are used when the investigator wishes to conduct a detailed study of the unique and particular experiences. Stake (1997) argues that case studies provide opportunities for "vicarious experience," and that because the case material adheres so closely to the actual experience of the study participant, readers feel as though they were there. This phenomenon is called naturalistic generalization (Stake & Trumbull, 1982).

The "group-individual" generalization issue has its roots in the writing of the German philosopher Wilhelm Windelband. Windelband (1961) labeled quantitative research as "nomothetic inquiry" because of the strict, lawlike assumptions that must be upheld in order to give the findings mathematical meaning. He associated quantitative research with the natural sciences. He labeled the study of "the singular" as "ideographic inquiry" and associated it with the human sciences. Windelband designated this nomothetic-ideographic dilemma as the central defining feature of the natural and human sciences, and noted that in order to have a more complete understanding of the meaning of any phenomenon of interest, both kinds of inquiry were necessary.

To successfully clear the generalizability hurdle, readers must understand that both quantitative and qualitative methods give rise to findings that are generalizable, but the meaning of generalizability is different. Quantitative studies focus on hypothesis testing and generalize to groups like the one studied. The information obtained through quantitative studies is true in the empirical sense because data are collected through experimentation. Qualitative studies focus on theory development and detailed description of phenomena and generalize to theoretical constructs and the essence of experience. Descriptive qualitative studies that are well done help the reader feel what the experience was like for the participant. In my view, all the studies discussed in this chapter are ready to be used in practice. The information obtained through the qualitative studies is true in the empirical sense because it is obtained through observation, but qualitative methods also provide opportunities to uncover ethical truth, as it was shown in the study by Dill (1995) discussed above.

The purpose of this chapter has been to illustrate the valuable information that can be gained when the findings of qualitative research are integrated into clinical practice. Qualitative research helps clinicians gain both empirical knowledge, as it relates to observation, and ethical knowledge, thereby "making sense" of their observations and solving practical problems.

Notes

1. For a more detailed discussion of the historical development of the positivist worldview and its limitations, see Lincoln and Guba (1985, pp. 14-128).

2. Cronbach (1975) argued that generalization is not ever really possible due to the influence of context. He said that the best an investigator could really do was to pay equal attention to both the variables that were "controlled" and those that were "uncontrolled," and to look carefully for things not seen before. From his point of view, generalizations one might make at the end of a study were simply "working hypotheses" rather than conclusions.

References

Aaronson, N., Ahmedzai, S., Bergman, B., Bullinger, M., Cull, A., Duez, N., Filiberti, A., Flechner, H., Fleishman, S., De Haes, J., Kaasa, S., Klee, M. N., Osoba, D., Razavi, D., Rofe, P., Schraub, S., Sneeuz, K., Sullivan, M., & Takeda, F. (1993). The European Organization for Research and Treatment of Cancer QLQ-C30: A quality-of-life instrument for use in international clinical trials in oncology. *Journal of the National Cancer Institute, 85*(5), 365-376.

Chase, S., Melloni, M., & Savage, A. (1997). A forever healing: The lived experience of venous ulcer disease. *Journal of Vascular Nursing, 15*(2), 73-78.

Coeling, H., & Wilcox, J. (1988). Understanding organizational culture: A key to management decision-making. *Journal of Nursing Administration, 18*(11), 16-23.

Cronbach, L. (1975). Beyond the two disciplines of scientific psychology. *American Psychologist, 30,* 116-127.

Dill, A. (1995). The ethics of discharge planning for older adults: An ethnographic analysis. *Social Science and Medicine, 41*(9), 1289-1299.

Drummond, N. (2000). Quality of life with asthma: The existential and the aesthetic. *Sociology of Health & Illness, 22*(2), 235-253.

Gould, J. (1999a). Truth is established by coherence. In J. Gould (Ed.), *Classical philosophical questions* (9th ed., pp. 367-374). Englewood Cliffs, NJ: Prentice Hall.

Gould, J. (1999b). Truth is established on pragmatic grounds. In J. Gould (Ed.), *Classical philosophical questions* (9th ed., pp. 375-383). Englewood Cliffs, NJ: Prentice Hall.

Hoffart, N., & Bradley, K. (1997). Using qualitative research in the management of health care. *Seminars for Nurse Managers, 5*(4), 173-181.

Hoffart, N., Schultz, A., & Ingersoll, G. (1995). Implementation of a professional practice model for nursing in a rural hospital. *Health Care Management Review, 20*(3), 43-54.

Hunt, L., Arar, N., & Larme, A. (1998). Contrasting patient and practitioner perspectives in type 2 diabetes management. *Western Journal of Nursing Research, 20*(6), 656-682.

Jackson-Frankl, K. (1990). The language and meaning of quality. *Nursing Administration Quarterly, 14*(3), 52-65.

Johnson, J. (1997). Generalizability in qualitative research. In J. M. Morse (Ed.), *Completing a qualitative project: Details and dialogue* (pp. 191-208). Thousand Oaks, CA: Sage.

Kerlinger, F. (1986). *Foundations of behavioral science* (3rd ed.). New York: Holt, Rinehart & Winston.

Kerr, D. (1996). The use of action research as an appropriate method of introducing and evaluating change in nursing care in an accident and emergency unit in Durban, Part 2. *Curationis, 19*(4), 7-12.

Killon, C. (1995). Special health care needs of homeless women. *Advances in Nursing Science, 18*(2), 44-56.

Kirkham, R. (1995). *Theories of truth: A critical introduction.* Cambridge, MA: MIT Press.

Lincoln, Y., & Guba, L. (1985). *Naturalistic inquiry.* Newbury Park, CA: Sage.

Magilvy, J., Congdon, J., & Martinez, R. (1994). Circles of care: Home care and community support for rural older adults. *Advances in Nursing Science, 16*(3), 22-33.

Marmoreo, J., Brown, J. B., Batty, H. R., Cummings, S., & Powell, M. (1998). Hormone replacement therapy: Determinants of women's decisions. *Patient Education and Counseling, 33,* 289-298.

McGuire, J. (1990). Putting nursing research findings into practice: Research utilization as an aspect of the management of change. *Journal of Advanced Nursing, 15,* 614-620.

Miller, W., & Crabtree, B. (1994). Clinical research. In N. Denzin & Y. Lincoln (Eds.), *Handbook of qualitative research* (pp. 340-352). Thousand Oaks, CA: Sage.

Morse, J. M., & Johnson, J. (1991). *The illness experience: Dimensions of suffering.* Newbury Park, CA: Sage.

Morse, J. M., Penrod, J., & Hupcey, J. (2000). Qualitative outcome analysis: Evaluating nursing interventions for complex clinical phenomena. *Journal of Nursing Scholarship, 32*(2), 125-135.

Olson, K., & Morse, J. M. (1996). Explaining breast self examination. *Health Care for Women International, 17*(6), 587-603.

Olson, K., Tom, B., Hewitt, J., Whittingham, J., Buchanan, L., & Ganton, G. (1998, October). *Development of supportive interventions for the management of fatigue experienced by patients with lung and selected gastrointestinal (GI) cancers.* Paper presented at the meeting of the Canadian Association of Nurses in Oncology, Regina, SK, Canada.

Pearcey, P., & Draper, P. (1996). Using the diffusion of innovation model to influence practice: A case study. *Journal of Advanced Nursing, 23,* 714-721.

Pederson, A. (1993). Qualities of the excellent head nurse. *Nursing Administration Quarterly, 18*(1), 40-50.

Rogers, E. (1983). *Diffusion of innovation* (3rd ed.). New York: Free Press.

Stake, R. (1997). Case Studies. In N. Denzin & Y. Lincoln (Eds.), *Handbook of qualitative research* (pp. 236-247). Thousand Oaks, CA: Sage.

Stake, R., & Trumbull, D. (1982). Naturalistic generalizations. *Review Journal of Philosophy and Social Science, 7,* 1-12.

Stephens, M. (1982). A question of generalizability. *Theory and Research in Social Education, 9,* 75-86.

Windelband, W. (1961). *Theories of logic.* New York: Citadel Press.

Dialogue:

Another Challenge

OLSON: I think this point is worth mentioning as an explanation for why so little is actually used. . . . First, you've got your theory, and then, you've got to operationalize it somehow, so that it can get out.

MORSE: It's tricky to use the word "operationalize." It's better to say, "Put it in a form that . . ." They want strategies and we're just giving them more theory. . . . The theory informs, but if you want them to do something, we have to provide them with the tools.

12

Research Utilization and Qualitative Research

CAROLE A. ESTABROOKS

While some bemoan an urgent need to increase the use of qualitative research findings, it also remains the case that despite the existence of thousands of clinical trials (in the area of pain, for example), quantitative research, even when plentiful, is notoriously poorly implemented in practice. The research utilization problem is this very gap between what we know (research) and what we do (practice). And much to the possible disappointment of many qualitative adherents, the process of *actually using* qualitative research findings is not essentially different from the process of using the findings of any kind of research. Qualitative findings may have an advantage because their *form* may be more appealing to clinicians. However, this is probably counterbalanced by the lack of familiarity with the criteria by which qualitative findings are judged adequate, the inherent mistrust many traditional scientists and practitioners have of qualitative work, and the relatively recent attention qualitative researchers and consumers of qualitative research have begun to pay to *the problem*.

This chapter is an overview of the complex field of research utilization and an invitation to treat this field more critically and with a greater appreciation of the science urgently needed to advance it. It is written with an attitude of optimism in hopes that the "doers" and "users" of qualitative research will take a more thoughtful approach to developing and understanding the science of research use.

In this chapter, I will (a) briefly trace the origins of the present-day evidence-based movement in order to locate the discussion, (b) outline a set of influential assumptions that operate in the literature on research utilization, knowledge utilization, innovation diffusion, and related fields, (c) describe kinds of research use, (d) describe two approaches to understanding the influences on practitioners' abilities to effectively use research, and (e) briefly discuss the role of research in influencing policy. The discussion will focus on the practices of nurses and physicians and will undoubtedly favor nurses, as this is the disciplinary perspective from which I derive; and as Thorne has illustrated in an earlier chapter, we are influenced and located by our disciplinary tradition.

This chapter, on the other hand, is not a collection of examples of qualitative research that clinicians, administrators, and other decision makers can use in their respective contexts. Such chapters and articles exist (e.g., Swanson, Durham, & Albright, 1997), and although helpful, none is ever complete or entirely satisfactory to the reader. Neither is this chapter a *how to use* qualitative research chapter. How to use any kind of research is so context dependent that it is unlikely such a recipe-driven approach is ever satisfactory. This chapter is not about how to use qualitative research to influence policy, although I will briefly address the policy problem toward the end. Policy is notoriously resistant to any research, no more or less so to qualitative research. Sometimes we confuse the current trend to "tell stories," that is, to create alternative *forms* for quantitative research findings, with the use of qualitative research because it is almost always presented in narrative form, and good narrative is compelling. Our enthusiasm for stories sometimes is translated into optimism that the story will be the thing that policy makers need.

Finally, this chapter is not a treatment of qualitative research as a *special case* of research requiring special research utilization techniques and approaches. Rather, I argue that to make this differentiation is a disservice to qualitative research that reflects an immaturity in our thinking in the field of research utilization. Although qualitative research possesses unique characteristics that in some cases advantage its potential users and in other cases disadvantage them, these (with the possible exception of *form*) are addressed in the preceding chapters and in many other texts and references now available on such topics as rigor and study evaluation, generalizability, and the synthesis of qualitative studies.

A repeating characteristic of the literature that addresses research utilization is its failure to differentiate prerequisite conditions for research utilization from research utilization itself. Examples of such prerequisite conditions include (a) research studies of sufficient quality to engender confidence in their findings, (b) existence of a sufficient critical mass of research studies in any given area to warrant synthesis or aggregation, (c) existence of appropriate synthesis methods for the body of research, (d) adequate dissemination of the research, and (e) sufficient *receptor capacity* in clinical and other decision-making settings.

Terminology, Origins, and Constructed Movements

Terminology

The literature is replete with terminology, often unique to particular disciplines, used to describe the general areas signified by such various terms as *innovation diffusion, technology transfer, knowledge utilization, research utilization,* and most recently, *Evidence-Based Practice.* These terms are not synonymous, and a failure to understand the origins of each has led in some instances to uncritical assumptions about the recent evidence-based movement in health care first described in medicine (Evidence-Based Medicine Working Group, 1992).

Dissemination refers to the spreading of knowledge or research that is done in scientific journals and at scientific conferences. It has its roots in library science and is concerned with getting information out to a wider audience (Backer, 1991). *Diffusion* also refers to the spreading of innovations, knowledge, and/or research to individuals, groups, organizations, and in some cases to society at large. *Diffusion* is a term usually used after there has been a decision to adopt an innovation. *Adoption* usually refers to the decision to adopt the innovation and has frequently been the dependent variable in innovation diffusion research. *Implementation* refers to the execution of the adoption decision when the innovation or the research is put into practice. *Utilization* is focused on assisting with the actual adoption process after dissemination and diffusion have occurred (Backer, 1991), and on the adaptation, implementation, and routinization processes discussed by Havelock (1986). *Routinization* is an "embedding" process and is also described as internalization, integration, incorporation, and institutionalization (Havelock, 1986, p. 25). Utilization most commonly implies an attendant behavior change. *Technology transfer* is the communication and practical use of information; that information is often scientific knowledge (Dearing, 1993; Glaser, Abelson, & Garrison, 1983). It is often used synonymously with dissemination and does not always include actual utilization.

Evidence-Based Medicine was defined in 1996 as

> the conscientious, explicit, and judicious use of current best evidence in making decisions about the care of individual patients. The practice of Evidence-Based Medicine means integrating individual clinical expertise with the best available external clinical evidence from systematic research. (Sackett, Rosenberg, Gray, & Haynes, 1996, p. 71)

Although not clearly articulated by proponents of Evidence-Based Medicine, it seems clear that Evidence-Based Practice is much broader than research dissemination, innovation diffusion, or research utilization, encompassing the use not only of research findings but other forms of practice knowledge as well. The term *Evidence-Based Practice* has crept into our language rapidly, and we have begun to use it without always paying attention to its origins or its meanings. I suspect that we often use it when we really intend to convey the narrower concept of research utilization.

Origins

Although we often proceed as if Evidence-Based Practice arose in the early 1990s with the publication of the important 1992 *New England Journal of Medicine* paper (Evidence-Based Medicine Working Group, 1992), in fact the origins of today's evidence-based movements can be traced at least to the early 20th century. Most authors trace the origin of diffusion research to the landmark 1943 study by Ryan and Gross on the diffusion of hybrid corn seed in Iowa. Rogers (1995) traces it to the 1903 work of French sociologist/social psychologist Gabriel Tardé. Rogers identified nine diffusion research traditions: anthropology, early sociology, rural sociology (the predominant one until the 1960s), education, public health/medical sociology, communication, marketing, geography, general sociology, and "other" (1995, chap. 2). Two studies from these nine traditions are frequently cited: the Ryan and Gross (1943) hybrid corn study and the 1955 Menzel and Katz study in which the diffusion of a new antibiotic was studied among New England physicians. Rogers's work (Rogers, 1962, 1983, 1986, 1988, 1995; Rogers & Agarwala-Rogers, 1976; Rogers & Shoemaker, 1971) has had a significant impact on the field of diffusion research. In fact, the 1962 work is credited with being the key factor responsible for the spread of the diffusion paradigm to other disciplines such as public health, economics, marketing, and political science (Valente & Rogers, 1995). Nursing has been a heavy importer of Rogers's concepts and theoretical positions, but this has not been the case with medicine or the Evidence-Based Medicine movement more generally.

The history of the field of knowledge utilization is less clear. The most often cited source from the knowledge utilization field is Glaser, Abelson, and Garrison's (1983) encyclopedic review of the literature on the topic. In addition, the work of Dunn (1983), Larsen (1980), Sunneson and Nilsson (1988), and Weiss (1979, 1980) are frequently drawn upon. Recently, Backer (1991) organized the evolution of knowledge utilization in three "waves": (1) 1920-1960, (2) 1960-1980, and (3) 1990 to the present. Beal (1986) attributes the growth of the field to the vigorous promotion of knowledge and technology as socially valuable in the post–World War II society, particularly in the United States. In this framework, science is accorded high social status, and significant resources are diverted into the scientific enterprise. Backer (1991) attributes the Reagan administration in the United States with a decade of drastic reduction in priority and resources to this field during the 1980s.

Innovation diffusion as a field of study is a precursor to knowledge utilization, rather than a separate entity. The increasing realization that diffusion is essentially a communicative and interactive social process (Rogers, 1995), the expansion of the diffusion tradition into disciplines beyond rural sociology, a growing interest in communication as an area of study, and a growing belief in such strategies as social marketing as being effective for bringing about mass change in behavior have resulted in the expansion of the innovation diffusion field to include more general theorizing. That more general theorizing now encompasses the field known as knowledge utilization.

Constructed Movements

Evidence-Based Practice and the developing evidence-based nursing movement are not synonymous with research utilization. Rather, they symbolize far-reaching programs in nursing and the health sciences more generally (Estabrooks, 1998, 1999a, 1999b, 1999c; Evidence-Based

Medicine Working Group, 1992; Kitson, 1997). Nursing has some 30 years of experience with one dimension of Evidence-Based Practice, research utilization (Estabrooks, 1998). This experience dates from the large and often cited Conduct and Utilization of Research in Nursing (CURN) project of the 1970s (Horsley, Crane, & Bingle, 1978; Horsley, Crane, Crabtree, & Wood, 1983) and from the first empirical studies into research utilization in the field of nursing (Ketefian, 1975; Shore, 1972).

At about the same time that nursing was experimenting with large research utilization initiatives such as CURN, Cochrane's influential book (1972) was published. It was not until 1993, however, that the Cochrane Collaboration was founded (Chalmers, 1993). Today, it is a global enterprise that is moving to infuse a new approach to teaching and practicing in medicine—Evidence-Based Medicine. Calls for evidence-based decision making, Evidence-Based Practice, evidence-based nursing practice, and/or evidence-based nursing arise from the Evidence-Based Medicine movement, and have received a recent boost in Canada from the National Forum on Health, which called for a culture of evidence-based decision making (Evidence-Based Decision Making Working Group, 1997). More recently, we see the beginnings of a transformation of Evidence-Based Practice into "best practices," as if somehow this eases the perceived and onerous expectations of Evidence-Based Practice. Or perhaps it is a genuine attempt to make explicit the broad and far-ranging conceptions of evidence, as well as the provisional nature of evidence, and the limitations of research to provide all or even most of the answers. Even more recent is the emergence of "knowledge management" terminology often associated with information sciences and with quality improvement programs.

Assumptions

At least six major assumptions, that is, positions or, in some cases, biases, are implicit in the conceptual and empirical work on research utilization and innovation diffusion. These assumptions serve to influence not only how we think of the field but also the kinds of inquiry we undertake. The first of these, a *pro-innovation* bias, dominates the literature both within and from outside the field of nursing. The pro-innovation bias position assumes that innovation is positive. It is addressed by Abrahamson (1991, 1993), Kimberley (1981), Rogers (1983, 1986), Romano (1990), Van De Ven (1986), Zaltman (1979), and others. One problem with such a bias is that it tends to preclude us from considering nonutilization as a viable alternative. Kimberley, over a decade ago, predicted that we would enter a phase of increased skepticism regarding innovation research.

The second assumption is made explicit by Rogers (1983, p. 106-107) and is implicit in the literature on nursing. It claims that *good workers (nurses) use research;* it resembles a "blaming the victim" stance, according to which nurses who do not use research are considered less than professional. This assumption discounts the multiple system factors that operate on micro and macro levels and form the context of nursing practice. The individual blame perspective probably came about because of the focus on individual innovativeness (Rogers, 1995) early in the development of innovation diffusion. Anyone trying to determine the extent of research utilization in juxtaposition with individual factors or trying to determine factors influencing research utilization faces the challenge of refraining from this perspective.

The third assumption and one that follows logically from a pro-innovation bias is that *research utilization results in an improved situation,* or, in the case of health care, in improved practices and improved patient outcomes. In nursing, the standard approach is to take a group of research studies that have been evaluated against a set of criteria for scientific merit and, judging them as sound, try to implement them in the practice setting, perhaps in the form of a clinical protocol.[1]

We assume that this will lead to improved outcomes. Apart from the difficulty inherent in identifying and measuring client outcomes, or in defining and measuring the intermediate dependent variable research utilization, this may be an unwarranted assumption. Although on a commonsense level, this is logical reasoning, it is probably too simplistic to be *necessarily* true in the complex practice setting. We should not be blinded to the possibility that improved outcomes demonstrated under experimental conditions may not necessarily hold when the intervention is implemented on a large scale in nonexperimental (i.e., naturalistic) conditions. Very few demonstration projects have been implemented to offer indications of the effects of larger-scale research utilization in the practice context. Concepts such as *transformation* (Orlandi, 1986), *reinvention* (Larsen, 1980; Lewis & Siebold, 1993; Rice & Rogers, 1980; Rogers, 1988, 1995), and *synergistic* interaction and diffusion, in which the adoption of one innovation facilitates or dampens the adoption of subsequent ones (Fennell, 1984; Kimberley, 1981), may occur between the context of the research study and the context of the practice setting.

The fourth assumption is the dominant *efficient-choice* perspective (Abrahamson, 1991). Within this perspective, it is assumed that adopters make rational choices guided by the tools of technical efficiency, and that free and independent choice is possible. This perspective assumes that (a) the planned change position discussed below is a valid one; (b) clinicians possess the autonomy to make choices in favor of research-based practice; and (c) if they do have the ability to control their choices, they will choose in favor of research-based practice. This perspective is somewhat similar to what Weiss (1979) characterizes as the *knowledge-driven* image of research utilization. This view originates with the natural sciences and has been the prevailing perspective on the development and use of "science" as knowledge. It assumes that "the sheer fact that knowledge exists presses it toward development and use" (Weiss, 1979, p. 427). It is equatable with a "push" model of utilization, in which science is "produced" and the clinician is expected to use it by virtue of its existence. Alternatively, a "pull" model would exist if clinicians demanded research that addressed problems with which they had to cope. Recently, Lomas (1999) has proposed that we are migrating from a predominately *pull* model to one of *partnerships,* in which linkage and exchange are the central forces.

The fifth assumption, and the one on which nearly all the work in the health sciences is premised, is that of *planned change.* The practice setting, in the way similar to most settings, grows increasingly unstable with the expansion of knowledge, advancement of technology, and the destabilization of our social, political, and economic world. Although it is true that models based rigidly on planned change need to be reconsidered in our work on research utilization, it is not true that alternative approaches to conceptualizing change have emerged and been examined.

The final assumption is that the primary *knowledge needed for practice is scientific in nature.* This theme has recently been taken up by critics of Evidence-Based Medicine and is apparent, for example, in recent exchanges in the *Journal of Evaluation in Clinical Practice* (Charlton, 1997; Norman, 1999). In nursing, Carper and others have made important contributions to our understanding of knowledge by offering us several forms of knowledge used in nursing. These included empires, aesthetics, personal knowledge, and ethics (Carper, 1978). While Carper's *empiric* form of knowledge is crucial to nursing practice, it is not appropriate to continue to focus on scientific knowledge to the exclusion of other knowledge forms. As Upshur demonstrates in Chapter 1, there is an increasing tendency to understand and include a much wider range of knowledge under the umbrella of evidence.

Kinds of Research Use

Some social scientists (Beyer & Trice, 1982; Dunn, 1983; Larsen, 1980; Rich, 1975, 1977; Sunneson & Nilsson, 1988, 1993; Weiss, 1979, 1980), social workers (Hasenfeld & Patti, 1992), and at least one nurse scholar (Stetler, 1994a, 1994b) have discussed instrumental, conceptual, and symbolic research utilization. Recently, I empirically demonstrated the presence of both an overall concept called research utilization and three distinct concepts—instrumental (direct), conceptual (indirect), and symbolic (persuasive) research utilization (Estabrooks, 1999a). This conceptual structure, although tested specifically in nurses, was not *nursing research* specific. Nurses were explicitly asked about their use of any kind of research.

Instrumental Research Utilization

Instrumental research utilization (Estabrooks, 1999c; Larsen, 1980; Rich, 1975, 1977; Stetler, 1994b; Weiss 1979) implies a concrete application of research, where the research has often been translated into a material and usable form such as a clinical protocol, clinical decision algorithm, or clinical practice guideline (CPG). In this case, the research is used to direct specific decisions and/or interventions. At the individual level, the research may be applied "directly" as an intervention without translation into another form such as a protocol. It may be applied fully, partially, or in modified form. It is this instrumental form of research use that has until now most commonly been referred to in discussions of Evidence-Based Practice or research utilization in nursing and most other fields.

Conceptual Research Utilization

In conceptual research utilization, research may change one's thinking but not necessarily one's particular action. In this kind of research utilization, research informs and enlightens the decision maker (Hasenfeld & Patti, 1992). Before Hasenfeld and Patti, Larsen (1980), drawing on the work of Rich (1975, 1977) and Weiss (1979), proposed that knowledge utilization can be classified as instrumental and conceptual. In nursing, Stetler (1994a, 1994b) is one of the few who have drawn upon this conceptual usage. In the Evidence-Based Medicine literature, as noted, we see a primarily instrumental treatment of use.

Symbolic (or Persuasive) Research Utilization

Symbolic utilization involves the use of research as a persuasive or political tool to legitimate a position or practice (Estabrooks, 1999c). There are many examples of *persuasive* research utilization in nursing; one of the most powerful is the work done by Florence Nightingale when she marshaled large volumes of epidemiological data in Scutari during the Crimean War. She used it to persuade the secretary of war and others of the need for radical reform in the British military and, in so doing, saved the lives of countless British soldiers. Although her work used the tools of epidemiology and statistics, her persuasive *use* of the data is not specific to quantitative data. Rather, it was her behavior and the processes of influence she used that defined the persuasive use of research.

The different kinds of research utilization are important to our understanding of how clinicians use research, including qualitative research, in their practice. It may be that qualitative research findings are more easily used conceptually and persuasively than instrumentally. It is also likely that clinicians in all health disciplines use research in their practices more commonly than it has been assessed to date, particularly when we consider the different ways in which research can be used.

Influences on Research Use

Scholars have struggled for some time now to isolate the particular influences that determine practitioners' use or nonuse of research.

Often, we have seen more certitude in the literature than is, upon closer inspection, warranted. For example, in nursing, we see assertions that education level, time spent reading professional journals, and adequate time for research utilization at work are important influences. However, the actual research evidence for these and other assertions is at best equivocal. Two bodies of literature from several disciplinary perspectives can be used to discuss the potential sets of influences determining research use. Although informative, they serve to illustrate the need for rigorous study in this area—study that originates from a number of different research paradigms.

Elements of the Diffusion Model

One approach to categorizing and understanding the multiple influences on clinicians' use of research in their practice is to categorize those influences as individual, organizational, or research specific (i.e., what diffusion researchers would describe as "attributes of the innovation"). This approach has been used by me (Estabrooks, 1999a, 1999b) and is briefly described below.

Individual Determinants Individual determinants of research utilization are those characteristics possessed by the individual that influence their use of research findings in their work. Examples of these factors include (a) a *positive attitude* to research (Bostrum & Suter, 1993; Champion & Leach, 1989; Lacey, 1994; Rizutto, Bostrum, Suter, & Chenitz, 1994); (b) *autonomy* (Funk, Champagne, Weiss, & Tornquist, 1991; Lacey, 1994; Rodgers, 1994; Walczak, McGuire, Haisfield, & Beezley, 1994); (c) *awareness of agency policy* and *educational level* (Michel & Sneed, 1995); (d) *conference attendance* (Coyle & Sokop, 1990); (e) *cooperativeness and self-efficacy* (Kim & Kim, 1996); (f) *job satisfaction* (Coyle & Sokop, 1990); (g) *involvement in nursing research activities* (Bostrum & Suter, 1993; Pettengill, Gillies, & Clark, 1994); and (h) time spent *reading professional journals* (Barta, 1995; Brett, 1987; Coyle & Sokop, 1990; Kirchoff, 1982). This body of research is, however, underdeveloped and offers little direction or certainty about what individual attributes might be important predictors of research utilization behavior. For example, when the individual determinants were assessed in one study (Estabrooks, 1999a), only a positive attitude to research, in-service attendance, and the ability to suspend strongly held beliefs remained in models as significant influencing factors.

Ongoing work (Estabrooks & Floyd, in progress) systematically assessing the influence of individual determinants on nurses' use of research reveals an underdeveloped and equivocal body of research in this area.

Organizational Determinants Organizational determinants are those characteristics of health care organizations, of units within those institutions, and of governance structures outside those institutions that facilitate the dissemination and uptake of research findings. We know even less about these than we do about individual determinants. Organizational size, administrative support, access to research, and time (Brett, 1987, 1989; Coyle & Sokop, 1990; Dunn, Crichton, Roe, Seers, & Williams, 1998; Funk, Champagne, Weiss, & Tornquist, 1991; Rutledge, Ropka, Greene, Nail, & Mooney, 1997; Varcoe & Hilton, 1995) have been examined. Other organizational determinants, such as complexity, centralization, presence of a research champion, traditionalism, and organizational slack, have not, for the most part, been addressed in the health literature, although others, such as organizational analysts, have studied these characteristics extensively (e.g., Chakrabarti, 1974; Damanpour, 1987, 1988, 1991, 1996; Downs & Mohr, 1976; Fennell, 1984; Kimberley, 1981; Kimberley & Evanisko, 1981; Mohr, 1969).

Perhaps most important, there are no published reports of studies whose investigators have examined organizational culture at the local (unit) level, or at multiple levels within the organization, and/or at regional levels. Unit and institutional culture undoubtedly constitute significant and multidimensional influences on research utilization behaviors. Elements such as unit norms, unit belief structures, local leadership and influence, rules of engagement, and interactions with other levels of the organization are likely embedded in the broader notion of organizational culture. In addition, organizational factors, such as a supportive administrative structure and adequate time to use research, can probably only be well understood within the context of local unit culture. A current systematic review of the influence of organizational determinants on research use by nurses shows that this area is seriously underdeveloped and the findings of studies at best equivocal. (Foxcroft et al., in progress).

Attributes of the Innovation Attributes of the innovation are those characteristics of the research findings and of the clinical phenomena that influence the uptake of relevant research. For example, the characteristics of the body of research on effective pain management, as well as the characteristics of the phenomenon of pain itself, will contribute to whether or not nurses make effective use of pain research in their practices. Unfortunately, although Rogers (1995) has outlined several essential attributes of innovations (e.g., complexity, relative advantage, compatibility, observability, and trialability), there is little if any understanding of the influence of attributes of the innovation on nurses' or other health professionals' research utilization behavior. Grilli and Lomas (1994) reviewed over a decade of MEDLINE entries addressing practice guidelines and evaluated them using complexity, trialability, and observability. They concluded that complexity and trialability were partial predictors of compliance. Although preliminary findings are not yet available, the potentially first systematic review to explicitly address innovation attributes in nursing is currently under way in Canada (Logan, Graham, & Pepler, in progress).

The Social Influences Model

Recently, social influence theory has been proposed as a useful framework for understanding physician behavior (Lomas, 1994; Mittman, Tonesk, & Jacobson, 1992). Social influence refers to the process in which one individual's behavior affects other people's behavior, feelings, or thoughts (Zimbano & Leippe, 1991). Mittman et al. (1992) propose social influence theory as building on traditional models of physician decision making. In traditional models, education, information, and financial incentives are viewed as key determinants of behavior (Eisenberg, 1986; Harris, 1990; Stafford, 1990). The social influences model does not abandon these types of incentives and influences but builds on them by arguing that, in addition to these, behavior change is also guided by (a) habit and custom; (b) assumptions, beliefs, and values held by peers; and (c) existing practices and social norms. The traditional model resembles the diffusion model in that dissemination of new information is often viewed as leading automatically to utilization if the appropriate incentives for the change are in place. Alternatively, the social influences model would predict that after exposure to new information, many physicians would be influenced by colleagues' judgments of the value and significance of the innovation (e.g., the CPG), or by their decisions to the contrary.

The rationale for the utility of the social influences model lies in the assessment that medicine is characterized by uncertainty, multiple perspectives, and a particular style of medical education and subsequent clinical practice (Mittman et al., 1992). The social influences model is especially predictive when uncertainty is high, as with the introduction of new guidelines for practice, the impact of which are not fully known. Clinical practice behavior is rooted in a system of social norms that are first developed during the medical education and socialization process, and which evolve through residency programs and ongoing interactions with colleagues and peers. Clinical practice is based not only on science and the best available evidence but also on shared consensus among peers and a system of traditions and conventions, some of which originate in one's training and many of which are locally defined. Therefore, a framework that suggests strategies beyond the dissemination of information is useful. In the social influences model, heavy emphasis is placed on local peer influence and on the recognition that habits, customs, norms, and conventions of practice are important sources of behavior.

Other determinants of physician behavior that have been identified and that support elements in both the innovation diffusion and the social influences models include (a) the characteristics of the CPG, the motivation of the practitioner, and clinical context (Kanouse & Jacoby, 1988); (b) characteristics of the physician and patient, peer opinion, tradition, organization of the physician's practice, financial incentives, and patient expectations (Leape, 1990); and (c) personalized feedback, opinion leaders, and the importance of local initiatives (Lomas, Enkin, Anderson, Hannah, Vayda, & Singer, 1991). Freiman (1985) found that physicians in solo practices had lower rates of adoption of innovations. Fox, Mazmanian, and Putnam (1989) found that purely professional motivations, such as a desire for increased competence and the belief that the clinical context demanded a change, drove the largest percentage of changes made by physicians.

Greer (1988) conducted an important study in which she interviewed 290 physicians and found strong support for the problem of uncertainty in clinical practice, the inadequacy of dissemination using journal articles alone, and the importance of conferences. She also found high levels of distrust for the usefulness of the scientific literature that was rooted in a distrust of the social structure of science, and a perceived insufficiency of scientific reporting in relation to practice

(Greer, 1988, p. 9). Her study locates technology decisions as embedded in the norms and relationships of local practice and underscores the importance of local consensus, local innovators, and idea champions as central to changing the behavior of physicians. Three terms from this study are important to subsequent discussion and need clarification. Greer identifies the importance of local opinion leaders, idea champions, and innovators. These three types of individuals are each different. *Opinion leaders* are not innovators but evaluators who are trusted to judge the "fit" between an innovation and their local situation. A *local innovator* introduces the innovation to his or her local community, modifying it as necessary to fit the situation. The *local idea champion* is an enthusiast whose persuasion and determination helps an innovation be adopted.

Finally, the work of Hill and Weisman (1991) and Tannenbaum, Sampalis, and Battista (1990) suggest that the strongest predictor of physician behavior after dissemination of CPGs is prior practice behavior that is compatible with the CPG recommendations. With this in mind, it becomes evident that it may be useful to try and incorporate strategies that focus on preparing target groups for an alternative approach. Continuing medical education (CME) and learning may be important in this by helping to predispose physicians to considering change and to reinforcing the change once it has occurred (Lomas, 1994). CME alone has not been demonstrated to be an effective strategy for changing physician behavior (Lomas & Haynes, 1988; Schroeder, 1987). However, as CME continues to evolve with the development of strategies, such as the primary and secondary ones described by Davis, Lindsay, and Mazmanian (1994), it holds potential as both a source of valuable strategies and a vehicle of influence on behavior.

Use in Practice and Policy

In the literature in this field, research utilization is often equated with the appraisal and critique of individual research reports, and of syntheses (often traditional meta-analyses) of these reports. Similarly, in undergraduate and graduate courses, we sometimes see "research utilization" and, more recently, "Evidence-Based Practice" courses that, when examined, would more accurately be titled "research critique and appraisal" courses. We see these patterns, I suspect, because we have been convinced that research utilization or Evidence-Based Practice is an individual responsibility, and we believe that if practitioners know the correct course of action, they will take the correct (evidence-based) decision. We subscribe implicitly and explicitly to a rational model of decision making.

This, of course, is not the case. Practitioners function in highly complex, dynamic environments—environments that are fundamentally political. They are affected by a host of personal, social, educational, professional, organizational, and environmental influences. To focus exclusively on research consumption and evaluation supposes that personal behavior and education are the primary influences determining whether research makes its way into action. It also supposes further that personal choices, even when the will is strong, are possible and, when taken, make a difference. In reality, we know this is not the case. Although we have little if any research yet to clarify the roles that environment, organizational climate, and organizational and group cultures play in facilitating or inhibiting the implementation of research (in whatever form it presents), we are increasingly aware that they factor centrally in determining the use of research in practice.

Creation of an Evidence-Based Practice (or best practice or research-based practice) that is systematic and comprehensive requires a collaborative effort on many levels, of which the individual is but one. It also requires that we appreciate how the real practice world functions. Jenkins-Smith and Sabbatier (1993) observed that the literature on knowledge utilization has evolved independently of the political science literature on the factors influencing the policy process. Were we to integrate these two literatures, we might find substantial improvements in our ability to understand and alter patterns of research implementation in the practice context. For example, relatively straightforward adjustments would result if we functioned with an understanding that in real-life contexts, the dominant approach to decision making is not a rational hypothetico-deductive one. Rather, decision making is much more likely to be influenced by bureaucratic and political processes. In a political model, for example, decisions are often the product of a negotiated compromise made to balance competing interests, rather than of rational decisions based on the best information (i.e., research) available.

Lomas (1997) describes a framework for understanding the context of decision making that divides the decision-making world into three interrelated domains: (1) formal and informal institutional structures for decision making, (2) values (ideologies, beliefs, interests), and (3) information (knowledge or research, its producers and its purveyors). Although it is beyond the scope of this chapter to explore the utility of such a framework for understanding research dissemination and uptake, it is worthwhile to consider Lomas's implicit assumption of decision making as a political process. For example, in his framework, ideologies represent those fundamental views formed through early socialization experiences that are minimally, if at all, amenable to change. Beliefs represent those assumptions that we hold about how the causal world operates, and interests represent responses to sets of incentives and rewards that coexist in any given system. With these perspectives in mind, it becomes clear that there is little advantage in attempting to change the ideological views an individual or group may hold—regardless of the power or eloquence of the research, ideology is resistant to its influences. Both the pro-life and the pro-choice sides of the abortion debate are the cases that demonstrate the unlikely prospect of changing ideological views using research or any other form of knowledge.

Beliefs are, on the other hand, amenable to the influence of change, although they tend to change slowly. Witness the enormous change in beliefs we have seen in the last decades regarding the effects of smoking and the attendant changes in formal and informal societal practices. Interests may be the most fruitful avenue to pursue in order to change behavior or practice—although not because the research immediately makes it so, but because incentive and reward systems can be changed to effect almost immediate changes in practice in some instances. For example, if nurses are denied the ability to practice in their chosen specialty unless they regularly certify (assuming practice in a chosen specialty is desirable), such regular certification can be readily mandated with a change in institutional practices to support it.

An understanding of these and other processes, addressed in frameworks such as that of Lomas or Sabbatier and Jenkins-Smith, would enable us, I believe, to make much more effective progress in implementing research into practice. Whether the research in question has been traditionally quantitative or more recently qualitative, the process of implementing it into practice is much the same. What may differentiate qualitative research is its *form*. It is often, if not usually, presented in narrative form, and as such is more readily comprehensible. One of Lomas's (1997) assertions is that research must be translated into common knowledge by its purveyors before it will be taken up readily. Because words are the everyday barter of clinicians, if Lomas's assertion is true, it places qualitative research perhaps in a position of privilege by virtue of its increased accessibility to readers who do not require sophisticated methods or statistical backgrounds to comprehend it. It also means that it may be more vulnerable to misuse and misinterpretation. Recently, among some Evidence-Based Medicine proponents, we have witnessed increased interest in "the story" as a desirable form of presentation of traditionally quantitative findings—because of its appeal to a wide range of clinicians. Whether this develops into a major thrust among dissemination experts remains to be seen. However, it is clear that qualitative research does not have proprietary rights over form.

Conclusions

The field of inquiry into the dissemination and utilization of research is complex and poorly understood. Ironically, what this field has to offer us has never been more urgently needed. As knowledge continues to expand at increasing rates, the challenges will increase, as will the need to get usable "best" information to clinicians and other decision makers. The following inquiries will be helpful: focused study of strategies that promote the dissemination and use of research, studies that evaluate whether the use of research improves health outcomes, and studies that broaden our understanding of what constitutes legitimate evidence for practice. What is clearly not helpful—from the perspective of someone engaged in the study of research utilization behaviors and processes—and in fact is unwarranted, is the belief that there is no longer any reason for pain to go unmanaged, or for pressure sores to develop, or for pregnant mothers to smoke, or for viral sore throats to be treated with antibiotics because we *know enough*.

We *knew enough* about scurvy 263 years before the British Merchant Navy introduced citrus as a routine dietary supplement to shipboard diets. If knowing enough were all it took, a goodly number of the diseases and social plagues of contemporary society would have been eradicated, and far greater resources would be dedicated to addressing the fundamental and social determinants of health than is currently the case.

Note

1. This phenomenon is not unique to nursing; in fact, it seems to be the preferred approach in the current CPG movement in Canada and the United States that is current among physicians as well as other health practitioners.

References

Abrahamson, E. (1991). Managerial fads and fashions: The diffusion and rejection of innovations. *Academy of Management Review, 16*(3), 586-612.

Abrahamson, E. (1993). Institutional and competitive bandwagons: Using mathematical modeling as a tool to explore innovation diffusion. *Academy of Management Review, 18*(3), 487-517.

Backer, T. E. (1991). Knowledge utilization. *Knowledge: Creation, Diffusion, Utilization, 12*(3), 225-240.

Barta, K. M. (1995). Information-seeking, research utilization, and barriers to research utilization of pediatric nurse educators. *Journal of Professional Nursing, 11*, 49-57.

Beal, G. M. (1986). A user-problem-need-driven model: Farming systems research and development. In G. M. Beal, W. Dissanayake, & S. Konoshima (Eds.), *Knowledge generation, utilization, exchange, and utilization* (pp. 183-208). Boulder, CO: Westview Press.

Beyer, J. M., & Trice, H. M. (1982). The utilization process: A conceptual framework and synthesis of empirical findings. *Administrative Science Quarterly, 27*, 591-622.

Bostrum, J., & Suter, W. N. (1993). Research utilization: Making the link to practice. *Journal of Nursing Staff Development, 9*(1), 28-34.

Brett, J. L. L. (1987). Use of nursing practice research findings. *Nursing Research, 36*, 344-349.

Brett, J. L. L. (1989). Organizational integrative mechanisms and adoption of innovations by nurses. *Nursing Research, 38*, 105-110.

Carper, B. A. (1978). Fundamental patterns of knowing in nursing. *Advances in Nursing Science, 1*(1), 13-23.

Chakrabarti, A. K. (1974). The role of champion in product innovation. *California Management Review, 17*(2), 58-62.

Chalmers, I. (1993). The Cochrane Collaboration: Preparing, maintaining and disseminating systematic reviews of the effects of health care. In K. S. Warren & F. Mosteller (Eds.), Doing more good than harm: The evaluation of health care interventions. *Annals of the New York Academy of Science, 703*, 156-163.

Champion, V. L., & Leach, A. (1989). Variables related to research utilization in nursing: An empirical investigation. *Journal of Advanced Nursing, 14*, 705-710.

Charlton, B. G. (1997). Restoring the balance: Evidence-based medicine put in its place. *Journal of Evaluation in Clinical Practice, 3*(2), 87-98.

Cochrane, A. L. (1972). *Effectiveness and efficiency.* London: Abingdon, Berks, Burgess.

Coyle, L. A., & Sokop, A. G. (1990). Innovation adoption behavior among nurses. *Nursing Research, 39,* 176-180.

Damanpour, F. (1987). The adoption of technological, administrative, and ancillary innovations: Impact of organizational factors. *Journal of Management, 13*(4), 675-688.

Damanpour, F. (1988). Innovation type, radicalness, and the adoption process. *Communication Research, 15*(5), 545-567.

Damanpour, F. (1991). Organizational innovation: A meta-analysis of effects of determinants and moderators. *Academy of Management Journal, 34*(3), 555-590.

Damanpour, F. (1996). Organizational complexity and innovation: Developing and testing multiple contingency models. *Management Science, 42,* 693-715.

Davis, D. A., Lindsay, E. A., & Mazmanian, P. E. (1994). The effectiveness of CME interventions. In D. A. Davis & R. D. Fox (Eds.), *The physician as learner: Linking research to practice* (pp. 245-280). Chicago: American Medical Association.

Dearing, J. W. (1993). Rethinking technology transfer. *International Journal of Technology Transfer, 8,* 478-485.

Downs, G. W., & Mohr, L. B. (1976). Conceptual issues in the study of innovation. *Administrative Science Quarterly, 21,* 700-714.

Dunn, V., Crichton, N., Roe, B., Seers, K., & Williams, K. (1998). Using research for practice: A UK experience of the BARRIERS scale. *Journal of Advanced Nursing, 27,* 1203-1210.

Dunn, W. N. (1983). Measuring knowledge use. *Knowledge: Creation, Diffusion, Utilization, 5*(1), 120-133.

Eisenberg, J. M. (1986). *Doctors' decisions and the cost for doctors' practice patterns and ways to change them.* Ann Arbor, MI: Health Administration Press.

Estabrooks, C. A. (1998). Will evidence-based nursing practice make practice perfect? *Canadian Journal of Nursing Research, 30,* 15-36.

Estabrooks, C. A.(1999a). Modeling the individual determinants of research utilization. *Western Journal of Nursing Research, 21*(1), 758-772.

Estabrooks, C. A. (1999b). Mapping the research utilization field in nursing. *Canadian Journal of Nursing Research, 31*(1), 53-72.

Estabrooks, C. A. (1999c). The conceptual structure of research utilization. *Research in Nursing & Health, 22,* 203-216.

Estabrooks, C. A., & Floyd, J. A. (in progress). *A systematic review of the literature addressing individual determinants of research utilization behavior in nursing.*

Evidence-Based Decision Making Working Group. (1997). *Creating a culture of evidence-based decision making in health.* Ottawa, ON: National Forum on Health.

Evidence-Based Medicine Working Group. (1992). A new approach to teaching the practice of medicine. *Journal of the American Medical Association, 268,* 2420-2425.

Fennell, M. L. (1984). Synergy, influence, and information in the adoption of administrative innovations. *Academy of Management Journal, 27*(1), 113-129.

Fox, R. D., Mazmanian, P. E., & Putnam, R. W. (Eds.). (1989). *Changing and learning in the lives of physicians.* New York: Praeger.

Foxcroft, D. R., Cole, N., Fulbrook, P., Johnston, L., & Stevens, K. (In progress). *Organizational infrastructures to promote evidence based nursing practice* [protocol].

Freiman, M. P. (1985). The rate of adoption of new procedures among physicians: The impact of speciality and practice characteristics. *Medical Care, 23,* 939-945.

Funk, S. G., Champagne, R. A., Weiss, R. A., & Tornquist, E. M. (1991). Barriers to using research findings in practice. *Applied Nursing Research, 4*(2), 90-95, (1), 39-45.

Glaser, E. M., Abelson, H. H., & Garrison, K. N. (1983). *Putting knowledge to use.* San Francisco: Jossey-Bass.

Greer, A. L. (1988). The state of the art versus the state of the science: The diffusion of new medical technologies into practice. *International Journal of Technology Assessment in Health Care, 4,* 5-26.

Grilli, R., & Lomas, J. (1994). Evaluating the message: The relationship between compliance rate and the subject of a practice guideline. *Medical Care, 32*(3), 202-213.

Harris, J. S. (1990). Why doctors do what they do: Determinants of physician behavior. *Journal of Occupational Medicine, 32,* 1207-1220.

Hasenfeld, Y., & Patti, R. (1992). The utilization of research in administrative practice. In A. J. Grasso & I. Epstein (Eds.), *Research utilization in the social services* (pp. 221-239). New York: Haworth Press.

Havelock, R. G. (1986). The knowledge perspective: Definition and scope of a new study domain. In G. M. Beal, W. Dissanayake, & S. Konoshima (Eds.), *Knowledge generation, utilization, exchange, and utilization* (pp. 11-34). Boulder, CO: Westview Press.

Hill, M. N., & Weisman, C. S. (1991). Physicians' perceptions of consensus reports. *International Journal of Technology Assessment in Health Care, 7,* 30-41.

Horsley, J. A., Crane, J., & Bingle, J. D. (1978). Research utilization as an organizational process. *Journal of Nursing Administration,* July, 4-6.

Horsley, J. A., Crane, J., Crabtree, M. K., & Wood, D. J. (1983). *Using research to improve practice: A guide.* New York: Grune & Stratton.

Jenkins-Smith, H. C., & Sabbatier, P. A. (1993). The study of public policy processes. In P. A. Sabbatier & H. C. Jenkins-Smith (Eds.), *Policy change and learning: An advocacy coalition approach* (pp. 1-6). San Francisco: Westview Press.

Kanouse, R. H., & Jacoby, I. (1988). When does information change physician behavior? *International Journal of Technology Assessment in Health Care, 4,* 27-33.

Ketefian, S. (1975). Application of selected nursing research findings into nursing practice. *Nursing Research, 24*(2), 89-92.

Kim, I., & Kim, M.I. (1996). The effects of individual and nursing-unit characteristics on willingness to adopt an innovation: A multilevel analysis. *Computers in Nursing, 14,* 183-187.

Kimberley, J. R. (1981). Managerial innovation. In P. Nystrom & W. Starbuck (Eds.), *Handbook of Organizational Design: Vol. 1* (pp. 84-104). Oxford: Oxford University Press.

Kimberley, J. R., & Evanisko, M. J. (1981). Organizational innovation: The influence of individual, organizational, and contextual factors on hospital adoption of technological and administrative innovations. *Academy of Management Journal, 24*(4), 689-713.

Kirchoff, K. (1982). A diffusion survey of coronary precautions. *Nursing Research, 31,* 196-201.

Kitson, A. (1997). Using evidence to demonstrate the value of nursing. *Nursing Standard, 11*(28), 34-39.

Lacey, E. A. (1994). Research utilization in nursing practice—a pilot study. *Journal of Advanced Nursing, 19,* 987-995.

Larsen, J. (1980). Knowledge utilization. What is it? *Knowledge: Creation, Diffusion, Utilization, 1*(3), 421-442.

Leape, L. L. (1990). Practice guidelines and standards: An overview. *Quality Review Bulletin, 16,* 42-48.

Lewis, R. K., & Seibold, D. R. (1993). Innovation modification during intraorganizational adoption. *Academy of Management Review, 18*(2), 322-354.

Logan, J., Graham, I., & Pepler, C. (in progress). A systematic review of innovation attributes and their influence on research utilization.

Lomas, J. (1994). Teaching old (and not so old) docs new tricks: Effective ways to implement research findings. In E. V. Dunn, P. G. Norton, M. Stewart, F. Tudiver, and M. Bass (Eds.), *Dissemination research/changing practice* (pp. 1-18). Thousand Oaks, CA: Sage.

Lomas, J. (1997, March). *Improving research dissemination and uptake in the health sector: Beyond the sound of one hand clapping.* Discussion document for Advisory Committee on Health Services (ACHS) to the Federal/Provincial/Territorial Conference of Deputy Ministers: Ottawa, ON.

Lomas, J. (1999, October 1-3). Proclaim, push, pull, participate: The four eras of research dissemination and uptake. *Closing the loop: Evidence into health practice, organization and policy.* The 3rd International Conference on the Scientific Basis of Health Services, Toronto, ON.

Lomas, J., Enkin, M., Anderson, G. M., Hannah, W. J., Vayda, E., & Singer, J. (1991). Opinion leaders vs. audit and feedback to implement practice guidelines. *Journal of the American Medical Association, 265,* 2202-2206.

Lomas, J., & Haynes, B. (1988). A taxonomy and critical review of tested strategies for the application of clinical practice recommendations: From "official" to "individual" clinical policy. *American Journal of Preventive Medicine, 4*(Suppl.), 77-94.

Menzel, H., & Katz, E. (1955). Social relations and innovation in the medical profession: The epidemiology of a new rug. *Public Opinion Quarterly, 19,* 337-352.

Michel, Y., & Sneed, N. V. (1995). Dissemination and use of research findings in nursing practice. *Journal of Professional Nursing, 11,* 306-311.

Mittman, B. S., Tonesk, X., & Jacobson, P. D. (1992). Implementing clinical practice guidelines: Social influence strategies and practitioner behavior change. *Quality Review Bulletin, 18,* 413-422.

Mohr, L. B. (1969). Determinants of innovation in organizations. *American Political Science Review, 63,* 111-126.

Norman, G. (1999). Examining the assumptions of evidence-based medicine. *Journal of Evaluation in Clinical Practice, 5*(2), 139-147.

Orlandi, M. A. (1986). The diffusion and adoption of worksite health promotion innovations: An analysis of barriers. *Preventative Medicine, 15,* 522-536.

Pettengill, M. M., Gillies, D. A., & Clark, C. C. (1994). Factors encouraging and discouraging the use of nursing research findings. *IMAGE: The Journal of Nursing Scholarship, 26,* 143-147.

Rice, R. E., & Rogers, E. M. (1980). Re-invention in the innovation process. *Knowledge: Creation, Diffusion, Utilization, 1,* 499-514.

Rich, R. F. (1975). Selective utilization of social science related information by federal policy makers. *Inquiry, 13,* 3.

Rich, R. F. (1977). Uses of social science information by federal bureaucrats: Knowledge for action versus knowledge for understanding. In C. H. Weiss (Ed.), *Uses of social research in public policy* (pp. 199-211). Lexington, MA: D.C. Heath.

Rizutto, C., Bostrum, J., Suter, W. N., & Chenitz, W. C. (1994). Predictors of nurses' involvement in research activities. *Western Journal of Nursing Research, 16,* 193-204.

Rodgers, S. (1994). An exploratory study of research utilization by nurses in general medical and surgical wards. *Journal of Advanced Nursing, 20,* 904-911.

Rogers, E. M. (1962). *Diffusion of innovations.* New York: Free Press.

Rogers, E. M. (1983). *Diffusion of innovations* (3rd ed.). New York: Free Press.

Rogers, E. M. (1986). Models of knowledge transfer: Critical perspectives. In G. M. Beal, W. Dissanayake, & S. Konoshima (Eds.), *Knowledge generation, utilization, exchange, and utilization* (pp. 37-60). Boulder, CO: Westview Press.

Rogers, E. M. (1988). Information technologies: How organizations are changing. In G. M. Goldhaber & G. A. Barnett (Eds.), *Handbook of organizational communication* (pp. 437-452). Norwood, NJ: Ablex.

Rogers, E. M. (1995). *Diffusion of innovations* (4th ed.). New York: Free Press.

Rogers, E. M., & Agarwala-Rogers, R. (1976). *Communication in organizations.* New York: Free Press.

Rogers, E. M., & Shoemaker, F. (1971). *Communication of innovations: A cross cultural approach.* New York: Free Press.

Romano, C. A. (1990). Diffusion of technology innovation. *Advances in Nursing Science, 13*(2), 11-21.

Rutledge, D. N., Ropka, M., Greene, P. E., Nail, L., & Mooney, K. H. (1997). Barriers to research utilization for oncology staff nurses and nurse managers/clinical nurse specialists. *Oncology Nursing Forum, 25,* 497-506.

Ryan, B., & Gross, N. C. (1943). The diffusion of hybrid corn seed in two Iowa communities. *Rural Sociology, 8,* 15-24.

Sackett, D. L., Rosenberg, W. M., Gray, J. A. M., & Haynes, R. B. (1996). Evidence-based medicine: What it is and what it isn't? *British Medical Journal, 312,* 71-72.

Schroeder, S. A. (1987). Strategies for reducing medical costs by changing physicians' behavior: Efficacy and impact on quality of care. *International Journal of Technology Assessment in Health Care, 3,* 39-50.

Shore, H. L. (1972). Adopters and laggards. *The Canadian Nurse, 68*(7), 36-39.

Stafford, R. S. (1990). Alternative strategies for controlling rising cesarean section rates. *Journal of the American Medical Association, 263,* 683-687.

Stetler, C. B. (1994a). Problems and issues of research utilization. In O. L. Strickland & D. L. Fishman (Eds.), *Nursing issues in the 1990s* (pp. 459-470). New York: Delmar.

Stetler, C. B. (1994b). Refinement of the Stetler/Marram model for application of research findings to practice. *Nursing Outlook, 42*(1), 15-25.

Sunneson, S., & Nilsson, K. (1988). Explaining research utilization. *Knowledge: Creation, Diffusion, Utilization, 10,* 140-155.

Sunneson, S., & Nilsson, K. (1993). Strategy and tactics: Utilization of research in three policy sector contexts. *The Journal of Applied Behavioral Science, 29*(3), 366-383.

Swanson, J. M., Durham, R. F., & Albright, J. (1997). Clinical utilization/application of qualitative research. In J. M. Morse (Ed.), *Completing a qualitative project: Details and dialogue* (pp. 253-282). Thousand Oaks, CA: Sage.

Tannenbaum, T. N., Sampalis, J. S., & Battista, R. N. (1990). Early detection and treatment of hyperlipidaemia: Physician practices in Canada. *Canadian Medical Association Journal, 143,* 875-881.

Van De Ven, A. H. (1986). Central problems in the management of innovation. *Management Science, 32*(5), 590-607.

Valente, T. W., & Rogers, E. M. (1995). The origins and development of the diffusion of innovations paradigm as an example of scientific growth. *Science Communication, 16*(3), 242-273.

Varcoe, C., & Hilton, A. (1995). Factors influencing acute-care nurses' use of research findings. *Canadian Journal of Nursing Research, 27,* 51-71.

Walczak, J. R., McGuire, D. B., Haisfield, M. E., & Beezley, A. (1994). A survey of research-related activities and perceived barriers to research utilization among professional oncology nurses. *Oncology Nursing Forum, 21*(4), 710-715.

Weiss, C. H. (1979). The many meanings of research utilization. *Public Administration Review, 39*(5), 426-431.

Weiss, C. H. (1980). Knowledge creep and decision accretion. *Knowledge: Creation, Diffusion, Utilization, 1*(3), 381-404.

Zaltman, G. (1979). Knowledge utilization as planned social change. *Knowledge: Creation, Diffusion, Utilization, 1*(1), 82-105.

Zimbano, P. G., & Leippe, M. R. (1991). *The psychology of attitude, change and social influence.* Philadelphia: Temple University Press.

Author Index

Subject Index

About the Authors

John D. Engel (PhD) is Vice President for Academic Affairs and Executive Associate Dean, Professor of Behavioral Sciences, and Director of the Center for Studies of Clinical Performance, Northeastern Ohio Universities College of Medicine. He is a Senior/Associate Editor for three international health profession journals. His research is focused on the areas of the sociology of the medical profession and qualitative research methodologies. He has been a Visiting Scholar at the National Endowment for the Humanities, The Hastings Center, and the Medical University of Pecs, Hungary. He received his PhD in research methodology and program evaluation in 1975 from the University of Delaware. He has over 20 years of academic experience in medical education.

Carole A. Estabrooks (RN, PhD) is Assistant Professor at the Faculty of Nursing, University of Alberta, in Edmonton, Canada. She is also a Canadian Institutes for Health Research (CIHR) Health Scholar and an Alberta Heritage Foundation for Medical Research (AHFMR) Population Health Investigator. She currently holds NHRDP- and AHFMR-funded grants examining the utilization of research within the context of pain management practices in adult and pediatric populations. Her program of research is focused on research dissemination and utilization. She has held clinical practice, clinical specialist, and management positions in critical care nursing, and senior administrative positions responsible for education, quality, and research. Her postdoctoral studies were completed at the Institute for Clinical Evaluative Sciences (ICES) in Toronto, Canada.

Ginger Gibson (MA) is Senior Research Associate at the Center for Environmental Communication, Rutgers University. Trained as an anthropologist, she has been a journeyman researcher working on issues related to stakeholder participation in environmental management in Canada and the United States.

She collaborates on projects on cross-cultural communication of risk information with First Nations communities in northern Canada, and stakeholder
involvement in watershed management in New Jersey. Her main research interests are in the areas of public understanding of science, cross-cultural risk
communication, community-based environmental decision making, and
participatory research methodologies.

Nancy Gibson (PhD) is Chair of the Department of Human Ecology, and Associate of the Department of Family Medicine, the Centre for Health Promotion Studies, and the International Institute for Qualitative Methods, University of Alberta, Canada. Her research program involves communities
undergoing transition resulting from relocation to a new environment or
from industrial intervention in their near environments. Her interests include
immigrant and aboriginal populations in Canada and displaced populations
in Sierra Leone, West Africa. Her research is collaborative, participatory, and
community based. The long-range goal of her research team is to identify a
model for community-based health care that accommodates the values and
coping strategies of ethnically diverse communities. Another of her research
interests is the ethics of participatory research. She has worked on international health projects in India, Guatemala, and Sierra Leone, and advised mu-
nicipal, provincial, and national governments on health programs.

Anton J. Kuzel (MD) is Associate Professor and Vice Chairman of the Department of Family Practice, Virginia Commonwealth University, in Richmond.
His introduction to qualitative research came in a class taught by John Engel,
and he has grown through collaboration with researchers from many disciplines but particularly in family practice and nursing. His particular interests
are in the application of qualitative methods to clinical questions and in the
evaluation of qualitative studies.

Ann C. Macaulay (MD, CFCP, FCFP) is Associate Professor of Family Medicine, McGill University. She is also a Fellow of the College of Family Physicians
of Canada, President of the North American Primary Care Research Group,
and Board Member of the Clinical and Scientific Section of the Canadian
Diabetes Association. She has spent 30 years as a family physician in the First
Nations community of Kahnawake, Quebec, and is principal investigator of
the Kahnawake Schools Diabetes Prevention Project, which is a participatory
research project with this Mohawk community promoting healthy lifestyles
for the primary prevention of Type 2 diabetes. Her other interests include

aboriginal health (for which she has served on Health Canada committees), ethics of participatory research, and promotion of diabetes clinical guidelines. She graduated from St. Andrews University, Scotland, before immigrating to Canada in 1969.

Irena Madjar (RN, PhD) is Professor of Nursing, University of Newcastle, Australia, with a background in medical, surgical, and critical care nursing. Her research interests are in the areas of pain and pain management, phenomenology of illness, and the cultural and ethical issues arising out of clinical practice. She is the author of *Giving Comfort and Inflicting Pain* and coeditor, with Jo Ann Walton, of *Nursing and the Experience of Illness: Phenomenology in Practice.*

Maria Mayan (PhD) is Project Director with the International Institute for Qualitative Methodology and an Alberta Heritage Foundation for Medical Research (AHFMR) Postdoctoral Fellow, studying the link between immigrant health and policy making. Her research interests include women and health, policy development, international development, and research methodology.

Lynn M. Meadows (PhD) is Assistant Professor at the Departments of Family Medicine and Community Health Sciences, University of Calgary, a Senior Population Health Investigator funded through the Alberta Heritage Foundation for Medical Research, Adjunct Assistant Professor at the International Institute for Qualitative Methodology, and Adjunct Assistant Professor in Sociology at the University of Calgary. Her program of work focuses on people's experiences of illness and well-being, with current populations under study including midlife women and seniors. Her research interests include articulation of how various determinants of health, health beliefs, and health experiences affect everyday well-being. She is a trainer for NUD*IST and Nvivo qualitative analytic software programs.

Janice M. Morse (PhD, Nursing; PhD, Anthropology; D. Nursing [Hon]) is the Director of the International Institute for Qualitative Methodology and Professor, Faculty of Nursing, University of Alberta. She has published extensively in the areas of comfort, suffering, and qualitative methods, and serves as editor of the bimonthly international, interdisciplinary journal, *Qualitative Health Research.*

Kärin Olson (PhD) holds an Alberta Heritage Foundation for Medical Research (AHFMR) Career Renewal Award in qualitative research methods and palliative care with a focus on fatigue at the International Institute for Qualitative Methodology. She was the Coordinator of Nursing Research at the Cross Cancer Institute in Edmonton, Canada, with responsibility for developing clinical research and implementing evidence-based nursing practice. She completed her PhD in educational psychology at the University of Alberta in 1990 with a dissertation that combined quantitative and qualitative research methods.

Lynne D. Ray (RN, PhD) is Assistant Professor at the Faculty of Nursing, University of Alberta. Her research focuses on families who are raising children with chronic health conditions. She has an interest in public policy that enables families in their caregiving roles. One of her current projects is development of an Internet-accessible resource database for families raising chronically ill children. Her qualitative research interests include hermeneutic inquiry and participatory research. She holds degrees from the University of British Columbia, Dalhousie University, and the University of Washington.

Janice M. Swanson (RN, PhD, FAAN) is Professor, Department of Nursing, Samuel Merritt College in Oakland, California. She serves as a consultant, both nationally and internationally, on the prevention of STDs, including HIV/AIDS in high-risk populations, and on the use of qualitative research methods. Her research and clinical interests over the past 26 years have focused on sexual and reproductive health issues in the community. She served as a member of the Nursing Research Study Section, Division of Research Grants, National Institutes of Health, 1991 to 1995. She received her BSN from Wayne State University in Detroit, Michigan, and her MS and PhD from the University of Maryland. She completed a postdoctoral research fellowship at the University of California, San Francisco, with the late Anselm Strauss.

Sally E. Thorne (RN, PhD) is Professor, School of Nursing, University of British Columbia. She conducts and publishes research on the influence of social context on illness experience, especially chronic illness and cancer. She is particularly interested in the philosophical and theoretical issues of how we know what we know in health care, and the bases upon which we make health-service delivery decisions. Her enthusiasm for these issues has led to an ongoing critical analysis of the implications of qualitative methodologies in the health sciences, and she has published widely in this area.

Ross E. G. Upshur (MA, MSc, MD) is the Director of the Primary Care Research Unit at the Sunnybrook Campus of the Sunnybrook and Women's College Health Sciences Centre, University of Toronto. He is also a Research Scholar and Assistant Professor, Departments of Family and Community Medicine and Public Health Sciences, at the University of Toronto. He is a member of The Royal College of Physicians and Surgeons of Canada, The Joint Centre for Bioethics at the University of Toronto, Associate Member of the Institute of Environment and Health at McMaster University, and Adjunct Assistant Professor of Geography and Geology at McMaster University His research interests include the concept of evidence in health care, medical epistemology, clinical reasoning, public health ethics, time series applications, and environmental epidemiology. He received his BA (Hons) and MA degrees in philosophy before receiving his MD from McMaster University in 1986. After 7 years of rural primary care practice, he returned to complete his MSc in epidemiology and fellowship training in Community Medicine at the University of Toronto.

Jo Ann Walton (RN, PhD) is Professor of Nursing at the School of Nursing and Midwifery, Auckland University of Technology, New Zealand, and Adjunct Professor at the Faculty of Nursing, the University of Newcastle, Australia. She has clinical nursing experience in a variety of settings, but her primary interest is in psychiatric mental health nursing. She is especially passionate about consumer rights, representation, and participation, and the ethical aspects of psychiatric/mental health care. Her current interests include work on youth suicide; on ethics and aesthetics in mental health nursing practice; consumer involvement in mental health care; and evaluation of mental health services.